PERGAMON INTERNATIONAL LIBRARY
of Science, Technology, Engineering and Social Studies

The 1000-volume original paperback library in aid of education, industrial training and the enjoyment of leisure

Publisher: Robert Maxwell, M.C.

Research Methods In Clinical Psychology (PGPS-130)

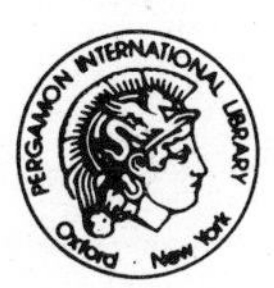

Pergamon Titles of Related Interest

Amabile & Stubbs PSYCHOLOGICAL RESEARCH IN THE CLASSROOM: Issues for Educators and Researchers

Barber PITFALLS IN HUMAN RESEARCH: Ten Pivotal Points

Barlow, Hayes & Nelson THE SCIENTIST PRACTITIONEER: Research and Accountability in Clinical and Educational Settings

Barlow & Hersen SINGLE CASE EXPERMENTAL DESIGNS: Strategies for Studying Behavior Change, Second Edition

Hersen & Bellack BEHAVIORAL ASSESSMENT: A Practical Handbook, Second Edition

Ollendick & Hersen CHILD BEHAVIORAL ASSESSMENT: Principles and Procedures

Walker CLINICAL PRACTICE OF PSYCHOLOGY: A Guide for Mental Health Professionals

Related Journals*

BEHAVIORAL ASSESSMENT
CLINICAL PSYCHOLOGY REVIEW
PERSONALITY AND INDIVIDUAL DIFFERENCES

***Free specimen copies available upon request.**

PERGAMON GENERAL PSYCHOLOGY SERIES
EDITORS
Arnold P. Goldstein, *Syracuse University*
Leonard Krasner, *SUNY at Stony Brook*

Research Methods In Clinical Psychology

Edited by
Alan S. Bellack
Medical College of Pennsylvania at Eastern Pennsylvania Psychiatric Institute

Michel Hersen
University of Pittsburgh School of Medicine

PERGAMON PRESS

NEW YORK · OXFORD · BEIJING · FRANKFURT
SÃO PAULO · SYDNEY · TOKYO · TORONTO

U.S.A.	Pergamon Press, Maxwell House, Fairview Park, Elmsford, New York 10523, U.S.A.
U.K.	Pergamon Press, Headington Hill Hall, Oxford OX3 0BW, England
PEOPLE'S REPUBLIC OF CHINA	Pergamon Press, Room 4037, Qianmen Hotel, Beijing, People's Republic of China
FEDERAL REPUBLIC OF GERMANY	Pergamon Press, Hammerweg 6, D-6242 Kronberg, Federal Republic of Germany
BRAZIL	Pergamon Editora, Rua Eça de Queiros, 346, CEP 04011, Paraiso, São Paulo, Brazil
AUSTRALIA	Pergamon Press Australia, P.O. Box 544, Potts Point, N.S.W. 2011, Australia
JAPAN	Pergamon Press, 8th Floor, Matsuoka Central Building, 1-7-1 Nishishinjuku, Shinjuku-ku, Tokyo 160, Japan
CANADA	Pergamon Press Canada, Suite No. 271, 253 College Street, Toronto, Ontario, Canada M5T 1R5

Second Printing 1987

Library of Congress Cataloging in Publication Data

Research methods in clinical psychology.
(Pergamon general psychology series)
Bibliography: p.
Includes Index.
1. Clinical psychology — Research. 2. Psychology, Pathological — Research. 3. Psychotherapy — Research. I. Bellack, Alan S. II. Hersen, Michel. III. Series.
[DNLM: 1. Psychology. 2. Research — Methods. BF 76.5 R432]
RC467.R466 1984 616.89'027 84-428
ISBN 0-08-029410-3
ISBN 0-08-029409-X (pbk.)

Printed in Great Britain by A. Wheaton & Co. Ltd., Exeter

Contents

Preface

For most new graduate students in clinical psychology the prospect of conducting their own research is both exciting and anxiety provoking. The excitement comes from the prospect of solving important problems and being involved in "Science." Research is, after all, something of an adventure: a cross between solving a challenging puzzle and being an explorer uncovering new territory. On the other hand, the novice is generally filled with apprehension. Like the explorer setting out on a voyage to uncharted territory with unknown equipment, an untrained crew, and an unknown goal, the new researcher does not know where to turn or how to proceed. How do you decide what to study? What are the critical procedures? How do you analyze the data? What controls are necessary? How many subjects do you need? What is the hypothesis? How do you get started?

To the experienced researcher, the above questions seem remarkably simple. When one has been conducting research for some time, hypotheses and questions evolve naturally from previous work. Controls and procedures are relatively straightforward, again being variations of earlier efforts. Yet the novice has no such background to fall back on. This situation is by no means unique to research. However, in contrast to many other endeavors, there generally is no systematic way for the beginning graduate student to learn research skills. Statistics courses typically teach statistics in the abstract, as if they are divorced from the rest of the research process. Such courses rarely deal with problems in hypothesis formation, design, and control. Students generally find themselves memorizing formulas that they cannot put into practice, and that they forget by the time they actually get to conducting their own theses and dissertations. Courses focusing on substantive topics (e.g., personality or therapy) generally focus on teaching existing knowledge and theory. Research is reviewed and criticized, but the emphasis is on learning about the overall literature rather than on learning how to conduct better work.

The most fortunate and industrious students learn research skills from their mentors. They work as graduate assistants or are otherwise apprenticed to faculty and advanced students. They have the good fortune to observe others developing research projects and get a gradual introduction to the process. Most others get a tougher introduction. They are forced into the fire with little preparation when they approach thesis or first-year project deadlines. The result is often marked by considerable distress and feelings of both futility and hostility. As a result, most students never do any systematic research after the dissertation.

This book is designed to deal with both the excitement and the apprehension of the novice researcher. We hope to facilitate the excitement by highlighting both some of the accomplishments and many of the remaining questions facing the field. We hope to reduce some of the apprehension by giving the novice some guidance and tools with which to begin his or her own research endeavors. Our contributors have discussed research methodology with a mind toward teaching students about the critical issues involved in planning, conducting, and evaluating a research project. The chapters on substantive topics are designed to identify issues and questions for future research, rather than simply summarizing the current state of the art. The authors have attempted to point out strengths and weaknesses of existing studies, so that the student is less awed by the fact that a study has been published. Too many students have the sense that if something appears in a journal it must be close to "truth and beauty." We have attempted to reflect the fact that other people make mistakes, and that most journal articles are stimuli for better research, rather than reflections of the fact that all important questions have already been answered. Overall, we hope that this book smooths the road for new researchers and helps them to retain the feelings of excitement that led them to clinical psychology in the first place. We hope that they become more sophisticated consumers of research, as well as more likely to produce meaningful (and enjoyable) research beyond graduate school.

Alan S. Bellack
Philadelphia, PA

Michel Hersen
Pittsburgh, PA

Part 1
INTRODUCTION

1

Research in Clinical Psychology

Michel Hersen
Alan S. Bellack

One of the most incessant questions asked of clinical psychologists by friends, relatives, and the general public is: What is the difference between a psychologist and a psychiatrist? There are two common answers: one reflecting a somewhat negative distinction and one a positive difference. The negative view, of course, is that psychologists are not "real doctors" and cannot prescribe medication. The positive view is that psychologists are trained as scientists as well as clinicians. Not only can they conduct meaningful research, but they have a more critical, empirical perspective on their clinical work. In fact, clinical psychology is unique in its scientist-practitioner orientation. While members of other practice-oriented professions sometimes seek supplemental research training and become excellent scientists, only clinical psychology makes research training a core feature of the discipline. Thus, even though most clinical psychologists never conduct publishable research after leaving graduate school, they all are trained to approach the clinical enterprise with a healthy, scientific skepticism.

The research tradition in clinical psychology dates back to the beginning of the profession and its roots in experimental psychology. The early experimental psychologists were primarily interested in the fundamental nature and processes of the mind: perception, sensation, reflex action, and so on. They developed highly precise methods and procedures for studying these phenomena, using the "hard" sciences, such as physics, for models. Clinical psychology began to develop in the late 1800s out of an interest in more functional or applied questions. Two lines of influence are especially notable (Bellack & Hersen, 1980; Korchin, 1983). The "psychometric tradition," with its emphasis on careful and specific measurement, spawned the development of "mental tests" and the *testing movement*. The signal milestone was the development of the first useful intelligence test by Alfred Binet in 1905. With this test, Binet (and his colleague, Simon) demonstrated that children could be compared and classified according to intellectual level, rather than simply catalogued as normal or retarded. This led to the development of new training programs for the educable mentally retarded, who previously had been thought unreachable. Early clinical psychologists became extensively involved in these programs because of their expertise in testing and test construction, as well as their knowledge of sensation, perception, and mental functioning.

The second major influence was the "dynamic tradition": the focus on human motivation, needs, and drives. The most significant force in this area was, of course, Sigmund Freud. But, his influence on clinical psychology was aided substantially by two American psychologists: G. Stanley Hall and William James. Curiously, Freud's initial impact was much greater on psychology than psychiatry, partly because he created an interest among early psychologists in the psychological basis of behavior, as well as in the potential uses of psychological approaches to change behavior. Rather than studying the limits of sensation and perception, clinically oriented psychologists began to consider why people behaved the way they did and how their feelings and needs affected their behavior.

Prior to World War I, the few "clinical psychologists" so labeled worked primarily in the area of testing and rehabilitation of children. With America's entry into the war, psychologists were called upon to develop procedures for assessing and classifying large numbers of recruits. Both intelligence and personality tests were developed to meet this need. The success of these instruments led to a marked increase in the use of testing. Over the next two decades, numerous tests were developed, including projective tests such as the Rorschach. During these years, clinical psychologists became increasingly involved in assessment and diagnosis of adult psychiatric patients. While the field gradually grew during this period, there was no specific training for clinical psychologists. They continued to be trained as experimental psychologists and received clinical training "catch as catch can." This situation continued until after World War II.

As with World War I, World War II was a marked stimulus for the development of the field. Not only did the armed forces require screening instruments, but they also had a tremendous need for clinicians. Until this time, psychologists were not permitted to conduct any type of psychological treatment. They served primarily as assessors on multidisciplinary teams. But, there were not nearly enough psychiatrists to treat the huge numbers of psychiatric casualties, so psychologists were pressed into service. Many were academic psychologists or graduate students who had had little prior clinical experiences, or even interest. This situation persisted after the war, with the establishment of the Veteran's Administration to care for discharged servicemen. Moreover, with the continuing great need for clinicians and with greater public awareness of the role of psychiatry and psychology, the United States government began to provide funds to train increasing numbers of mental health professionals. Also, many of the former "experimental" psychologists pressed into service as clinicians found they liked their new roles, and upon returning to civilian life retained their new-found clinical focus. These research-trained clinicians served as the core of the teaching faculty for this mushrooming discipline over the next 25 years.

However, there still was no systematic training plan for clinical psychologists at that time. In response to government requests, the American Psychological Association convened a committee of leading psychologists to address this problem. The resulting Shakow Report (American Psychological Association, 1947) has served as a blueprint for the field ever since. It was quickly adopted by most existing programs, and was reaffirmed in 1949 at a national training conference in Boulder, Colorado, where it became known as the *Boulder Model* (Raimy, 1950). Based upon the scientific heritage of the field, the model mandates that clinical psychologists be trained as scientist-professionals. This combined focus was seen as essential for assuring the unique and meaningful contribution of the discipline. The specific balance of the two aspects of training is not mandated, and programs vary considerably in the emphasis placed on one or the other, yet all Boulder Model programs attempt to provide an integrated approach. Students do not simply take a few isolated research (or clinical) courses. Rather, all courses are taught from an empirical perspective, and research courses (e.g., statistics, experimental design) generally focus on applied topics (e.g., research on treatment, personality, and so on). The Boulder Model has been increasingly criticized in the past decade for being unresponsive to the "clinical" interests of most students. A number of schools have developed new degree programs (e.g., Psy D.) which focus almost solely on professional practice. Nevertheless, the scientist-professional model remains the preeminent approach to training clinical psychologists and promises to continue to dominate for the foreseeable future.

THE SCIENTIFIC METHOD

Although it is categorized as a social science (as opposed to a "hard" science such as biology), psychology in general has emulated its more precise sister disciplines and has followed the scientific method. The sub-branch of psychology known as clinical psychology also has, in the last two to three decades, made a valiant effort to shed its more mystical qualities and begun to pursue the scientific method with considerable vigor. This relatively new direction has been seen equally well in the study of personality, assessment and diagnosis, and psychotherapeutics. Whereas the clinical journals once were filled with theoretical and clinical accounts, they now abound in the dissemination of tables, graphs, and reports of statistical inference. Overall, this trend has been welcomed by the field, particularly those who are empirically-minded, but at times it has caused distress among the die-hard clinicians. The time for the empirical clinician, despite being heralded (cf. Barlow, 1980), is not quite yet a reality. But increasing numbers of clinical psychologists are involved in the research enterprise (cf. Bellack & Hersen, 1980; Kazdin, Bellack, & Hersen, 1980).

What, then, is the scientific method as it applies to the research endeavor in the field of clinical psychology? Is it merely a "cut-and-dried" process in which experimental hypotheses are exposed, put into experimental form, and then tested? Or is the process a more fluid one in which there is considerable interplay between clinical practice, clinical hunch, and strategies applied to confirm or disconfirm such hunches? In essence, we are raising the question as to whether there is some artistry that goes into the development of good research in clinical psychology.

With regard to the rhetorical questions posed above, we believe that the following quote, taken from what Edwards and Cronbach (1952) wrote over three decades ago, fully applies today:

> Every research worker has to have two personalities if he is to get the most good from his data. He must be the rigorous tester who believes nothing without conclusive evidence, when he is deciding what relations are to be admitted as proven facts . . . after the tough-minded half of the investigator's personality has accepted what it will from the study, he must turn loose the inquiring, speculative, and tender-minded half which is willing to entertain doubtful ideas. If this tender-minded soul is gullible, *believing* in what has met no significance test, he will end with a science stuffed with superstitions. But if he holds these yet-unproven ideas in the air, as notions which may guide him in the next experiment or the treatment of the next patient, he is more likely to be correct than the man who casts the idea from his mind as soon as one experiment fails to provide significant confirmation. (p. 57)

It should be crystal clear, then, that the innovative clinical researcher needs to maintain a healthy balance between theoretical speculation, clinical lore, and empirical data. When these are placed in correct juxtaposition, the likelihood of posing and answering penetrating questions is enhanced.

Let us now consider in some detail the process of clinical inquiry. To do so we have arbitrarily divided the process into eleven categories: (1) Primary Aims, (2) Speculation, (3) Work of Others, (4) Independent and Dependent Variables, (5) Hypotheses, (6) Research Strategies, (7) Population and Sampling, (8) Randomization and Matching, (9) Statistical Evaluation, (10) Ethical Considerations, and (11) Dissemination of Results.

Primary Aims

Since clinical psychology is a social science involving the study of human behavior, its three primary aims are: (1) to order and classify behavior, (2) to predict behavior, and (3) to modify behavior. The *first* aim, of course, is concerned with the orderly classification of behavior (i.e., diagnosis). Included in the aim are the systems of classification (e.g., DSM-III: American Psychiatric Association, 1980) and the methodology for making nosological decisions (e.g., interviews, scales, observational techniques, and tests). The *second* aim concerns the study of personality and the specific conditions that will determine the consistency of behavior across time, settings, and interpersonal situations. In recent years, however, there has been considerable interest in the situational specificity of behavior (e.g., Eisler, Hersen, Miller, & Blanchard, 1975), as applied to trait conceptualizations of behavior (cf. Eysenck & Eysenck, 1968). The *third* aim involves the specific modification of behavior, whether it be individual, family, or group therapy, or whether the approach is psychoanalytic, humanistic, or behavioral. In recent years the emphasis here has been on determining the most effective approach for a given patient of a given diagnosis of a particular age. That is, one no longer asks the generic question as to whether treatment works, but rather for whom and under what circumstances (i.e., therapist characteristics, patient characteristics, and specifics of the treatment). Thus, the evaluation of treatment has gained precision with an ultimate goal of ascertaining the specificity and limitations of a particular therapeutic strategy.

Speculation

Given the three primary aims of research in clinical psychology, it is most likely that a particular research project will be subsumed entirely or at least in part under the three categories we have outlined. In some instances the study may embrace all three categories, or two when the differential effectiveness of treatments is being determined for, say, two diagnostic groupings. In any event, irrespective of the eventual breadth or scope of the project, it first emanates as an idea. As noted by Kendall and Norton-Ford (1982), "Research ideas typically arise from an interest in solving a clinical problem or testing some aspect of a particular theory. This can come from personal experiences, group discussion, or issues raised in the research literature" (pp. 86–87).

Indeed, very good research ideas have emanated from the careful clinical observation of patients. Consider, for example, the therapist who has seen a long series of school-phobic children during the course of his clinical practice. He may have noted, when interviewing the parents of such children, that father is either absent or weak and that mother is overprotective and overindulgent. This, then, might lead him (or her) to conceptualize the problem as one in which mother reinforces avoidant behavior (i.e., the child remaining at home). But is the pattern of the overprotective mother and absent father peculiar to school phobia, or is this seen in other examples of child psychopathology (e.g., the socially anxious child who is able to attend school)? Of course, this second question posed by the clinical researcher leads to further speculation and undoubtedly will contribute to the type of research design to be ultimately carried out.

Work of Others

As we have noted in the previous section, theoretical and clinical speculation is a most fruitful cognitive endeavor that may lead to the generation of testable research ideas. However, before any idea can be tested empirically it behooves the scholarly researcher to examine both the theoretical and empirical work of others. Many more junior researchers unfortunately have plunged "head first" into the research operation without first perusing the relevant work of others. The problems with this approach are threefold: (1) the study, or some variant, may have already been performed, (2) our impetuous researcher is quite likely to commit errors (design and procedural) that could have been avoided if a careful literature search had been accomplished, and (3) an entirely different research tack, based on previous findings, might be taken if the work of others were to be meticulously examined.

We also might note that clinical descriptions of patients should not be disdained as a source for stimulating research ideas. Some of our most elegant treatment procedures have been based on the careful study of the single case (see Hersen & Barlow, 1976).

To do a careful search of the critical work of others, the clinical researcher needs to be aware of the relevant sources. He/she should recognize those specialty journals in which certain areas are covered. Periodicals such as *Psychological Abstracts, Index Medicus,* and *Biological Abstracts* which abstract journal articles are an invaluable source. Moreover, given key words or phrases, the age of the computer has now made it possible to retrieve long lists of source material.

Independent and Dependent Variables

Surprising as it may seem, many clinical researchers do not give sufficient attention to the variables that they are manipulating and measuring before they develop the experimental hypothesis. This, therefore, tends to result in muddy conceptualizations and unclear outcomes. Irrespective of the type of research strategy that eventually is employed (correlational, experimental, single case, group comparison, factor analysis), a precise determination of all variables is warranted. The *independent* variable is the one that is under the experimenter's direct control in order to determine its effect. For example, institution and removal of a token economy in a ward of chronic schizophrenics to determine the effect of activity level is a clear instance of the application of an *independent* variable. By contrast, the dependent measure is *activity* level as determined through nurses' ratings of patient behavior. Thus, the dependent *measure* is the strategy through which one assesses the outcome of the *independent* variable. With the possible exception of self-monitoring (which can serve both as an independent and dependent variable) these two operations are clearly distinguishable.

Although the following issue will be discussed to some extent in the section on Randomization and Matching, it is critical for the experimenter to ensure that his operation (i.e., the independent variable) is the agent responsible for change and not some extraneous (perhaps correlated) variable that is associated with its implementation. This is nicely illustrated in a study by Bloom, Weigel, and Trautt (1977) showing how the "credibility" of the therapist was affected by the decor of his or her office.

Hypotheses

Development of testable hypotheses follows from the clinical researcher's speculatory efforts, examination and evaluation of the work of others, and a clear delineation of the independent and dependent variables as well as their possible confounds. Once this preliminary stage of the clinical-experimental endeavor has been reached, the researcher can begin to operationalize his definitions and procedures. That is, he is able to define hypothetical concepts entirely through the operations followed in their measurement. Although seemingly a bit circular, this serves to clarify functions and allows for suitable replication by others in the future. For example, in the case of our school-phobic child, an operational definition of mother's overprotectiveness could be her keeping him home upon his presentation of a minor physical complaint (fever of 99°, stuffed nose, minor discomfort in the abdomen, minor headache).

Again using the school phobia example, one could develop a testable hypothesis that mother's overindulgence results in school phobic behavior and that a parental retraining procedure to reduce such overprotectiveness will result in elimination of the school phobia. This would lead to a treatment outcome study in which the parental retraining procedure is evaluated in controlled fashion. However, for experimental purposes, the hypothesis is stated in negative terms (i.e., there is no relationship between the treatment and improved school attendance). This is referred to as the *null hypothesis*, and the objective of our clinical researcher is to reject this null hypothesis on statistical grounds.

Research Strategies

There basically are four research strategies (with numerous variants) that are followed by researchers in clinical psychology. We will only briefly allude to them here inasmuch as they will be given detailed emphasis in the body of this volume. The *first* we refer to as the *description and observational* strategy. The primary objective here is to tally, code, quantify, and observe existing behavior (e.g., a nurses' observational scale, or a family interaction measurement system). Although this strategy can be accomplished on a clinical-intuitive basis, the empirical clinical researcher prefers the use of reliable and valid scales, interview procedures, and rating systems.

Our *second* strategy is the *correlational* approach. The major objective is to determine the relationship between two or more variables (e.g., unassertiveness and depression). Thus, the strength of the relationship can be determined as well as the *direction* of the relationship (i.e., positive or negative). For example, there exists a moderate negative relationship between assertiveness and depression. That is, those ranking high in depression are more likely to be low on assertiveness. It is most important to note that the correlational approach *does not* allow one to conclude cause-and-effect relationships, but only that the two or more variables are related.

Our *third* strategy is *factor analysis*, which is a close, albeit more complicated, relative of the simple, correlational approach. Given the advanced development of computer analyses, the factor analytic strategy allows the researcher to evaluate the simultaneous interrelationship among a large number of variables. This is of particular importance in identifying items that cluster together (i.e., factors) within scales. Although a statistical procedure, the researcher still has to provide a suitable label for each factor.

The *fourth* strategy is termed *experimental* and includes between and within group designs, factorial designs, and the many single case research strategies. In each of these design strategies the independent variable is manipulated by the clinical researcher, thus resulting in his/her ability to make cause-and-effect statements on the basis of resulting data.

Population and Sampling

In the course of conducting clinical research it behooves the experimenter to precisely describe the population of interest. This can be done behaviorally through clear description (see Hersen & Bellack, 1981) or through use of the much improved psychiatric diagnostic system (DSM-III: American Psychiatric Association, 1980). In either case the experimenter studies a sample of the population and must insure that it is a *representative* sample of that particular population. This is most critical with regard to the generality of statements that can be reached about the population on the basis of the more limited sample studied. Moreover, precise description and adequate samples not only allow for generalization of results, but also facilitate inter-study comparison.

Randomization and Matching

A major aim of clinical research is to isolate relevant variables, test their efficacy or power, and render conclusions about their controlling influences. However, an obstacle to achieving that end is the possible interference of uncontrolled variables. Let us consider the following possibility. Two separate therapies (A + B) are applied to two presumably similar groups of anxious subjects (1 + 2). But unbeknownst to the clinical researcher, subjects in Group 1 are more highly motivated to improve than those in Group 2. When the study is complete and it appears that Therapy A (applied to Group 1) did better than Therapy B (applied to Group 2), can one assume the superiority of Therapy A over B? The answer obviously is no; there is a major confound in that the two groups of anxious subjects were not matched on the motivational factor.

The careful clinical researcher generally ensures that all uncontrolled variables are *randomly* distributed across the two or more groups that will be contrasted. Or, if he/she knows that a given variable may interact with the procedure (thus leading to erroneous conclusions), an attempt may be made to match that variable (e.g., age or IQ) across the groups. With an increased number of uncontrolled variables it becomes more difficult to match carefully, and the random assignment of subjects to groups is followed. But irrespective of the attempt to randomize, it often pays to do midpoint and post-hoc checks to determine the success of such random assignment.

Statistical Evaluation

With the exception of some of the single case strategies (cf. Hersen & Barlow, 1976), the results of both correlational and experimental research are evaluated statistically. (Indeed, there now is increasing emphasis on performing statistical analyses even in the single case study. Edgington, in press.) In doing statistical analyses, of course, the experimenter is interested in disconfirming the null hypothesis. That is, he or she is interested in documenting a significant statistical relationship between variables or between his technical operations and their product.

Unfortunately, in many clinical research studies use of statistical analysis is an afterthought, with the statistical expert consulted on a post-hoc basis. However, this does not represent the scientific method at its best. By contrast, the meticulous clinical researcher makes statistical analysis an integral part of the experimental procedure and ensures that the design selected is able to accommodate a viable statistical procedure. In short, we are saying that the statistical analysis is a central feature of the design and, as such, deserves much forethought. For example, in outcome studies, the careful attention to statistical matters at the design stage may dictate the absolute number of subjects required per condition in order to be able to obtain significance between and across groups. This is referred to as the power statistic. If this is neglected and the N is too small, statistical significance may not be achieved, leading perhaps to potentially useful data being discarded. Thus, the message is clear: If you need a statistical consultant, consult him or her during the planning stages of the project. Later may be too late!

Ethical Considerations

We will not dwell on this subject since it is covered in detail in Chapter 13. However, we should note that in recent years ethical considerations in the conduct of clinical research have become increasingly intertwined with the scientific method. As in the previous section on use of statistical methodology, ethical considerations are to be accorded attention during the planning stages of experimentation and not as an afterthought to be sent to the institutional human use committee at some later date. We therefore are recommending the integrated rather than the piecemeal approach to planning and executing clinical research.

Dissemination of Results

Although the anonymity of the individual subject is one of the ethical guarantees of the clinical research enterprise, specific and group findings derived from such research become public domain once reports appear in the scientific periodicals and books (see Chapter 15). Since clinical psychology is one of the helping professions, results of clinical research have the potential of being of considerable use to other psychologists (psychiatrists, social workers, etc.) working with similar clinical populations. Thus, it becomes a professional obligation of the clinical researcher to share his or her findings with the largest possible audience of peer professionals. This is accomplished through presentations at local and national professional associations, articles in relevant clinical publications, chapters in books, and comprehensive monographs on the subject. Important findings in our field should not remain stored in file cabinets in the form of computer printouts, but should be made public as soon as the relevant statistical analyses have confirmed or disconfirmed the experimenter's favorite hypotheses.

In light of the fact that professional advancement often is contingent on publication of results, withholding of findings is rarely a problem. On the contrary, some clinical researchers err in the other direction and publish prematurely before the "whole story is in." In any event, either extreme is to be avoided.

SCOPE OF RESEARCH POSSIBILITIES

Research in clinical psychology covers a tremendously diverse range of subjects. The discipline is often described as an applied research field, and distinguished from so-called "experimental" psychology. Yet, in reality the borders are quite blurred. Many clinical researchers focus on such clearly applied issues as developing new therapies or considering the etiology of schizophrenia. But others are studying topics such as brain function or subtle aspects of learning which have, at best, a remote relationship to clinical practice and psychopathology. The distinction between basic and applied research probably depends more on whether the researcher thinks about the ultimate relevance of the study than on the study itself. Clinical psychologists are much more likely to go from applied questions to basic research studies, while their "experimental" colleagues are more likely to think about the applications of their work afterwards, if at all.

The most prominent areas of clinical psychology research are described in Chapters 6–12. Chapter 6, on personality, reflects the continued influence of the "dynamic tradition." This broad area deals with the nature of human behavior, motivational forces, and individual differences: How do people behave? Why do people behave the way they do? How and why do they behave differently from one another? The following titles of articles in a recent issue of the *Journal of Personality and Social Psychology* illustrate the diversity of this broad topic: "Alienation and drinking motivations among adolescent females" (Carman, Fitzgerald, & Holmgren, 1983); "A cross-cultural exploration into the meaning of achievement" (Fyans, Salili, Maehr, & Desai, 1983); and "Measuring loneliness in different relationships" (Schmidt & Sermat, 1983).

Chapters 7 and 8, on psychopathology and psychotherapy, respectively, most clearly reflect the applied aspect of clinical psychology research. The term psychopathology refers to all aspects of disordered behavior and psychological functions. Given the difficulty of distinguishing what is "normal" from what is "abnormal," research in this area often entails studying non-disordered subjects and behaviors in order to better identify and understand the nature of psychiatric disorders. The title of Chapter 8, Psychotherapy, may imply *verbal* psychotherapy, which is one specific approach to psychological treatment. But clinical psychologists are involved in research on a host of diverse treatment approaches, including: behavior therapy, family therapy, psychopharmacology, educational remediation, rehabilitation of psychiatric patients and individuals with neurological impairments, and specialized treatments such as sex therapy and programs for cigarette smoking, obesity, alcohol, and drug abuse.

Chapter 9, on Assessment and Test Construction, continues the "psychometric tradition." Measurement procedures needed for research run the gamut from simple frequency counts to complex tests or rating scales of personality, intelligence, psychopathology, and neurological functioning. Just about every clinical and research endeavor requires some measurement system. Research in this area encompasses development and construction of new tests and measures, evaluation of existing measures, and studies on the testing or assessment process per se (e.g., how to make a procedure more reliable, how to measure reliability).

Chapter 10 details research on epidemiology. Probably as a result of the community mental health movement and community psychology, over the past decade epidemiology has been increasingly recognized as a vital area of study. Loosely, it deals with the incidence, prevalence, and course of disorders. It is a systems or population approach to the study of psychiatric disorders, in contrast to the individual or small group approach. It is an approach which tends to look more at the forest than the trees, and hence gives a broader perspective. It often exposes patterns, such as the overall impact of deinstitutionalization of chronic psychiatric patients, which would not be discerned by traditional small group studies.

Behavioral Medicine, discussed in Chapter 11, is one of the most rapidly developing subspecialties of clinical psychology. It deals with the interface of psychological and physical functioning. Just about any medical disorder in which psychological factors play a prominent role in etiology, treatment, recurrence, or rehabilitation may be the subject of behavioral medicine research. Topics covered range from the more obvious psychosomatic disorders, such as obesity and hypertension, to such apparently "physical" problems as kidney disease, coronary heart disease, and cancer, where psychological intervention may play a key role in rehabilitation and the prevention of relapse.

Chapter 13 describes some of the major areas of research with children. Increasing attention is being paid to the role of childhood problems in later adult disorders. It appears that the stage for adult problems is often set in childhood. Also, it is becoming increasingly apparent that prevention and early intervention (e.g., in childhood) may often be more effective than trying to treat adults once their problems are ingrained. This chapter also highlights the unique impact of the developmental process. Research must take into account the fact that children change dramatically over the course of childhood: They do not simply "grow up," but they think and perceive things differently at different stages.

These seven chapters provide an overview of the major research areas. By no means do they cover all areas of clinical psychology research. Through their multifaceted training, clinical psychologists are prepared for diverse areas of specialization. They are seemingly limited only by their imaginations and by continued exposure to the current literature. The latter is especially important as the field is constantly changing (e.g., behavioral medicine did not exist 10 years ago!). Some of the other promising areas for continued and future research include: geriatrics, neuropsychology, forensic psychology (legal and ethical issues), sports psychology, prevention, and space psychology (e.g., psychological factors affecting astronauts). Clearly, the "sky is the limit!"

PROGRAMMATIC NATURE OF RESEARCH

In our discussion of the scientific method we already have argued that important clinical research involves a healthy balance between theory, clinical findings, and empirical data. This, of course, results in a comprehensive approach. We have labeled such an approach as *programmatic*, in contradistinction to isolated and unrelated studies that may be carried out in any given area. In the present section we therefore will briefly illustrate the nature of programmatic research with the work that has been accomplished in systematic desensitization over the last 30 years. Our discussion will document the relationship and interplay between basic animal research, theoretical speculation, pure clinical application, confirmation of clinical success via therapy analogue studies with sub-clinical populations, further confirmation of therapeutic success in controlled clinical trials, and a return to analogue studies to identify the active ingredients in systematic desensitization. The most amazing aspect of programmatic research in systematic desensitization is how it has been implemented in many laboratories by hundreds of researchers in many different countries and continents.

Wolpe's (1948, 1952, 1958) original experimentation in developing and treating neuroses in cats was carried out in South Africa.

> In the neuroses produced in cats . . . by administering high voltage, low amperage shocks to them, while confined in a small cage, it was found that the anxiety responses conditioned to the cage and related stimuli and to an auditory stimulus that had preceded the shocks were extremely resistant to the nominal process of extinction. Neither prolonged nor repeated exposure of the animals to the environment of the cage led to decrements in the intensity of these responses even though the animals were never again shocked. The animals, however hungry, could not be tempted to eat attractive food scattered in the experimental cage. However, because they showed milder anxiety on the floor of the experimental laboratory and still less in a series of other rooms, graded to their degree of resemblance to the laboratory, they were offered food in these various places in descending order of similarity. When, in a particular room, the evocation of anxiety was not great enough to inhibit feeding, successive offerings of food were eaten with increasing readiness while all signs of anxiety receded to vanishing point. The room next in resemblance to the experimental laboratory could then be dealt with. After a series of similar steps, eating behavior was eventually restored in the experimental cage itself, and this made possible the total elimination of all signs of anxiety even there. In parallel piecemeal fashion, anxiety was deconditioned from the auditory stimulus that had preceded the shocks. (Wolpe & Lazarus, 1966, pp. 56–57)

The above led Wolpe, a psychiatrist, to search for those elements resulting in production of human neuroses and strategies for their deconditioning. Thus, the original work with cats, theoretical speculation combined with clinical observation and application, and Wolpe's reading of Salter's (1949) *Conditioned Reflex Therapy* and Jacobsen's (1938) *Progressive Relaxation* led to the formulation of systematic desensitization as a treatment for phobia (Wolpe, 1958). It does not require considerable imagination or particularly high Miller Analogy scores to see the parallel between the graduated approaches inherent in systematic desensitization (deep muscle relaxation, development of hierarchy, graded exposure, etc.) and the earlier animal model of reconditioning.

Soon thereafter, large series of phobic patients were treated with desensitization by Wolpe (1958) and Lazarus (1963). Of 210 patients so treated, Wolpe (1958) evaluated the success rate at 90%, whereas Lazarus (1963) considered 70% of some 408 patients he had treated as having derived "marked benefits." However, these were *clinical* evaluations beset by the usual biases held by proponents of one's favorite therapeutic strategy.

Interestingly, the first empirical evidence of the treatment's success was to come from the short-term analogue therapy studies conducted in psychological clinics by graduate students and their professors (e.g., Davison, 1968; Lang & Lazovik, 1963; Lang, Lazovik, & Reynolds, 1965; Paul, 1966). In these short-term treatment studies with mildly fearful (e.g., of snakes) and anxious (e.g., public speaking) college students, data confirmed that systematic desensitization was superior to comparable short-term insight-oriented treatment, waiting list controls, no contact controls, attention-placebo controls, and pseudotherapy controls. An important finding was that "non-believers" in behavior therapy could be trained to conduct systematic desensitization therapy with excellent results. But, criticism was leveled in that subjects were "sub-clinical" and solicited, and insight-oriented therapy was too brief.

The rather spectacular effects of systematic desensitization therapy found in clinical reports and analogue studies have not quite held up in protracted clinical trials with "real" phobics (cf. Marshall, 1981). However, in the oft-quoted clinical trial by Sloane, Staples, Cristol, Yorkston, and Whipple (1975) contrasting behavior therapy, dynamic psychotherapy, and minimal contact, results for behavior therapy (of which systematic desensitization was one of the more frequently used techniques) were superior to the control condition and equal or better to psychotherapy on all dependent measures. An important feature of this study is that each of the therapies was administered by a senior proponent of its application (e.g., Joseph Wolpe). At this point in time systematic desensitization is considered to be the treatment of choice for simple phobia (and some complex phobias) by most practicing clinicians.

The studies in the early and mid 1960s by Peter Lang and his colleagues (Lang & Lazovik, 1963; Lang, Lazovik, & Reynolds, 1965) set the stage for a spate of similar studies in the 1970s to evaluate the components of systematic desensitization. Using sub-clinical college subjects experiencing moderate fear of small animals, many behavioral researchers gave the clinical world the impression that snake, rat, and spider phobia epidemics were rampant on campus (see Hersen, 1979). But whatever their shortcomings (see Kazdin & Wilcoxon, 1976), these research efforts raised important questions about the process of systematic desensitization, such as: (1) the nature of the therapist-patient relationship, (2) the role of relaxation, (3) the importance of standard versus mixed hierarchies, and (4) the validity of Wolpe's theoretical account for why the therapy works.

Many aspects of systematic desensitization still are open to debate (see Bellack & Hersen, 1977, Chap. 2 and 3). And it is unlikely that these will be resolved in the near future. However, its very existence as a treatment strategy has had a marked impact on the clinical world and has stimulated much exciting research of a most comprehensive nature at several levels of inquiry. Moreover, it remains, in our estimation, the classic example of how programmatic research in clinical psychology emerges and continues to bear fruit. Thus, we see its evaluation as the model for programmatic evaluation.

MULTIDISCIPLINARY ISSUES: OR THE TEAMWORK APPROACH

The old adage that "too many cooks spoil the broth" definitely *does not* apply to the current scene in clinical research. Whereas years ago the clinical research endeavor may have been controlled by individual "sultans" and their respective followers, today's norm reflects collaboration and teamwork within and across specific disciplines. Especially in large-scale clinical trials conducted over a number of years, the expertise of many individuals is required to draw the most out of resulting data. Moreover, when psychotherapeutic and pharmacological approaches are contrasted and combined, medical and psychological investigators work hand-in-hand.

We can best illustrate the above points by considering a long-term clinical trial that we have just completed in evaluating treatments for unipolar depressed women (cf. Hersen, Bellack, Himmelhoch, & Thase, in press). The basic design of the study was as follows. Four treatments for 120 female unipolar (nonpsychotic) outpatients were contrasted: (1) social skills plus placebo, (2) social skills plus amitriptyline, (3) amitriptyline, and (4) psychotherapy plus placebo. Experienced clinicians conducted 12 weeks of initial treatment and then 6 months of maintenance therapy at reduced frequency. A large variety of self-report, behavioral, and observer-rated scales served as the dependent measures.

The research team for our study has varied in its membership over some five years, but has mainly consisted of clinical psychologists, psychology interns, post-doctoral fellows, psychiatrists, and psychiatric residents. For example, M. Hersen and A. S. Bellack, clinical psychologists, administered the grant and trained the behavioral therapists. Jonathan Himmelhoch, a psychiatrist, administered the medical aspects of the grant, while Homer V. Capparell, a psychiatrist, conducted "blind" evaluations of patients at various points in the study.

Illustrative of our teamwork approach is how publications reflect particular areas of interest. Let us briefly present a synopsis of the relevant publications emanating from this work. Karen Wells, then a psychology intern, did initial pilot work in the social skills area (Wells, Hersen, Bellack, & Himmelhoch, 1979). Hersen presented clinical results of five cases receiving social skills training during the early part of the study (Hersen, Bellack, & Himmelhoch, 1980). Bellack developed the treatment manual for the social skills approach (Bellack, Hersen, & Himmelhoch, 1980) and presented the initial findings of the study (Bellack, Hersen, & Himmelhoch, 1981). Hersen has described the overall findings for initial and maintenance treatment (Hersen, Bellack, Himmelhoch, & Thase, in press), whereas Bellack has reported specific findings for behavioral measures (Bellack, Hersen, & Himmelhoch, 1983). Hersen has looked at differences between solicited and nonsolicited subjects (Hersen, Bellack, & Himmelhoch, 1981), and this has been followed up with regard to outcome by Cynthia Last, a post-doctoral fellow (psychologist) (Last, Thase, Hersen, Bellack, & Himmelhoch, 1983). Deborah Greenwald and Sander Kornblith (psychologists administering social skill treatment) evaluated differences between social skill therapists and psychotherapists (Greenwald, Kornblith, Hersen, Bellack, & Himmelhoch, 1981). In addition, Michael Thase (a post-doctoral fellow: psychiatrist) has been most interested in evaluating endogenous aspects of depression both from the vantage point of assessment (Thase, Hersen, Bellack, Himmelhoch, & Kupfer, in press), and with regard to differential treatment effectiveness (Thase, Hersen, Bellack, Himmelhoch, Kornblith, & Greenwald, 1982). And finally, Scott Monroe, a clinical psychologist, has examined life events, symptom course, and outcome in our unipolar depressive patients (Monroe, Bellack, Hersen, & Himmelhoch, in press).

In short, our publication endeavors truly mirror the collaborative spirit of our research endeavor.

CLINICAL PSYCHOLOGY WITHIN CONTEXT

Whether or not one can or does work on a multidisciplinary team, it is clear that clinical psychology research cannot be conducted in an intellectual vacuum. The information explosion in the past 10–20 years has made it difficult to keep up with the current literature in one's own field, let alone be current in other disciplines. This is a troublesome situation as it leads to narrow thinking and a tendency to ignore or discount anything that does not seem to be clearly relevant to one's own work. This phenomenon is no less true for clinical psychology than for other disciplines. To produce really meaningful research, the clinical psychologist must stay abreast of progress in related fields both within psychology (e.g., learning, psychobiology, cognitive psychology) and outside of psychology (e.g., medicine, sociology). A good example of this issue is the area of health psychology or behavioral medicine. Here, progress in medicine and physiology have a direct impact on psychological interventions and research. The clinical psychologist working on treatments for headaches or insomnia who is not at least roughly familiar with the physiology of pain and sleep can only produce naive and potentially harmful work (e.g., by failing to differentiate clearly physical disorders from those with substantial psychological components).

The importance of this issue is illustrated in a project one of us (ASB) is conducting on the etiology of essential hypertension. The term "essential" hypertension is taken to mean high blood pressure with an unknown physical cause, and therefore probably a psychological problem. It has long been hypothesized that a critical factor predisposing patients to essential hypertension involved problems handling anger. Either the person is too easily angered, or cannot express anger outwardly and thus "bottles it up" or "represses it" (Weiner, 1979). While this general notion has received widespread support from clinicians working with hypertensives, it has not received much empirical confirmation. This is partly because it really is a rather vague idea, which is impossible to measure objectively (How do you know when someone "represses" anger?).

In an effort to test this hypothesis scientifically, we reconceptualized the anger problems in terms of concrete, measurable deficits in the social skill of assertiveness. Specifically, we hypothesized that individuals with essential hypertension lack the ability to make appropriate assertive responses (e.g., refuse unreasonable requests) when frustrated or treated unfairly. Thus, the problem is not anger per se, but an inability to act assertively, which leads to a variety of unpleasant emotions (e.g., anger, frustration, anxiety), the consequence of which is elevated blood pressure.

This is a nice, testable hypothesis, but there are three problems with it. *First*, it does not account for the fact that many people who are unassertive do not develop essential hypertension. *Second*, it does not explain how frequent blood pressure elevations due to frustration lead to a state of chronic elevation. *Third*, it does not account for the fact that some people with essential hypertension do *not* have problems with assertiveness. Currently, most experts in medicine, physiology and psychology believe that the answers to the first two questions lie in inherited predispositions to develop hypertension. Some people are physiologically susceptible and others are not. Further research on the pathophysiology of hypertension will undoubtedly identify these predisposing factors.

Our own research is focusing on the third issue. Negative emotions can produce elevated blood pressure by their impact on the Autonomic Nervous System (ANS). But, there are a host of other biochemical factors which can produce high blood pressure that are not connected to ANS reactions (e.g., problems in the elasticity of blood vessels). Perhaps, unassertiveness only leads to essential hypertension in individuals whose elevated blood pressure results from ANS overactivity? To answer this question we must somehow be able to distinguish high ANS active hypertensives from non-ANS active hypertensives. How can this be done? One possible way is to measure renin, a biochemical substance produced by the kidney. There are some suggestive data from medical and physiological laboratories (e.g., Esler, Julius, Zweifler, Randall, Harburg, Gardiner, & DeQuattro, 1977; Harburg, Blakelock, & Roeper, 1979) that renin production is a marker for ANS activity: the more renin produced, the more ANS activity. Thus, we have been comparing assertive skills in hypertensives who are high and low in renin production. Preliminary findings support our hypothesis. More important, we never could have *developed* this hypothesis by only reading the clinical psychology literature.

ETHICAL ISSUES

No discussion of research is complete without mention of the ethical issues involved in conducting research with human subjects. (There are substantial issues involved in conducting research with animals as well, but as most clinical psychology research employs human subjects, we will limit our discussion accordingly.) Until recently, scientific ethics were given scant attention. It was simply assumed that scientists were ethical: that they were honest about their data, accurately reported what they did and what they found, and treated subjects with due concern. These assumptions are no longer tacitly accepted either within the scientific community or in the community at large. The vast majority of scientists are honest and do treat their subjects in a responsible and appropriate manner. However, there are some who are not ethical, and there are now well-documented cases of data being forged and subjects being exposed to unsafe and/or needlessly unpleasant conditions. As a result, most research is now subject to oversight and review by some outside group or agency.

At first glance, it might seem unreasonable that all researchers should be penalized by the misdeeds or poor judgement of a few individuals. But, it should be recognized that an investigator does not really have an objective view of his or her own work. Even with the best of intentions, the investigator may underestimate the effects of a particular manipulation on a subject, or conclude that a certain amount of distress is reasonable due to the "great" importance of the experiment. For example, someone investigating the physiological effects of embarrassment might assume that it is reasonable to deceive subjects in order to make certain that they are very embarrassed in front of a group of opposite sex peers. An objective observer, on the other hand, might conclude that the study would not yield sufficiently important information to justify the distress caused subjects, or might be able to suggest a better way to conduct the research.

Another frequent argument against the use of outside review groups is that potential subjects should be able to decide for themselves whether or not they want to participate. In most cases, they can, and they are the final authority on whether or not the study can be conducted. (After all, if no one volunteers the study cannot be run.) However, potential subjects are not always able to make a free and informed choice. Certainly, they cannot give informed consent if the study involves deception: By definition, the experimenter must mislead subjects about the nature of their participation in order to carry out the study. There are also many situations in which potential subjects are unable to make a free choice even when they are informed. Prison inmates often feel that refusing to "volunteer" will result in harsh treatment, or that volunteering may speed their release. Children and psychiatric patients often do not understand what they are volunteering for, or cannot realistically evaluate the risks involved. Finally, even when researchers strive diligently to provide necessary information, they frequently underestimate the complexity of the issues for the naive subject (naturally it seems simple to the researcher as he/she designed the study), and/or take shortcuts in providing information because they have so much invested in the more exciting aspects of conducting the study.

Space does not allow us to present all of the arguments for and against outside review of research. We also cannot consider all of the ethical issues involved in conducting psychological research on human subjects. (Many of the most significant issues will be discussed in the remaining chapters of this book.) In concluding this section, we will present a brief overview of the review procedures involved in submitting a research grant application to the National Institutes of Health (NIH) (the source of most support for clinical psychology research); their requirements are representative.

First and foremost, someone applying for a grant must be affiliated with an organization that has an institutional review board. This is a committee of people who are qualified to evaluate the appropriateness and safety of the experimental procedures. The committee is empowered to develop standards for research conducted at the agency and to provide ongoing oversight of all research conducted there (i.e., they do not simply approve projects; they also insure that the researcher does what he/she promised). Generally, these committees, referred to as Human Use or Human Subject committees, consist of researchers from a variety of scientific disciplines. They are purposefully heterogeneous, so every study is evaluated from diverse perspectives and values. In addition to establishing a review procedure and standard for such things as the Informed Consent Form, they must sign a document certifying that they have approved the research before it can be conducted (with or without grant support). In addition to securing approval from the committee within his or her own institution, the researcher applying for a NIH grant must also indicate to the grant review committee that he/she is familiar with all of the risks and human use issues involved in the study, and justify the procedures accordingly. Every application must contain a discussion of the following points, which should serve as a set of guidelines for *planning* research as well as criteria for evaluating it (United States Public Health Service, 1982, p. 17):

1. Describe the characteristics of the subject population, such as their anticipated number, age ranges, sex, ethnic background, and health status. Identify the criteria for inclusion or exclusion. Explain the rationale for the use of special classes of subjects, such as fetuses, pregnant women, children, institutionalized mentally disabled, prisoners or others who are likely to be vulnerable.
2. Identify the sources of research material obtained from individually identifiable living human subjects in the form of specimens, records, or data. Indicate whether the material or data will be obtained specifically for research purposes or whether use will be made of existing specimens, records, or data.
3. Describe plans for the recruitment of subjects and the consent procedures to be followed, including the circumstances under which consent will be sought and obtained, who will seek it, the nature of the information to be provided to prospective subjects, and the method of documenting consent. State if the institutional review board has authorized a modification or waiver of the elements of consent or the requirement for documentation of consent. The consent form, which must have institutional review board approval, should be submitted to the PHS only on request.
4. Describe any potential risks—physical, psychological, social, legal, or other—and assess their likelihood and seriousness. Where appropriate, describe alternative treatments and procedures that might be advantageous to the subjects.
5. Describe the procedures for protecting against or minimizing any potential risks, including risks to confidentiality, and assess their likely effectiveness. Where appropriate, discuss provisions for insuring necessary medical or professional intervention in the event of adverse effects to the subjects. Also, where appropriate, describe the provisions for monitoring the data collected to insure the safety of subjects.
6. Discuss why the risks to subjects are reasonable in relation to the anticipated benefits to subjects and in relation to the importance of the knowledge that may reasonably be expected to result.

OVERVIEW OF THE BOOK

This book is designed to give the student a basic understanding of the nature of research in clinical psychology. It is not designed to teach basic research skills, but rather to highlight the most significant research issues, methodologies, and topics. This first chapter has examined the central role of research in the definition of the discipline and training of clinical psychologists. The chapters in Section II, *Research Methods*, describe the most common and fundamental methodologies. Chapter 2 discusses reliability and validity. These are basic requirements of sound research, as well as specific factors affecting the quality and utility of assessment procedures. Reliability and validity serve as a backdrop to other aspects of solid research design. Chapters 3, 4, and 5 examine the most widely used research designs: single case designs, group designs, and correlational studies. In addition to highlighting basic design issues, these chapters consider some of the primary controls and procedural requirements to be considered in designing experiments as well as providing examples of well-designed studies.

As indicated above, Section III on *Research Topics* describes the most frequent topics studied in clinical psychology research. Section IV, *General Issues*, deals with two accessory topics which are germane to the research enterprise. In Chapter 13 it becomes clear that one of the best ways to learn how to *design* quality research is to become an effective critic of other people's published studies. Thus, Chapter 13 discusses the critical evaluation of research from the editorial perspective. In addition, one important requirement of the skilled researcher is to be able to obtain sufficient funds to conduct meaningful research. This typically depends on the ability of the investigator to write clear and persuasive grant applications. Therefore, Chapter 14 considers the techniques and strategies for writing effective grant applications as well as the political issues involved.

REFERENCES

American Psychiatric Association. (1980). *Diagnostic and statistical manual of mental disorders* (3rd ed.). Washington, DC: Author.

American Psychological Association. (1947). Recommended graduate training program in clinical psychology. *American Psychologist, 2,* 539–558.

Barlow, D.H. (1980). Behavior therapy: The next decade. *Behavior Therapy, 11,* 315–328.

Bellack, A.S., & Hersen, M. (1977). *Behavior modification: An introductory textbook.* New York: Oxford University Press.

Bellack, A.S., & Hersen, M. (1980). *Introduction to clinical psychology.* New York: Oxford University Press.

Bellack, A.S., Hersen, M., & Himmelhoch, J.M. (1980). Social skills training for depression: A treatment manual. *JSAS Catalog of Selected Documents in Psychology, 10,* 92. (Ms. no. 2156).

Bellack, A.S., Hersen, M., & Himmelhoch, J.M. (1981). Social skills training, pharmacotherapy, and psychotherapy for unipolar depression. *American Journal of Psychiatry, 138,* 1562–1567.

Bellack, A.S., Hersen, M., & Himmelhoch, J.M. (1983). A comparison of social-skills training, pharmacotherapy and psychotherapy for depression. *Behaviour Research and Therapy, 21,* 101–107.

Bloom, L.J., Weigel, R.G., & Trautt, G.M. (1977). "Therapeugenic" factors in psychotherapy: Effects of office decor and subject-therapist sex pairing on the perception of credibility. *Journal of Consulting and Clinical Psychology, 45,* 867–873.

Carman, R.S., Fitzgerald, B.J., & Holmgren, C. (1983). Alienation and drinking motivations among adolescent females. *Journal of Personality and Social Psychology, 44,* 1021–1024.

Davison, G.C. (1968). Systematic desensitization as a counterconditioning process. *Journal of Abnormal Psychology, 38,* 91–99.

Edgington, E.S. (in press). Statistics and single case analysis. In M. Hersen, R. M. Eisler, & P. M. Miller (Eds.), *Progress in behavior modification: Vol. 14.* New York: Academic Press.

Edwards, A.L., & Cronbach, L.J. (1952). Experimental design for research in psychotherapy. *Journal of Clinical Psychology, 8,* 51–59.

Eisler, R.M., Hersen, M., Miller, P.M., & Blanchard, E.B. (1975). Situational determinants of assertive behaviors. *Journal of Consulting and Clinical Psychology, 43,* 330–340.

Esler, M., Julius, S., Zweifler, A., Randall, O., Harburg, E., Gardiner, H., & DeQuattro, V. (1977). Mild high-renin essential hypertension: Neurogenic human hypertension? *New England Journal of Medicine, 296,* 405–411.

Eysenck, H.J., & Eysenck, S. (1968). *The Eysenck Personality Inventory.* San Diego: Education and Industrial Testing Service.

Fyans, L.J., Jr., Salili, F., Maehr, J.L., & Desai, K.A. (1983). A cross-cultural exploration into the meaning of achievement. *Journal of Personality and Social Psychology, 44,* 1000–1013.

Greenwald, D.P., Kornblith, S.J., Hersen, M., Bellack, A. S., & Himmelhoch, J. M. (1981). Differences between social skills therapists and psychotherapists in treating depression. *Journal of Consulting and Clinical Psychology, 49,* 757–759.

Harburg, E., Blakelock, E.H., & Roeper, P.J. (1979). Resentful and reflective coping with arbitrary authority and blood pressure: Detroit. *Psychosomatic Medicine, 41,* 189–202.

Hersen, M. (1979). Limitations and problems in the clinical application of behavioral techniques in psychiatric settings. *Behavior Therapy, 10,* 65–80.

Hersen, M., & Barlow, D.H. (1976). *Single-case experimental designs: Strategies for studying.* New York: Pergamon Press.

Hersen, M., & Bellack, A.S. (Eds.). (1981). *Behavioral assessment: A practical handbook* (2nd ed.). New York: Pergamon.

Hersen, M., Bellack, A.S., & Himmelhoch, J.M. (1980). Treatment of unipolar depression with social skills training. *Behavior Modification, 4,* 547–555.

Hersen, M., Bellack, A.S., & Himmelhoch, J.M. (1981). A comparison of solicited and nonsolicited female unipolar depressives for treatment outcome research. *Journal of Consulting and Clinical Psychology, 49,* 611–613.

Hersen, M., Bellack, A.S., Himmelhoch, J.M., & Thase, M.E. (in press). Effects of social skills training, amitriptyline, and psychotherapy in unipolar depressed women. *Behavior Therapy.*

Jacobsen, E. (1938). *Progressive relaxation.* Chicago: University of Chicago Press.

Kazdin, A.E., Bellack, A.S., & Hersen, M. (Eds.). (1980). *New perspectives in abnormal psychology.* New York: Oxford University Press.

Kazdin, A.E., & Wilcoxin, L.A. (1976). Systematic desensitization and nonspecific treatment effects: A methodological evaluation. *Psychological Bulletin, 83,* 729–758.

Kendall, P.C., & Norton-Ford, J.D. (1982). *Clinical psychology: Scientific and pro-*

fessional dimensions. New York: John Wiley & Sons.

Korchin, S.J. (1983). The history of clinical psychology: A personal view. In M. Hersen, A.E. Kazdin, & A.S. Bellack (Eds.), *The clinical psychology handbook.* New York: Pergamon.

Lang, P.J., & Lazovik, A.D. (1963). Experimental desensitization of a phobia. *Journal of Abnormal and Social Psychology, 66,* 519–525.

Lang, P.J., Lazovik, A.D., & Reynolds, D.J. (1965). Desensitization, suggestibility, and pseudotherapy. *Journal of Abnormal Psychology, 70,* 395–402.

Last, C.G., Thase, M.E., Hersen, M., Bellack, A.S., & Himmelhoch, J.M. (1983). Treatment outcome for solicited vs. nonsolicited unipolar depressed female outpatients. Unpublished manuscript.

Lazarus, A.A. (1963). The results of behaviour therapy in 126 cases of severe neurosis. *Behaviour Research and Therapy, 1,* 69–80.

Marshall, W.L. (1981). Behavioral treatment of phobic and obsessive-compulsive disorders. In L. Michelson, M. Hersen, & S.M. Turner (Eds.), *Future perspectives in behavior therapy.* New York: Plenum Press.

Monroe, S.M., Bellack, A.S., Hersen, M., & Himmelhoch, J.M. (in press). Life events, symptom course, and outcome for female unipolar depressives receiving treatment. *Journal of Consulting and Clinical Psychology.*

Paul, G.L. (1966). *Insight versus desensitization in psychotherapy: An experiment in anxiety reduction.* Stanford, CA: Stanford University Press.

Raimy, V. (Ed.). (1950). *Training in clinical psychology.* New York: Prentice-Hall.

Salter, A. (1949). *Conditional reflex therapy.* New York: Creative Age Press.

Schmidt, N., & Sermat, U. (1983). Measuring loneliness in different relationships. *Journal of Personality and Social Psychology, 44,* 1038–1047.

Sloane, R.B., Staples, F.R., Cristol, A.H., Yorkston, J.J., & Whipple, K. (1975). *Psychotherapy versus behavior therapy.* Cambridge, MA: Harvard University Press.

Thase, M.E., Hersen, M., Bellack, A.S., Himmelhoch, J.M., Kornblith, S.J., & Greenwald, D.P. (1982). Social skills training and endogenous depression. Unpublished manuscript.

Thase, M.E., Hersen, M., Bellack, A.S., Himmelhoch, J.M., & Kupfer, D.J. (in press). Validation of a Hamilton Scale for endogenous depression. *Journal of Affective Disorders.*

U.S. Public Health Service. (1982). *Grant application Form 398.* Washington, DC: U.S. Government Printing Office.

Weiner, H. (1979). *The psychobiology of essential hypertension.* New York: Elsevier.

Wells, K.C., Hersen, M., Bellack, A.S., & Himmelhoch, J.M. (1979). Social skills training in unipolar nonpsychotic depression. *American Journal of Psychiatry, 136,* 1331–1332.

Wolpe, J. (1948). An approach to the problem of neurosis based on the conditioned response. Unpublished M.D. thesis, University of Witwatersrand, South Africa.

Wolpe, J. (1952). Objective psychotherapy of the neuroses. *South African Medical Journal, 26,* 825–829.

Wolpe, J. (1958). *Psychotherapy by reciprocal inhibition.* Stanford, CA: Stanford University Press.

Wolpe, J., & Lazarus, A.A. (1966). *Behavioral techniques: A guide to the treatment of neuroses.* New York: Pergamon.

Part 2
RESEARCH METHODS

2
Reliability and Validity

Lee Sechrest

INTRODUCTION

The acts of measurement are unavoidable, whether in science or in everyday life. I define measurement as the assignment of quantitative statements to phenomena according to rules devised in a way so as to have some likelihood of reflecting the characteristic of interest. Assigning quantitative statements (e.g., numbers) haphazardly or randomly or in ways that do not imply quantity is not measurement. Statements of quantity may be as crude as "a lot of" or "small," or they may even be binary in nature (exists or does not exist). Since to exist at all implies some value of a characteristic above zero or some other threshold, there is no reason not to consider a binary designation as measurement.

A special case of binary assignment involves what is sometimes called "nominal" measurement. In that type of "measurement," phenomena are assigned to categories (e.g., apples may be designated as "red," "yellow," or "green"). It is possible, however, and I think useful, to regard such designations as a series of binary assessments (e.g., red, yes or no; yellow, yes or no; green, yes or no). (The similarity to dummy coding of categorical variables in statistical analysis is obvious.) Thus, a red apple can be thought of as having a binary-system "score" of 100, a yellow apple one of 010, and so on.

Measurements differ, of course, along a dimension of precision, and some are made with a high degree of precision, or at least implied precision. When a nurse records a patient's oral temperature as 100.4 degrees Fahrenheit or when a highway patrolman clocks a speeder at 78 mph, that at least implies a substantial degree of precision. This is easily seen by contrasting the numerical statements with more mundane language, such as "has a low-grade fever" or "driving very fast." Even more precise, again implicitly, are statements such as that the membership of the American Psychological Association (APA) in 1982 was 54,282. That highly precise statement is open to such questions as: Can 54,000 things really be counted that accurately? Did no one resign or die on the day the count was made? Were no new applications processed that day? Is it possible that someone might have been listed twice under different names? It is of interest to consider what happens if the estimate is given as "about 54,300," or even as "about 54,000." The fact that we *can* report measures with high precision does not necessarily mean that we should do so, since such implied precision may be spurious and misleading.

We all regularly make quantitative statements about phenomena in everyday life and are not so much different from scientists in doing so; George Kelly (1955) thought it useful to view Everyman as scientist. We say, "It is a warm day." Or we say, "That is a great team." Or, "That is a beautiful dress." We may become more numerical in such statements as "I am sure it is over 90 degrees," or, "On a scale of 1 to 10, that dress is a 9." In making such statements we follow our own or some consensually accepted set of rules. That is, we do not make such statements without reason, or haphazardly.

Science does not differ in its measurement processes from other exact, or aspiring to be exact, fields or disciplines. Science does proceed by following relatively exact rules that can be explicated if necessary. But so do other enterprises. For example, the number of members in the APA is arrived at by a rule (if implicit) something like: Identify each separate listing on the membership roster and increment the count by one for each listing. (Duplicates are eliminated, all members count equally, and so on.) A bank counts its money, down to the penny, in much the same way and with a high degree of exactness. It should be clear, though, that exactness may imply far more precision than is actual (e.g., computers will calculate answers to many more decimals than are warranted by most of our data).

The rules for scientific measurement should be clear and explicable, but they do not necessarily have to produce precision in the usual sense. A rule for measuring psychopathology, for example, might be: Accept the judgment of a trained clinician who will have had contact with the subject for at least 2 hours. Assuming terms such as "trained clinician" to be definable, the rule is clear, communicable, and replicable. It is just as good a rule, from a scientific standpoint, as "use an oral thermometer reading provided by a nurse" or "use the score from the XYZ scale." Scientists may, albeit often with reluctance, measure by means of black boxes as long as they believe that the black boxes, by whatever unknown processes, produce dependable information.

RELIABILITY, VALIDITY, AND GENERALIZABILITY

When we measure something, we want to obtain a value (score) that is generalizable or dependable[1] (Cronbach, Gleser, Rajaratnam, & Nanda, 1972). The value we obtain has to have a meaning that transcends its specific occurrence. If you are told that a prospective student has an IQ score of 140, you may

[1]In this chapter the term *dependability* will be preferred, following Cronbach, Gleser, Rajaratnam, and Nanda, but it will be used interchangeably with reliability and should be understood to refer to generalizability of a score or value.

have some interest in that score because of your anticipations about what it may mean. But if you are told that the score should not be taken as an indicator of performance on any other test, under any other circumstances, at any other time, or in relation to any other behavior, your interest in the score will be reduced to wondering why anyone bothered to obtain it, let alone tell you about it. Scores generated by a table of random numbers would not be of any interest. To the extent that scores are not generated randomly, they may be of interest because they may generalize to some other performance.

Some scores largely reflect the characteristics of the instruments used to produce them. For example, a time produced by an electronic timer used in a race reflects almost solely the characteristics of the instrument: how accurate it is, how sensitive it is, how dependable it is. Other values represent the conjunctions of instrument and user within a system. Thus, the value of representing "how high off the ground are we" as determined by an altimeter may reflect both the characteristics of the altimeter and the person reading it. A faulty altimeter may produce readings that both pilot and co-pilot would agree on but that might or might not be correct at any given moment. By contrast, a poorly designed altimeter might give highly accurate information if properly read, but might be so difficult to read that a pilot and co-pilot might sometimes disagree about their altitude.

Upon obtaining an altitude estimate, we will be interested in its generalizability to many different circumstances. For example, here are some:

- To another user: Will the co-pilot make the same estimate?
- To other times: Will the reading be the same on the return trip?
- To other weather conditions: Does it matter that it is raining now?
- To other terrain: If there is a lake below instead of land, is the reading still OK?
- To other altimeters.
- To altitude measured in other ways: Does the reading agree with radar?

These do not exhaust the possibilities (e.g., if we were going to move the altimeter to another airplane, we would want to know whether the value would generalize across that move). All of these are important considerations if we are asked to put our faith in an altimeter. We would not want an altimeter that varied considerably under different weather conditions even if, on the average, it was correct. Nor would we want an altimeter that was dependable across many conditions if it always overestimated altitude by 200 feet.

Some of these types of generalizability are often called reliability, a useful term, although, in my opinion, somewhat superceded by the notion of generalizability. It is often said, somewhat unthinkingly, that a measure cannot be valid if it is not reliable. Reflection on the example of the altimeter will show that that is not so. If I am the sole user of my altimeter, and it is dependable in other respects, I may not care that another person reading it would not agree with me. And I would not want an altimeter that did not vary over time if I believed that my veritable altitude was changing over time. I might not even care if my altimeter overestimated altitude as long as it did so systematically in some simple way (e.g., requiring only the subtraction of 200 feet from every estimate).

It also is clear that the various types of dependability (or generalizability) are not intersubstitutable. Assurances that the altimeter is not affected by weather conditions will not be relevant to the question of whether it is dependable without respect to the nature of the terrain over which one flies. Similarly, the dependabilities of psychological and behavioral measures are not intersubstitutable. Harrell (1981) claimed, for example, that a measure of remorsefulness in criminal offenders inferred from probation officer reports was "reliable," because when he scored the material on two separate occasions, he obtained the same values. It is common to find references to the reliability of measures based solely on the fact that two judges agree in scoring them. Such uses of the term completely ignore the many facets of the problem of establishing dependability.

To take a measure that is more psychological/behavioral in nature, consider the assessment of snake phobia by an approach test (i.e., a test that determines how closely a subject will approach a snake, usually encased in a glass cage within a laboratory room). Let us say that an approach score of three feet is obtained on the occasion of measurement. We would, or ought to, then want to know whether the score would generalize to:

- other occasions,
- other examiners,
- other rooms,
- other snakes,
- other instructions,
- other situations, e.g., zoos,
- uncaged snakes in the grass, or
- willingness to go on picnics in the woods.

The number and complexity of these issues stand in stark contrast to usual efforts to assess "reliability" of behavior in such situations.

Universe Scores

Classical test theory depended heavily on the notion of a *true* score assumed to be characteristic of a subject (although the idea is readily extended, for example, to scores descriptive of objects or situations).[2] Every observed score was then regarded as a true score plus some random error. Thus, an observed

---

[2]In this chapter, whenever the term "subject" is used, it should be understood that the notions would apply as well to objects, situations, or other things being measured.

IQ score of, let us say, 140, could be regarded as a reflection of a true, but unknown, IQ plus error, which could, of course, have either a positive or a negative value. Since, however, the errors involved were assumed to be random, just as likely to be positive or negative, any observed score was assumed to be an unbiased estimate of the true score. And with only one observed score, as on an IQ test, the observed score was considered to be the best estimate of the true score.

Cronbach et al. (1972) thought it more useful to think in terms of *universe* scores (termed *generic true scores* by Lord & Novick, 1968). Every observed score can be thought of as a sample from a universe of scores that might have been obtained under the prevailing conditions of measurement. An IQ score of 140 would be one of a universe of IQ scores that might have been obtained for the person in question, the universe to be defined by the conditions of measurement and the interpreter of the score. Universes can be defined quite broadly or very narrowly. For example, the following are two descriptions of universes that might be (explicitly or implicitly) the bases for interpretation of the IQ score:

- Scores obtained on the Epsilon test administered in careful adherence to standard directions by Examiner X in a laboratory setting during the morning hours of a weekday with the subject strongly motivated to perform well.
- Scores obtained on standardized IQ tests administered by trained examiners.

The latter universe is more nearly the one usually assumed in interpretation of IQ scores, but note that it assumes that the Epsilon test that was actually used, the examiner (E) actually involved, the conditions of testing, and so on are representative of the universe. The reasonableness of the interpretation depends on the reasonableness of those assumptions.

An even broader universe of performances is involved in the interpretation that "This person with an IQ score of 140 is a really smart person who will do well in classes." That interpretation assumes that the IQ testing situation is representative of a very wide range of intellectual performances.

Components of Variance. A straightforward extension of the idea of the universe score is that any given score may (theoretically) be decomposed into sources of variance. True score theory postulates that, in effect, all variance not attributable to the true score itself is random error. Generalizability theory, which is what Cronbach and his associates have called their theory of test scores, postulates that an observed score is the result of a number, perhaps a large number, of factors, some perhaps known, with the residual, otherwise termed error, better regarded as unexplained variance. As implied previously, a snake phobia score is attributable to the particular conditions, the examiner, the instructions, the particular snake, and so on.

If the appropriate studies are done, it is possible to estimate the variance in scores attributable to what Cronbach et al. call *facets* of the measurement process. One could, for example, determine either for a particular subject or across subjects how much of the variance in snake approach scores is attributable to: (1) the type of snake used, (2) the specific instructions, or (3) the interaction of type of snake and instructions. In such a study, the variance attributable to the examiner might be eliminated by using only one examiner, albeit at the possible cost of limiting the interpretation of the findings, or might be allowed to enter the unexplained variance term by employing multiple examiners without systematically estimating that effect.

It should be clear from the preceding discussion that there is no one "reliability coefficient" for any test or measure (nor any one "validity coefficient"). There are as many reliability coefficients as there are conditions of measurement or as there are universes from which to sample. The appropriate value to use will reflect the universe to which one wishes to generalize. If one wishes to generalize across examiners, then it is not appropriate to use an estimate of dependability (reliability) based on results obtained by one examiner. Suppose one wanted to show, for example, that students exposed to an intervention designed to increase assertiveness would, in fact, become socially more assertive. If in a post-intervention in vivo test, one used three different situations but only a single confederate, one should not use the reliability coefficient calculated for the three situations in a later claim that the performance is dependable across different stimulus persons or across time as in a test-retest measurement.

Classical Concepts of Reliability

Discussions of reliability have usually referred to three or four forms of dependability that are somewhat narrow, delimited aspects of generalizability. In effect, the various forms each represent one facet of a universe. From the standpoint of generalizability, there is nothing particularly special about any one of the concepts, but the failure to understand the generalizability problem and the possible confusion stemming from the use of the same term—reliability—to refer to them all, has led to serious misuses in the research literature, primarily the tendency to consider them as intersubstitutable with the consequent frequent use of the wrong type of reliability estimate.

In classical test theory, *parallel forms reliability* represents a key concept (Gulliksen, 1950; Lord & Novick, 1968). Underlying this notion is the assumption that agreement between parallel forms of a test, defined as yielding identical true scores and independent errors with the same variances (Lord & Novick, 1968), should provide a good estimate of the reliability of a performance. In effect, if a Form A and a Form B of a test are carefully constructed so that the items on the two forms are equivalent, then the correlation between the two forms should be a good estimate of the reliability of measurement. A problem immediately arises in that it is difficult to know that two forms are equivalent if they do not correlate highly, and unless the two forms are administered simultaneously, or at least quite near in time, the correlation may be reduced because of changes over time as well as because of unreliability of measurement. It is, of course, difficult in many areas to construct parallel measures, and the use of parallel forms has been largely limited to achievement and ability testing.

In any case, when placed in the context of generalizability theory, parallel forms address only the question of generalizability across the universe of test items. All other facets (e.g., examiners, are either fixed so that they have no effect or are varied unsystematically so that their effects become part of the unexplained [error] variance).

Test-retest reliability avoids the problems involved in trying to produce parallel forms of a measure on two occasions, and thereby limits the generalizability question to one of time and such incidental situational changes as occur with two test administrations. The question of the appropriate time interval across which test-retest reliability ought to be established always arises and has never been quite satisfactorily resolved. As Lord and Novick (1968) point out, there are three difficulties with test-retest reliability estimates: practice effects, fatigue effects, and genuine changes in what is being measured. Practice (and memory) effects tend to produce errors that are correlated—not random—over occasions and may, therefore, inflate estimates of reliability. Fatigue effects may increase the random element on the second occasion and reduce apparent reliability. Genuine changes would be expected to reduce reliability unless there is some sort of constant change across all subjects. Memory and fatigue effects should be relatively short-lived and, hence, affect reliability only over brief intervals. But the longer the intervals, the greater the likelihood of real change. One may say that the appropriate interval between tests is that over which generalizability is an issue. In measuring bodily processes such as temperature and blood pressure, for example, only brief intervals of the order of minutes would appear appropriate if one wanted to determine the stability of a reading obtained with a particular instrument. More psychological characteristics such as trait anxiety, phobic responses, and social assertiveness ought to be demonstrably stable over days or weeks. Intelligence is usually thought to be highly stable; it would not be unreasonable to use a much longer time interval to demonstrate temporal stability, since the generalizations we are inclined to make have a relatively long time frame.

Internal consistency can be seen as a special case of parallel forms since the interest is in generalizability across the universe of test items and not across time, examiners, situations, and so on. The various coefficients estimating internal consistency, although varying somewhat in specific assumptions, address the question of whether the specific items chosen from the universe of items make a difference in the scores obtained.

Agreement between judges, or *judge reliability,* although not part of classical test theory, is often encountered in the literature. Obviously the issue of agreement between judges has to do with the question of whether the particular judges selected from the universe of judges, which may be broadly or narrowly defined, make a difference in the values that are obtained from the judging process. It should be obvious why a correlation between judges cannot be substituted for other forms of reliability.

"Items" in Psychological/Behavioral Research. If we were to measure self-assertiveness by means of a typical self-report questionnaire or inventory, we might well include an item such as: "I do not have any difficulty resisting requests to do things that I would rather not do." But we would certainly recognize that that one item comes nowhere close to exhausting the definition of the concept of social assertiveness, and that it is susceptible to idiosyncratic interpretations that would make us unwilling to use it as a single item test. So we would create other items from an imagined, even if poorly specified, universe (domain) of possible items. Similarly, we ought with other kinds of measures to recognize that single instances of behavior may not be sufficiently dependable to be of great value in either research or clinical work. How much confidence ought we to have in a single observation of whether a subject takes a near or a far chair when invited to enter a room and take a seat? But as Epstein (1979, 1980) has argued both cogently and with data, when aggregated across enough instances, behavioral observations may show quite useful consistency. Rushton, Brainerd, and Pressley (1983) provide a number of instances in which aggregation resulted in impressive overall dependability of measurement.

Errors of Measurement

Errors of measurement are of two kinds: constant and random. Only the latter play an important role in theory measurement, but it is important to understand constant errors. A constant error is one that is the same for every subject with a particular score. If the error is the same for all scores within the sample, and if the error is detected, it is a relatively simple matter to deal with by either adding or subtracting the appropriate correction. For example, if using a female confederate in an assertiveness assessment study results in a somewhat higher assertiveness score for all subjects in a known category, say for all males, then the scores of those subjects can be corrected by subtracting a constant from the scores of all males. Of, if there is an average loss from fatigue of four points on a test, four points can be added to all the scores to estimate the true effect of any intervention. The problem is considerably more complicated, but still resolvable, if constant errors are a function of the original scores (e.g., practice effects are larger for subjects with initially higher scores). The problem is to detect and correct the error by a correction related to the scores.

Random errors are those that are uncorrelated from person to person, occasion to occasion, test to test, and so on. The magnitude of random error (including unexplained variance) may be estimated and used to establish ranges (standard errors of measurement) within which true scores have a probability of lying. The standard error of measurement is given by:

$$\sigma = \sigma\sqrt{1 - r_{tt}}$$

where σ is the standard deviation of the set of scores, and r_{tt} is the reliability of the measure. The value obtained represents an estimate of the limits within which it is .67 probable that the true score lies. The *probable error of measurement* is .6745 of the standard error and is an estimate of the limits within which it is .5 probable that the true score lies. For example, the standard deviation of IQ scores from individually administered tests of intelligence is usually about 15, and the reliability of such tests is around .85. Thus, the standard error of measurement is about 6 (5.8). Therefore, if a youngster obtains an IQ score of 115 on a test, there is about a two-out-of-three likelihood that his true IQ score is between 109 and 121, and there is about a 50/50 probability that it is between 111 and 119.

Note that the standard error of measurement depends heavily on the estimate of reliability that is used. The interpretation of the standard error of measurement should *always* be couched in terms of the specific concept of reliability that is used in the formula. If the reliability estimate is of internal consistency, then the interpretation would be that with a different, randomly chosen set of items from the same universe of items, the probability is .67 that the score would lie within the calculated limits. If the estimate were for test-retest reliability, then the interpretation would be that upon retesting after some interval but with the same items the score would be within the obtained limits. It ought to be evident why an internal consistency coefficient should not be used to estimate the standard error associated with retesting. If the reliability were for agreement between judges, the interpretation would be in terms of the likelihood of obtaining a score within the calculated limits with a different judge (e.g., scorer).

Asymmetrical Errors of Measurement. The previous discussion of errors of measurement assumes that errors of measurement are symmetrical around the observed score (i.e., that for any given score, the likelihood and magnitude of errors is equally likely on either side of the observed score). That is, for example, equally likely that an observed IQ score of 115 is too high by 6 points as too low by 6 points. That assumption may be challenged, and the implications are important.

The logic of the challenge is that the direction and magnitude of error is related to the extremeness of the observed score because error contributes to extremeness. Random errors are uncorrelated across occasions, and so on, but observed scores represent only single observations. If we think of the things that might be favorable to obtaining a high score other than ability, we would come up with such factors as trying particularly hard, being lucky in being asked the things one happens to know, having scoring errors be in one's favor, feeling extra good at the time, and so on. The more of these things in one's favor on any occasion of measurement, the higher one's score would be likely to be for any given level of ability. Conversely, the higher one's observed score, the more likely it is that one or more of these things did operate and that the effects were large. If a runner is to break a world record, then everything has to be going well for him or her at the same time. Similarly, very low scores tend to occur when everything goes poorly at once. It is not that a low score does not reflect low ability, but it is also likely to have in it a component of particularly poor luck unlikely to be repeated on some subsequent occasion. This logic suggests, then, that errors of measurement are both biased and relatively large for extreme scores and least biased and smallest for scores in the middle of a distribution.

The detailed arguments for regression to the mean cannot be given here (see Cook & Campbell, 1979), but it is both a statistical and empirical certainty that observations that are extreme on one occasion are likely to be less so on subsequent occasions. That is so because the observed extreme observations include a lot of luck that will not occur on subsequent occasions. The 10 highest scoring teams one week will almost certainly not score as many points the next week, and the 10 lowest scoring teams will score more. The students at the top of the grade distribution on the first quiz will not do as well on the second quiz. Especially short fathers will have sons that are, on the average, taller than they, and a year that is rainier than usual is likely to be followed by one that is relatively drier.

The phenomenon of regression to the mean is a function of reliability of measurement—or, more accurately—of unreliability. Because highly reliable measurements have smaller error components, it follows that extreme scores will be less inaccurate and that regression will be less. If the 10 highest scoring teams this week were also among the highest scoring last week and were similarly high scoring last year, we may suspect that our measure of scoring potential is fairly dependable and that little regression is likely. If a student has scored high on several different tests, reliability of measurement can be assumed to be substantial, and little regression toward the mean will occur. On the other hand, if performance is determined largely by chance (i.e., has a large error component), regression will be substantial. If a group of novices are asked to hit one golfball each and are then asked to hit another, we would expect a great deal of regression toward the mean on the second shot (i.e., the shortest hitters would get better and the longest hitters would appear to deteriorate).

The amount of regression expected for any performance is equal to $1 - r_{tt}$, i.e., 1 minus the reliability of the measure. Thus, if an IQ score is measured with a reliability of .85, we would expect that upon remeasurement it would regress toward the mean by about .15 of the difference between the observed score and the mean. An IQ score of 115 would be expected to regress by about $.15 \times 15$, or about 2 points. Classical test theory postulates that the best estimate of the true IQ of a person scoring 115, in the absence of other information, is 115. This more sophisticated test theory that incorporates considerations of reliability of measurement (Lord & Novick, 1968) suggests that the best estimate of the true IQ of a person scoring 115 is about 113 (assuming that reliability is .85). Since the correlation between heights of fathers and sons is about .5, the best estimate of the likely height of a son of a father who is about 4 inches shorter than average is that he will be about 2 inches shorter than average. This variation of test theory should help us to keep from being surprised on occasion by inconsistencies in performance. We should understand why, for example, a student who scores 1300 on the SATs may not really do all that much better than a student who scores 1200. At least a part of the advantage of the higher scoring student is likely to be attributable to error of measurement.

It is not invariably the case that any repeated observation will regress toward the mean of the most obvious sample or population. Regression will be in the direction of the mean from which the observed score is a departure. For example, if we knew that a student came from a highly intelligent family, that the student was a graduate student in mathematics, and that the student had been selected for a prestigious fellowship, then we might expect that an observed IQ score of 115 resulted from measurement error actually driving it downward. That is, we would think it likely that the student was really brighter than IQ = 115 would indicate.[3] We would expect the student on any subsequent occasion to score higher than 115. Or, if a professional golfer and a complete novice each drove a golfball 175 yards on one try, we might well expect the professional to hit it further on the next try and the novice to have a shorter drive. Each would regress toward the mean of the appropriate comparison group. Knowing a student's background provides information about intelligence, and likely IQ score, that causes us to think that the observed score must be low. And knowing that a golfer is a professional or a novice gives us information upon which to base an expectation of performance. Ordinarily, the more information we have, the more reliable our measurement, and the less regression we may expect.

---

[3]James Watson, the Nobel Prize winner, claimed (Watson, 1968) that his measured IQ was only 106! We can be sure that a lot of measurement error was involved in that score.

It is important to recognize that seemingly irrelevant information may actually constitute "measurement" of a sort. *Any* item of information that is correlated with a variable of interest is, in effect, a measurement. For example, if one had to guess which of the following sentences is most likely an erroneous description, the choice is obvious: He is 6 feet, 3 inches tall./She is 6 feet, 3 inches tall. That is because knowledge of sex enables us to say something about expected height. One of my friends (Turner, 1980) once diagnosed a person as not mentally retarded, although the person had actually been diagnosed as retarded and had himself accepted as fact that he was retarded. The basis for the revised diagnosis was that the person wrote a cogent, literate, and sensitive letter to a newspaper editor. Anxiety may, at least across persons, be assumed in persons who are in psychotherapy; being in therapy is, then, in some sense a measure of anxiety. These considerations become important in the design of research. For example, a group of persons who both score high on an anxiety scale *and* are in psychotherapy are probably dependably more anxious than a group who score the same on the scale but do not seek therapy. The scale and enrollment in psychotherapy give us two measures of anxiety that are likely to be more reliable than the scale alone.

CLASSICAL CONCEPTS OF VALIDITY

Several different concepts have usually been presented in discussions of validity. These concepts have been written about as "types" of validity, as if they were separate. More recently, however, validity has come to be accepted as a single concept, and these types of validity are more properly regarded as components of validity and as types of evidence that might be adduced in favor of validity (Committee to Develop Joint Technical Standards for Educational and Psychological Testing, 1983). There are three components that appear to be distinguishable: content, criterion-related, and construct. Only two of these are, in my view, true validity concepts, but all three merit mention, along with the old but still useful notion of face validity.

Content and Face Validity

As indicated earlier, the issues of validity of measurement have to do with the generalizability of performances on one measure to performances on some other measure. Tests or other measures are valid for whatever they generalize to and to the extent that they generalize. Neither face nor content components of validity are necessary nor sufficient conditions for generalization to occur. They may, however, be necessary for acceptance of measures by those who are to use them or to whom they may be applied, and they may contribute to other validity components.

Face Validity. If a test appears to measure what it purports to measure, it may be said to have face validity. A test lacking in face validity may tend to be unacceptable to some part of a community exposed to it. For example, when I was in graduate school, a question once asked on prelims required students to list the colors of the covers on various psychological journals. Some of the students were upset with the question on the grounds that it had no connection with what the prelims were supposed to be about. The question lacked face validity, at least for some students. State and national legislators, newspaper columnists, and so on have on occasion attacked behavioral scientists for using measures that did not have obvious connections to the characteristics that were purportedly being measured. Cronbach (1970) has indicated that face validity is especially important in employment testing, and it will probably become even more so as demands for obvious job relevance increase.

On the other hand, for some purposes face validity seems to have negative value, since if subjects know what is being measured, they can easily distort their responses. Such measures are highly *reactive* (Webb, Campbell, Schwartz, Sechrest, & Grove, 1981). That has led some investigators to attempt deliberately to develop scales or other measures *lacking* face validity. Some scales of this type are called "subtle" (e.g., Wiener, 1948). This is not the place to review the literature on subtle scales, but the evidence suggests that attempts to develop subtle personality scales have not been successful. They are both poor predictors of other behavior and are insufficiently subtle, since they are susceptible to faking despite efforts to ensure otherwise (Holden, 1982). The case for nonreactive (including unobtrusive) measures has been put strongly by Webb et al. (1981), but there is still not an abundance of evidence for their general usefulness.

Although face validity may be important for the acceptance of measures and may even be a characteristic of most good personality measures (Holden, 1982), it is not certain that face validity should be sought for its own sake. Measures may have a high degree of face validity with little additional advantage for measurement purposes. What can be stated firmly is that face validity is not at all a sufficient ground for presuming any type of generalizability.

One final point is that there is no standard method for assessing face validity and no metric in which it may be expressed if it is studied. We do not know quite how to measure face validity, how much of it we have got, and how much of it we ought to have.

Content Validity. Every measure, including individual items, can be considered a sample of some universe of related measures. To use another term common in measurement, our measures aim, or ought to aim, to sample some *domain* of behaviors or characteristics that is the focus of our interest. Content validity refers to the adequacy with which a universe or domain is sampled. For example, an arithmetic test made up solely of problems involving division of fractions might be considered to lack content validity even though division of fractions might require the separate operations of addition, subtraction, and multiplication. Similarly, a test of attitudes toward authority that had items referring only to supervisor-worker relationships might be thought to lack content validity; the domain of attitudes toward authority is broader than that.

The idea of content validity can be extended to responses required as well as to stimuli. A measure of social assertiveness that tapped only the ability to refuse intrusive requests would be lacking in content validity. Not only is the stimulus of intrusive requests too narrow, but the response of refusing does not well represent the universe of responses that need to be sampled in studying social assertiveness. In part, the processes involved in social validation (Kazdin, 1977) can be seen as an attempt to assure content validity, since the attempt is to show that changes in the targeted behaviors are associated with more general changes in the broader domain.

As with face validity, we have no standard procedures for studying, producing, or assessing content validity. Even for such a simple domain as arithmetic, for example, no one can say exactly how many of just what kinds of problems ought to be in an arithmetic test to ensure content validity. For a test of attitudes toward authority, how many "father" items should there be in relation to "boss" items and "political leader" items and "legal authority" items? What is done, in fact, when the issue of content validity is considered at all, is that a domain or universe is roughly defined and then an attempt is made to see that each of the major parts of the domain is represented by some items.[4] If that is done, the measure is pronounced satisfactory unless it is subjected to criticism by someone else.

Criterion-Related Validity

In academic and employment testing, criterion-related, or empirical, validity looms as a large problem. Empirical validity has also been a substantial problem in the attempts of psychologists and others to predict recidivism of criminal offenders and, to a lesser extent, of mental patients. It is looming larger and larger in relation to the alleged inability of psychologists (and psychiatrists) to predict violent behavior. It will likely become a problem in the

[4]Some universes might be defined by ecological analysis, determining what items or behaviors occur with what frequency under natural circumstances and representing them proportionately in samples. For example, people probably add more often than they divide in doing everyday arithmetic. That approach might not, however, let behaviors be represented in terms of their criticality. If inability to divide properly is more likely to result in critical errors, then division items might need to be overweighted in relation to the frequency of their occurrence.

field of mental disorder more generally as clinicians are asked to make predictions about response to deinstitutionalization, to discontinuation of treatment, and so on.

Criterion-related validity lies in the size of the correlations between our measures and some behavior of interest in its own right. Thus, for example, a measure of predicted violent behavior, which may utilize the clinician as a "black box" predictor, is validated against the occurrence or nonoccurrence of violent behavior. The criterion must itself be of interest and not be simply a sign or indicator of something else. In that case, one begins to get into the realm of construct validity. In employment testing, the criterion should be success on the job, however that is defined. In prediction of recidivism, the criterion should be rearrest, reconviction, return to prison, or some other measure of failure to maintain good behavior.

One potential threat to estimates of empirical validity is the possibility that knowledge of test scores or other measures may affect the criterion, in which case the criterion is said to be *contaminated.* If, for example, probation officers know the recidivism risk scores of delinquent youths, that knowledge may affect their decisions about which youths to return to institutions. That would increase the apparent validity of the predictor. On the other hand, if a prisoner is labeled as potentially violent, that may lead to extra-careful treatment that would reduce the likelihood of violence and, hence, decrease the apparent validity of the predictor. My very first publication (Hemphill & Sechrest, 1952) demonstrated a relationship between ratings by superiors of the skill of bomber crews; a relationship that was attributable to the fact that the superiors had access to the bombing accuracy scores of the crews. And those accuracy scores proved to have a (test-retest: i.e., across missions) reliability of .00! Bomber crews were building reputations on chance variations in performance.

At one time, criterion measures were assumed to be measured without error; in fact, the concepts of validity and reliability were said to be irrelevant to criteria. One determined, after all, just what it was that one wanted to predict, and there was no point then in asking whether it was in principle predictable. It is now accepted that all measures, including criterion and dependent measures, are measured with some error and that findings are better interpreted if that measurement error is taken into account. Correction for unreliability (attenuation) must be done with care lest the results be misleading, but measurement error ought not to be ignored.

It may be instructive to consider what is meant by measurement error for instances in which it may not be obvious. In the first place, in nearly all instances the actual behaviors or characteristics we observe are only surrogates for the psychological/behavioral phenomena in which we are interested. Take, for example, income. When we use it as an independent variable, we are unlikely, as psychologists, to be interested in dollars per se. Rather, we are interested in a set of attitudes or a cluster of experiences that we believe go along with income at differing levels. Income is likely to be only a fairly pale shadow of those attitudes or experiences, and however precisely we may count the dollars, we need to recognize that the underlying variable(s) of interest is (are) at best poorly measured. People will have arrived at given income levels in different ways, will have varying demands on income that alter its meaning, and so on.

Recidivism and violence provide good examples of seemingly objective criteria that are not what they seem. We might be inclined to think that recidivism is clear cut: Delinquents either go back to institutions or they do not. But we are not really likely to be interested in the literal fact of reincarceration. We use recidivism as a sign of continuing criminal tendencies. We would not, for example, be particularly happy with a program that simply made delinquents more clever so that they were less likely to be caught. And we would not be very happy about delinquents reincarcerated for purely technical violations of parole taken advantage of by vindictive or overly strict parole officers. And we would, if we thought about it, realize that decisions about reincarceration are often razor's-edge-type decisions, with some delinquents barely escaping reincarceration and others barely falling into it. Similar concerns occur for violence as a criterion. Surely, some "missed" predictions of violence occur because the offender is not detected in the behavior. Other predictions may go awry because the behavior is just not quite violent enough to fall into the category (e.g., a fistfight may not be termed assault by a police officer). And in still other instances a violent act may be accidentally averted (e.g., a potential victim successfully escapes or a passing patrol car makes a mugging too risky). We use known violent acts as an index of continuing propensity toward violence, but those acts do not capture the propensity with more than modest accuracy.

Criterion-related validity does offer the advantage that we can quantify it and express it in reasonably well understood terms. That advantage, however, can also make painfully clear how limited the validity of our predictions often is. Consider, for example, the current disparagement of the ability of psychologists to predict violence (Monahan, 1980) and the recommended limitation on courtroom testimony on that matter. Contrast this recommendation with the confident and uncontested testimony that psychologists regularly give on such matters as mental disorder, competency, and fitness of parents. It is unlikely that predictions in the latter cases are in fact any more valid than predictions of violence, but the latter has a clear criterion (even if flawed) that makes it evident how poor—or how good, depending on one's point of view—the predictions are.

Under some circumstances even very small correlations between a predictor and a criterion may be useful (e.g., when only a small number of persons need to be selected from a large pool and when the decision is either critical, as in selection of pilots, or when an adverse decision has no serious consequences to the person not selected).

The validities to which we are accustomed (i.e., correlations in the range of from .25 to .45) may be satisfactory for use in research involving sizable groups, for assignment of subjects on the basis of such correlations guarantees a reasonable difference in mean scores between groups. If a test correlates with college grades to the extent of .40 and subjects are divided into a high and low group on the basis of the test, the two groups should differ by about one standard deviation. If the test were an IQ test, the groups would, then, differ by about 15 IQ points, surely enough to expect some substantial mean difference in grades.

But for individual selection, validities in the range of .25 to .45 offer serious possibilities for injustice. For example, if the validity of a measure is .35, there is about a 25% chance that a person scoring in the lowest 10% on the predictor will score in the upper half of the distribution on the criterion (Peters & Van Voorhis, 1940).[5] That means, therefore, that about one out of every four persons deselected for scoring so low would have succeeded reasonably well if permitted to try whatever was involved. How one feels about such substantial inaccuracies in predictions about individuals depends on the degree of disadvantage conferred on those for whom predictions would have been erroneous and on the justification for selection at all (i.e., as opposed to letting everyone have a try at whatever it is that is being selected for or to selecting randomly if there are not enough places for all).

Construct Validity

Assuming that a performance is not completely random (i.e., that there is some dependability to it), it follows that something, or some set of things, is determining the performance. What determines the performance is the *construct* underlying the test or measure. So that, for example, if performance on a treadmill is determined by physical fitness, then "physical fitness" is the construct underlying the treadmill test. Or if scores on the Beck Depression Inventory are determined by depression, then "depression" is the relevant construct (i.e., the construct being measured by the test). Of course, if scores on the Depression Inventory are determined in some other way, then depression is not the construct being measured.

But if depression is not being measured, then presumably something else is, and that something else is then the construct being measured. It follows, then, that *all dependable measures have construct validity.* The problem is that we may be mistaken about the nature of the construct. An examination of the stream of research related to the construct validity of almost any test

[5]This book contains a series of highly useful tables relating predictive accuracy to magnitude of correlation.

or instrument will show that the question running through all the research is: "What is it that this test measures?" Various investigators may pose hypotheses about what it is that a test measures and then attempt to test those hypotheses. The answers about what a test measures may even shift from time to time. In fact, the appropriate metaphor for "validating" a test, which sounds rather active and affirmative, is more likely "discovery." A test has a mind of its own; it measures whatever it measures, and we do not change that by our research efforts. Our research efforts do, however, change our notions about what it is that a test measures (or at least our notions ought to change). If research shows that a given measure is heavily saturated with social desirability, then obviously what we have is a new measure of social desirability, although we may not want or need one.

Construct validity should not be thought of as either unidimensional or constant. To the extent that any measure is multidimensional, then it has construct validity for more than one construct. It may not be a particularly good measure of any of the constructs, but nevertheless it is a measure. Construct validity may vary with the populations to which the measures are applied. A measure may have good construct validity for males but not for females, for English-speaking subjects but not for non-English speakers, for college students and not for blue-collar workers. Construct validity may also vary with conditions of measurement. A scale to measure psychological distress may have good construct validity if administered in a way designed to reduce subjects' concerns about self-presentation. The same scale may be no more than a good measure of defensiveness if administered in some other way. Construct validity once established does not just sit there.

There are no prescriptions for determining construct validity. The results of construct validation cannot be summarized in one handy coefficient. Construct validation is a gradual, incremental process as evidence builds toward a coherent and persuasive case for linking the measure and the construct. In general, construct validity is established by showing that a measure is related in a systematic way to other measures and performances as would be expected from the theoretical nature of the construct. Ideally, one defines the construct carefully and from that definition derives predictions about relationships to other measures or about the behavior of persons high and low on the measured construct. Then these hypotheses are tested. That sort of systematic exploration does occur, but more common is the building up of a case from findings that make sense gathered from here and there.

Convergent and Discriminant Validity. Campbell and Fiske (1959) did advance both the concepts and methods pertinent to construct validity by proposing the complementary terms called *convergent* and *discriminant* validity, and the method of studying them called a multitrait-multimethod matrix. Convergent validity represents the proposition that a measure ought to correlate with other measures of the same construct. For example, a proposed new measure of anxiety ought to correlate at least reasonably well with other measures of anxiety. On the other hand, a measure of a given construct ought not to correlate very well with measures of other constructs. For example, a measure of anxiety ought not to correlate too well with a measure of hostility or with a measure of need for approval. Finding that measures do not correlate with other measures with which they should not correlate is divergent validity. Although the concepts of convergent and divergent validity are not, even together, synonymous with construct validity, they are useful in suggesting directions for thinking and research. The multitrait-multimethod matrix need not be further considered here, but it is based on the idea that correlations between measures will be greater if they involve common rather than different methods. The research strategy involves measuring two or more traits by two or more methods and then examining all the intercorrelations to determine whether they exceed what would be expected by overlapping methods of measurement.

Construct validity is at once a highly important and frustrating concept. Since our interest in various measures is not satisfied by examining piecemeal correlations with specific criteria, and since we lack any clear criterion for a large proportion of our measures, we need a way to think about validating our measures that takes patterns of relationships and findings into account. On the other hand, construct validity is somewhat slippery as a concept. It is difficult to know how to look for it, often difficult to recognize it when we encounter it, difficult to tie down once and for all, and difficult to know when we have enough of it. Mark Twain is reported once to have said: "When it comes to good bourbon, too much is barely enough." The same could be said for evidence of construct validity.

Incremental Validity

In many situations, particularly practical ones, we use measures in ways that imply a type of validity that they may not have. Experimental tests of the validity of measures are usually carried out in such a way that evidence for validity is established if the use of a measure produces a correlation significantly different from zero. In practice, however, we often have a great deal of information before a measure is factored into our mental processes. Clinicians, for example, know the details of patients' socio-demographic descriptors, know many biographical facts, and are aware of diagnosis, symptoms, and other behaviors. When all that is known, the addition of test information (e.g., from the Rorschach) may not add much. A test may lack *incremental validity*; its use does not improve on the predictions that may be made without it (Sechrest, 1963).

As Lord and Novick (1968) noted, the idea underlying the concept of incremental validity is quite familiar in applying such procedures as multiple regression. A measure may be significantly related to a criterion to be predicted, but if it is too highly related to other measures, it will be redundant and will not end up with a significant regression coefficient. Two measures are not invariably better than one.

PURPOSES OF MEASUREMENT

Generally speaking, we usually have one or the other of two purposes in mind when we undertake measurement (occasionally both). A common aim of measurement is to be able to differentiate between instances of the person, object, or situation being measured. A second aim of measurement is to determine whether the value observed on the measure for the person, object, or situation being measured surpasses some previously established value. Occasionally we may be greedy and hope to perform both kinds of measures at once.

Differentiating Between Instances

When we measure something we often want to distinguish it as clearly as possible from other similar things. For example, when we measure physical attractiveness, it is usually with the aim of differentiating between persons with respect to attractiveness. If our measure, say judges' ratings, is undependable, it will fail us by producing attractiveness scores that do not clearly distinguish between persons. If we then want to study responses in relation to attractiveness, we may split the group at the median to form high and low attractiveness groups, or we may use correlational methods to study the variable along its entire range. It would not make any difference if a careless research assistant accidentally added 10 to everyone's score. Similarly, we may use a set of test items, as for extraversion, to differentiate among people on that characteristic. If we were studying the outcome of two therapeutic interventions, we would like to have a measure that would be highly sensitive to differences between persons so that we would maximize our chances of finding differences between treatments.

When our aim is to differentiate between persons (or objects or situations), what we care about is that we have a dependable *ordering* of those persons. We want two judges rating photos for physical attractiveness to rate them in such a way that they end up on the same order. It would not matter if one judge consistently gave more favorable ratings. Or, if we are testing children for assertiveness and desire to know that our measure is stable over time, we would be satisfied if the children were ordered the same way on the two occasions even if they were generally more assertive on the second than on the first occasion.

When our measurement aim is to differentiate, requirements for reliability are satisfied if different measures preserve the order of scores. A correlation coefficient is sensitive only to changes in order of scores and not to changes in their absolute magnitude or to their spread. For the purpose of differentiating, a correlation of 1.00 would be highly satisfactory no matter what the means or standard deviations of two sets of scores might be. Averaging the scores would take care of mean differences if it were important to do so, and they could be standardized to correct for unequal variances.

Cutting Scores

There are many circumstances in which we establish on some basis a critical value for some measure: a threshold above which people pass, objects are judged satisfactory, and so forth. In taking a driver's test, one must perform above some threshold, but there is no interest in differentiating between people above that threshold, nor, indeed, below it. In effect, the only scores for which dependability is of interest are those on either side of the cutting score. There is no entirely satisfactory way of estimating the reliability of one particular score, but methods are available. The standard error of measurement can be used as an approximation if one assumes that errors of measurement are equal and symmetrical around observed scores throughout the distribution. The standard error of measurement would be a good approximation of the limits within which the true score is likely to lie if the cutting score is reasonably close to the middle of the distribution. If it is much toward either extreme, a correction of some sort would be required (Dick & Hagerty, 1971). An extension of generalizability theory to procedures used in establishing cutting scores has been achieved by Brennan and Lockwood (1980).

Absolute Measures

There are occasional instances in which we may have an interest in the absolute value of a score and in which differentiating among instances is not sufficient. A good example is the comparison of sentencing decisions made by judges. It is fundamental to our legal system that like cases should be treated the same. It does not satisfy our sense of justice to know that the correlations between sentencing decisions of judges is high if there are substantial mean differences between them. If rape and armed robbery result in stiffer sentences than assault and burglary for all judges, but some judges give sentences of 15 years to life while others give sentences of from 5 to 10 years, we would not necessarily think that the judges were in satisfactory agreement.

Arguments have been waged in the literature concerning the necessary conditions for asserting that measures are reliable, with some writers insisting that measures should not be termed reliable unless identical scores are obtained from separate measures (e.g., judges should give exactly the same sentences). Other writers insist that high correlations between measures are sufficient. The argument appears to me to be resolvable if we distinguish between the aims of our measurement efforts. Correlations will be sufficient if we are interested only in the relative positions of measured persons. Exact comparability of scores is required if we are interested in absolute scores. The reliability of a cutting score is best estimated by determining the bounds within which the true score most likely resides.

STATISTICAL DEFINITIONS OF RELIABILITY

Since observed scores are made up of true score plus error (or explained variance plus unexplained variance), the variance of observed scores must, of necessity, always be greater than the variance of true scores. That is, errors of measurement will ensure that observed scores have a wider range than true scores. The amount of error can be estimated by comparing the variance of true scores with the variance of observed scores. Reliability, then, can be defined as the ratio of true score to observed score variance. All that remains is to estimate true score variance, no small task.

For many types of reliability, the statistical coefficient is calculated directly by means of a product-moment correlation (e.g., between test and retest, between Form A and Form B, between scores obtained in Situation 1 and scores obtained in Situation 2). The resulting correlation may be interpreted as the proportion of variance in the measure that is reliable (dependable).

Estimating the internal consistency of a test based on only a single administration has been a more formidable challenge, in part because a formula that can actually be calculated usually requires numerous assumptions. The most commonly encountered internal consistency coefficient currently is almost certainly coefficient alpha (so named by Cronbach), but also known as Kuder-Richardson Formula 20, a useful formula for calculation when test items are binary in form. If we had a set of perfectly reliable items, then all of the variance in observed scores would be attributable to differences between persons. Since, however, items are not perfect, some of the variance in observed scores is attributable to the peculiarities of individual items (e.g., specific wording of an item causes responses to it to be inconsistent with responses to another item). By calculating the variance between items and expressing it as a proportion of the total variance and then subtracting that proportion from 1.0, we arrive at an estimate of the variance attributable to persons, the dependable variance. One formula for alpha is:

$$\alpha = \frac{n}{n-1}\left[1 - \frac{\Sigma_x^2}{\sigma_T^2}\right]$$

In words, one sums the variances across individual measures (e.g., items), divides by the total variance, and subtracts that dividend from 1. There is an additional correction factor reflecting the number of measures. When items of a binary nature are involved, the computational formula is known as Kuder-Richardson Formula 20. A computationally even simpler formula is Kuder-Richardson 21:[6]

$$\alpha_{21} = \frac{n}{n-1}\left[\frac{\sigma_T^2 - \bar{X} + \frac{\bar{X}^2}{n}}{\sigma_T^2}\right]$$

That is, one begins with the total variance, subtracts the mean of the distribution, adds the square of the mean divided by the number of measures, and divides the sum by the total variance. (Again, there is a correction factor for number of measures.) Both alpha and K-R21 are considered to yield lower bound estimates of reliability since they involve assumptions that are unlikely to be completely justified. K-R21 is especially likely to underestimate reliability, and its use probably should be limited to quick, exploratory estimates (Lord & Novick, 1968). An old way of estimating internal consistency was to split a test into two halves, usually into odd and even items, and to calculate the correlation between the halves. That was not completely satisfactory since there are many ways of splitting a test of any length. Alpha yields an estimate of the average correlation between all possible splits of a set of measures. In fact, one computational form for alpha is:

$$\alpha = \frac{n\bar{r}_{ii}}{[l + \bar{r}_{ii}(n-1)]}$$

where n is the number of items and $\bar{r}_{ii}$ is the mean interitem correlation.

Test Length and Reliability

It should be obvious that, other things being equal, longer tests should be more reliable than shorter ones. There is, in fact, a lawful relationship between test length and reliability that is expressed by the *Spearman-Brown prophecy formula.* The equation is simple and easy to calculate. It is often given in the form used to estimate the effect of doubling the length of a test and is:

[6]There are several computational forms of K-R20 and K-R21 that are algebraically equivalent. The one given here is arbitrarily chosen.

$$\text{reliability of } 2n \text{ items} = \frac{2r_{tt}}{1 + r_{tt}}.$$

The equation is generalizable to any changes in length of a test by the equation:

$$\text{reliability of } kn \text{ items} = \frac{kr_{tt}}{1 + (k-1)r_{tt}}.$$

So, if we have a brief test of 10 items that has an α coefficient of .40, and we want to know what would happen if we quadrupled the number of items:

$$\alpha_{.40} = \frac{4(.40)}{1 + (4-1)(.40)} = .72.$$

One can use the formula as well to estimate the effect of shortening a test.

An important caution about the Spearman-Brown formula is that, among the other things that must be equal, items that are used to increase test length must be considered to have been drawn randomly from the same universe as the original items. It often proves to be the case that the first 10 items one writes for a scale are relatively easy to write and then it becomes progressively difficult to think up additional items. If that is the case, then one may actually dilute a scale in such a way that increasing the length of a scale will decrease its reliability.

The Spearman-Brown formula can be applied to measures other than test items, of course (e.g., to observers, raters, tasks, and so on). The same cautions apply (i.e., any new observers, raters, etc., must be as good as those already used). But the effects of increasing numbers of raters or observers can be quite useful. If a single rater has a reliability of only .20 (much too low to be useful), it is helpful to know that if 10 raters can be employed, the reliability of the aggregate ratings should be .71.

The Relationship Between Reliability and Validity

It is often thought that a reliability coefficient represents the limitation on the validity of a measure, but that is not the case. Remember that the reliability coefficient is the *reliable* variance in a measure (i.e., the variance that can be accounted for). From that, it follows that the maximum validity of a test is actually the *square root of the reliability,* just as a correlation is the square root of the variance it accounts for (r squared). Thus, a test with a very modest reliability of only .5 *could* have a validity as high as .7 or so. That does not mean that it will have validity that high; only that it could.

Another important insight is that if any measure correlates significantly with any other measure, assuming that the correlation is not the 1 in 20 significant by chance, the measure is perforce reliable. Since correlations are symmetric in their interpretation, if a measure can account for variance in another measure, it in turn has dependable variance that can be accounted for. At the very least, the reliability of a measure must be equal to the square of any correlation that it has with another measure. If one can demonstrate that a measure has good validity, its reliability can be assumed and becomes a secondary issue.

Correction for Attenuation

Merely increasing test reliability will, however, have only a very small, sometimes disappointing, effect on validity. The relationship between test validity and reliability is (Gulliksen, 1950):

$$\frac{r_{xy}}{\sqrt{r_{xx}}}.$$

Thus, the ratio of the validity coefficient to the index (square root) of reliability is a constant and not dependent on test length. For example, if a test width reliability of .6 has a correlation with another measure of .35 (validity), then the constant is:

$$\frac{.35}{\sqrt{.60}} = .45.$$

Then improving the reliability to .70 will increase validity to .38, i.e.,:

$$\frac{.45}{(\sqrt{.70}})$$

and increasing the reliability to .80 will increase validity to .40. One can see that there are only limited gains to be achieved in validity solely by increasing test reliability. When one considers the substantial cost in time required for testing and the great risk in writing additional test items that will not represent the universe well, the slight increases to be achieved in validity are especially disappointing. It is for such reasons that in an especially cogent discussion of "band width versus fidelity," Cronbach and Gleser (1965) argued that for a given amount of effort (e.g., testing time) we are likely to be better off measuring several things less well than by trying to measure one thing really well.

Two additional points should, nonetheless, be noted. First, small gains in validity, when squared, may represent considerably larger gains in proportion of variance accounted for. Thus, if validity is .3, then the predictor accounts for 9% of the variance in the criterion. If validity is increased to only .35, variance accounted for goes to 12.5% when viewed in one way: a one-third increase. That increase may or may not be worth the effort involved. A second point is that there may well be ways of achieving important increases in reliability without increasing test length. In fact, improved internal consistency can very often be achieved by shortening a test (i.e., by removing items that correlate only minimally with others). Bell and Lumsden (1980) found that by purifying scales by removing "bad" items, they often can be shortened considerably without important effects on validity. Improved reliability may also be achieved by improving conditions of test administration, by increasing sample heterogeneity, and in other ways that may not be costly and that might be worthwhile even if gains in validity were small.

Sometimes it is desirable to know what the "true" correlation between one variable and another might be (i.e., what the correlation would be if one or both variables were measured without error). The correction for measurement error is known as the *correction for attenuation* and is a more general case of the formula just given for relating validity to reliability:

$$r_{xy} = \frac{r_{xy}}{\sqrt{r_{xx} r_{yy}}} .$$

In other words, the correlation between two variables when corrected for attenuation is calculated by dividing the observed correlation by the square root of the product of the two observed reliabilities. If the correlation between two measures is .30, and one has a reliability of .6 and the other .7, then the attenuation-corrected correlation is .46. Such information may be useful for theoretical purposes since it may be important to know the degree of relationship between two variables at some theoretical level without intrusion of measurement problems. Correction for attenuation may also suggest which of two tests would be the best prospect for improvement. A test with a validity of .3 and a reliability of .4 might in the long run be a better prospect than a test with a validity of .35 and a reliability of .8. Correction for attenuation would indicate that the maximum validity of the first test would be about .47 and that of the second only about .39. Everything would depend on the difficulty expected in increasing the reliability of the first test from .4 to .8 or so.

Correction for attenuation should be used only with considerable caution. The outcome is highly sensitive to the reliability estimates used, and those estimates that tend to be low can result in inflated corrected correlations. A correlation of .3 associated with a reliability of .3 becomes .55 if corrected for attenuation, but if reliability is estimated to be .6, correction increases the correlation only to .38.

Effects of Differential Reliability of Measures on Research Outcomes

Imagine being given the task of assessing the effects of a training program devised to improve "guessing ability," the ability of people to anticipate outcomes of events. Let us suppose that the outcome measure chosen is the ability to guess the face of a die that will turn up when it is rolled down a chute onto a table. What would we find? Well, we would certainly find no effect of the training program because the die face that would turn up would be a random (unpredictable, unreliable) event. Suppose the outcome measure were to be the outcomes of horse races. Well, those are not random, and people trained to use a racing form could well improve initial naive ability to predict which horse would win each race (but not necessarily how to beat the parimutuel betting odds). We can expect interventions of whatever kind to have an effect only on dependable measures.

It follows from the preceding that if measures are differentially dependable over time, or if they are differentially dependable over samples, we may get quite misleading results from the statistical analyses of the effects of interventions. Measures may be differentially dependable over time for a number of reasons, but the most likely is the maturation of subjects and a change in their ability levels. If a test is too difficult for children of an average age of 4 years old, their scores will tend to be random. If, when they are tested again at age 6, the test is at the right difficulty level, their scores will be dependable. If we attempt to determine which children have "changed" most, we will get nonsense results, although we may not know it. For we would be subtracting an initial random value from a later dependable value. The result would be an outcome of almost certainly very low, if not zero, dependability.

The dependability of measures may also differ substantially across types of measures with similar consequences for our evaluations of outcomes. We can expect substantial effects from efforts to teach children to play checkers; we cannot expect any effects from efforts to teach them to roll large numbers with dice. If some subtests in an ability battery are less dependable than others, we cannot expect the effects of training on those abilities to be as great.

The same problem holds when samples differ with respect to the dependability of their performances on measures. If, for example, males and females differ in the dependability of their performances on tasks, then comparisons of them over time or interventions may produce misleading results. Campbell and Erlebacher (1970) showed how differential reliability between groups can produce differential regression toward the mean, which, in the case they analyzed, may have made children exposed to Head Start programs look as if they had been disadvantaged by being in the program.

One can only issue the caveat that attempts should always be made to assess the dependability of all measures being employed in a study, and that any evidence of differential reliability between measures, groups, and so on should be grounds for extreme care in both analysis and interpretation of findings.

Change Scores

In many studies of developmental processes and interventions, we want to determine whether change has occurred. But we usually want to know whether change has been differential between groups differently identified or in different circumstances. For example, we want to know whether boys gain more in mathematics scores than girls, whether children in a special reading program improve more than those in another program, whether children who watch certain TV programs become more aggressive than those who do not watch those programs. The concept of change is appealing; we can sense it regularly and everywhere. Unfortunately, its *measurement* is one of the most problematic tasks faced by social science researchers.

The problem is not, obviously, the measurement of absolute change. We know when children's scores improve, when they grow in height, when they come to be more aggressive. We also know by about how much children improve, grow, and become aggressive. The problem arises from the fact that our interest is in *differential* change. We want to know whether children in Group A improved *more* than children in Group B, whether children receiving the nutritional supplement grew *more* than those not receiving the supplement, whether children who watch violent TV increase *more* in aggressiveness than those who watch other programs. It has been known for quite some time that the measurement of differential change poses problems (Harris, 1962). Awareness of the problem became acute, however, when Cronbach and Furby (1970), in a penetrating article, concluded that accurate measurement of differential change may be nearly impossible and that the aim should be abandoned. Cronbach and Furby had excellent statistical arguments on their side, but the force of common sense has kept social scientists devoted to the task. No matter what the statisticians say, there *must* be something to the notion that people change in differing amounts.

Since the Cronbach and Furby attack on measurement of change, there has been some softening in the anti-change-measurement position, and, at any rate, social scientists have continued to infer differential change regularly by using difference scores, gain scores, covariance analyses, and so on. It may help, however, to note the problems that are inherent in attempts to measure differential change.

One of the simpler but better accounts of the problems is given by Magnusson (1966). The problems begin with the fact that the reliability of a change (or difference) score depends on the reliabilities of *both* scores that enter into the calculation, which are never higher, and usually lower, than the reliability of the least reliable measure. The reliability of a difference score drops off quite rapidly as the reliability of either measure involved diminishes from 1.00.

The second problem, one less intuitively clear, is that the reliability of a change score is an inverse function of the correlation between the two measures involved. That is, the higher the correlation between the two measures, the lower the reliability of the differences between them. To take the limiting case, if the correlation between two scores is 1.00, then the differences between them will be .00 plus (perhaps) some constant. Since all the differences are .00, those differences obviously have no reliability. At the other extreme, if two variables correlate .00, then any differences between them must be dependable to the extent that the separate measures are dependable. What a paradox! In selecting a pretest measure we usually want one that is substantially related to our posttest measure. But in making such a selection, we guarantee that the detection of dependable change will be difficult.

The problems have not been resolved and the arguments in the literature continue. The best that can be recommended at present is still the admonition of Cronbach and Furby (1970) to avoid the problem if possible (e.g., by using research designs that permit an analysis based only on posttest scores). The problem usually arises, however, because a quasi-experimental design must be used, and difference scores are wanted because groups were unequal from the beginning. In that case, it is by now widely known, but not widely enough, that analysis of covariance based on raw scores is to be avoided. Some advantage may inhere, however, in an analysis of covariance based on estimated (regressed) true scores, that is, estimates of initial true scores that take into account the differential measurement error in different parts of the distribution of scores (Judd & Kenny, 1981).

REFERENCES

Bell, R., & Lumsden, J. (1980). Test length and validity. *Applied Psychological Measurement, 4,* 165–170.

Brennan, R.L., & Lockwood, R.E. (1980). A comparison of Nedelsky and Angoff cutting scores procedures using generalizability theory. *Applied Psychological Measurement, 4,* 219–240.

Campbell, D.T., & Erlebacher, A. (1970). How regression artifacts in quasi-experimental evaluations can mistakenly make compensatory education look harmful. In J. Hellmuth (Ed.), *The disadvantaged child* (Vol. 3). New York: Brunner/Mazel.

Campbell, D.T., & Fiske, D.W. (1959). Convergent and discriminant validation by the multitrait-multimethod matrix. *Psychological Bulletin, 56,* 81–105.

Committee to Develop Joint Technical Standards for Educational and Psychological

Testing. (1983). *Joint Technical Standards for Educational and Psychological Testing*. Draft, American Educational Research Association, American Psychological Association, and National Council on Measurement in Education.

Cook, T.D., & Campbell, D.T. (1979). *Quasi-experimentation: Design and analysis issues for field settings.* Chicago: Rand McNally.

Cronbach, L.J. (1970). *Essentials of psychological testing* (3rd ed.). New York: Harper and Row.

Cronbach, L.J., & Furby, L. (1970). How we should measure change—or should we? *Psychological Bulletin, 74,* 68–80.

Cronbach, L.J., & Gleser, G.C. (1965). *Psychological tests and personnel decisions* (2nd ed.). Urbana, Ill.: University of Illinois Press.

Cronbach, L.J., Gleser, G.C., Rajaratnam, N., & Nanda, H. (1972). *The dependability of behavioral measures: Theory of generalizability for scores and profiles.* New York: John Wiley.

Dick, W., & Hagerty, N. (1971). *Topics in measurement: Reliability and validity.* New York: McGraw-Hill.

Epstein, S. (1979). The stability of behavior: On predicting most of the people some of the time. *Journal of Personality and Social Psychology, 37,* 1097–1126.

Epstein, S. (1980). The stability of behavior: Implications for psychological research. *American Psychologist, 35,* 790–806.

Gulliksen, H. (1950). *Theory of mental tests.* New York: John Wiley.

Harrell, W.A. (1981). The effects of alcohol use and offender remorsefulness on sentencing decisions. *Journal of Applied Social Psychology, 11,* 83–91.

Harris, C.W. (1962). *Problems in measuring change.* Madison, WI: University of Wisconsin Press.

Hemphill, J.K., & Sechrest, L. (1952). A comparison of three criteria of aircrew effectiveness in combat over Korea. *Journal of Applied Psychology, 36,* 323–327.

Holden, R.R. (1982). *Item subtlety, face validity, and the structured assessment of psychopathology.* Unpublished doctoral dissertation, University of Western Ontario, London, Ontario.

Judd, C., & Kenny, D. (1981). *Estimating the effects of social interventions.* Cambridge: Cambridge University Press.

Kazdin, A.E. (1977). Assessing the clinical importance of behavior change through social validation. *Behavior Modification, 1,* 427–452.

Kelly, G.A. (1955). *The psychology of personal constructs* (Vol. 1). New York: W. W. Norton.

Lord, F.M., & Novick, M.R. (1968). *Statistical theories of mental test scores.* Reading, MA: Addison-Wesley.

Magnusson, D. (1966). *Test theory.* Reading, MA: Addison-Wesley.

Monahan, J. (1980). *The clinical prediction of violent behavior.* Washington, DC: U.S. Government Printing Office.

Peters, C.C., & Van Voorhis, W.R. *Statistical procedures and their mathematical bases.* New York: McGraw-Hill, 1940.

Rushton, J.P., Brainerd, C.J., & Pressley, M. (1983). Behavioral development and construct validity: the principle of aggregation. *Psychological Bulletin, 94,* 18–38.

Sechrest, L. (1963). Incremental validity: A recommendation. *Educational and Psychological Measurement, 23,* 153–158.

Turner, J. (1980). Yes, I am human: Autobiography of a retarded career. *Journal of Community Psychology, 8,* 3–8.

Watson, J.D. (1968). *The double helix: A personal account of the discovery of the structure of DNA*. New York: Atheneum.

Webb, E., Campbell, D.T., Schwartz, R.D., Sechrest, L., & Grove, J.B. (1981). *Nonreactive measures in the social sciences.* Boston: Houghton-Mifflin.

Wiener, D.N. (1948). Subtle and obvious keys for the Minnesota Multiphasic Personality Inventory. *Journal of Consulting Psychology, 12,* 164–170.

3

Case Study and Single-Case Research in Clinical and Applied Psychology

Thomas R. Kratochwill
Stacey E. Mott
Cecilia L. Dodson

INTRODUCTION

Case study methods and single-case research methods are frequently used in clinical and other applied areas of psychology. Although many areas of psychology and related fields rely on large-*N*-between-group designs for their empirical knowledge base, clinical psychology has employed case study and single-case designs in research for many years. Increasingly, researchers and other scholars in the field are recognizing the importance of case study and single-case investigations for the development of a knowledge base in the field. Many important methodological and conceptual advances in this area of research have occurred over the past few years. The advances that have been made are worthy of examination by clinical psychologists for a number of reasons (Kratochwill & Mace, 1983).

First of all, both case study and single-case research designs provide an important knowledge base that is unobtainable through traditional large-*N*-between-group designs in therapy research. Although single-case methodologies are not limited to a single client, they are uniquely suited to evaluation of treatments involving a single client—a primary interest in clinical psychology. This characteristic takes on special importance when consideration is given to the fact that it often is impossible to conduct group comparative outcome studies due to the limited number of subjects for a particular type of disorder or problem. For example, sometimes certain rare disorders, such as cases of multiple personality, schizophrenia, and phobic reactions, are unavailable for group investigations. In this regard, there is a great deal of interest in conducting research on clinical problems that do not always match the type of clients recruited for comparative group outcome studies. In fact,

The authors express their appreciation to Mildred A. O'Brien and Glen I. Nicholson for their suggestions on the role of practice in generating hypotheses for research.

many research studies on clinical problems have been an analogue to some of the rare disorders that clinical psychologists and others working in applied settings actually see (Ross, 1981). Thus, rather rare clinical disorders can be studied through case study and single-case research procedures, making these strategies sometimes less analogous than some typical investigations in the clinical psychology field.

Another major advantage of case study and single-case research designs is that they provide an alternative to traditional large-*N* group designs about which various ethical and legal considerations are often raised (e.g., Hersen & Barlow, 1976). Concerns in group research have centered around the ethical objections of withholding treatment from clients in the no-treatment control group. Both case study and single-case designs provide an alternative in that treatment can often be implemented immediately.

Fourth, both case study and single-case research designs have promoted the development of a measurement technology that can be used repeatedly over the therapeutic process. For example, various outcome measures such as direct observation, rating scales and checklists, and self-monitoring, as well as various psychophysiological recordings, can be used as ongoing measures of client functioning over the course of therapy. Such repeated measures taken on a client over time allow for an analysis of individual variability as well as monitoring of potential response covariation within a single client. Such covariation in client functioning can be represented on measures of cognitive, behavioral, and physiological content areas. Perhaps the most important aspect of this repeated measurement technology is its flexibility in the modification of treatment if the data indicate that it has not been successful.

Finally, to some extent both case study and single-case research strategies have provided options for practitioners to be involved in research. Although carefully designed case study and single-case research designs are usually difficult to implement in practice (Kratochwill & Piersel, 1983), some forms of case study investigation have provided this option under several conditions. For example, as will be discussed below, the clinical replication case study provides an important step in testing the generalizability of research findings in practice. Thus, under some conditions, case study and single-case research designs enable practitioners to conduct research.

Case study and single-case research methodology can make important contributions to therapy research in clinical and other applied areas of psychology. In this chapter we provide an overview of case study and single-case research and methodological and conceptual issues surrounding their use in the clinical psychology field.

CASE STUDY METHODS

Case study methods have played an important role in investigations in diverse areas of psychology, education, and related fields. As traditionally conceived, the case study has involved the intense study of the individual; however, case study methods have in no way been limited to therapeutic or applied work. In fact, case study investigation has taken many different forms, including investigations of non-therapeutic areas, providing examples of assessment strategies, as well as their more common role in clinical and applied areas of psychology as a method of evaluating therapeutic programs. Table 3.1 lists several different types of case study investigations that can be distinguished.

Non-Therapeutic Case Study

Sometimes case study investigations are used to provide information to the researcher interested in non-clinical topics, such as developmental, educational, or biological issues. Indeed, throughout the history of psychology a number of classic case studies have provided such data (Dukes, 1965). One area where case study data have set precedence for future work is in the study of physical growth. Between the years of 1759–1771 Count Philbert de Monteillard gathered data on his son's height, measured every 6 months from birth to 18 years. The data were published by Buffon in a supplement to the *Histoire Naturelle*. The Count was able to provide information in this case study that demonstrated the increments in height from one age to the next expressed as a rate of growth per year. The data represent, even today, one of the most famous records of human growth and can be considered one of the best records in existence (Tanner, 1970). In his review of physical growth data, Tanner (1970) cites several other classic studies of human growth that are based on the data of a single case (e.g., measurements by R. H. Whitehouse of a girl from age 3½ to age 10 in the Harpeden Growth Study [see Israelsohn, 1960] and growth curves for identical twins [see Tanner, 1962]).

Another pioneering effort in the study of human performance was made

Table 3.1. Types of Case Study Investigations.

Type	Characteristics
Nontherapeutic Case Study (1) descriptive/uncontrolled (2) biography/autobiography	Researcher is interested in non-clinical investigation. Such areas as developmental or educational psychology would be representative. Includes traditional baby biographies.
Assessment/Diagnosis Case Study (1) descriptive case	Researcher employs various psychometric instruments for diagnosis or description of cognitive or social behavior.
Therapeutic/Intervention Case Study (1) uncontrolled (2) pre-experimental (3) clinical replication case	Researcher is primarily interested in a clinical disorder and may either describe natural course of disorder or develop intervention to treat client's problem.

Source: Adapted from Kratochwill, T.R. (in press). *Time-series research.* New York: Academic Press.

by Herman Ebbinghaus, wherein the principles of learning developed from his analyses of individual performance were applied to the population in general. The work most often cited is his quantitative study of the loss of retention with the lapse of time (Ebbinghaus, 1886). Having reviewed several theories regarding the cause of forgetting, he believed that none were very good, and decided that the best program was to leave theories aside and initially develop a knowledge base of facts that explained them (Woodworth & Schlosberg, 1954). The way he accomplished this task was through the intensive study of individuals, including both himself and others. For example, using himself as a subject, he learned over 1,000 lists of nonsense words, each containing 13 syllables. Ebbinghaus found that learning efficiency differed at different hours of the day. For example, it took him 12% longer to memorize a list at 6 to 8 p.m. than it did at 10 to 11 a.m. This series of studies by Ebbinghaus represents a classic contribution to measurement that is still recognized today.

In addition to descriptive and uncontrolled non-therapeutic case studies, individuals have written their autobiographies or have developed biographies of other famous individuals. These kinds of case study contributions have served the useful purpose of elucidating various factors that contributed to the development of certain work in psychology and child development, among other areas.

It can be observed that case study methods have traditionally provided important information and data about significant issues that have influenced contemporary psychology and education. Although these procedures have often been described as limited due to the lack of scientific strategies, they do indicate how data gathered through case study methods have made a significant impact on various fields.

The Assessment Case Study

Assessment case studies can be distinguished from more traditional therapeutic interventions in that their primary purpose is to provide an example of the application of various psychometric instruments for either diagnosis or description of cognitive and social behavior. Such case studies, due to either theoretical or conceptual biases regarding the focus of assessment efforts, are typically designed to elucidate aspects of a case where certain forms of measurement might be as desirable. For example, Hartledge (1981) argued that a neuropsychological evaluation can provide precise measurement of discrete abilities subserved by given cortical regions, as well as a systematic assessment of substrates of learning relevant to school settings. Such data are primarily gathered to assist individuals (e.g., school psychologists, child clinical psychologists) in understanding learning problems that may have important implications for interventions. Hartledge (1981) describes the case of James, a 9½-year-old boy who had average reading achievement scores, but who was nevertheless having difficulty in school. In fact, the child's teacher requested a psychoeducational evaluation to determine whether or not the child had a major learning disability. Based on this referral, a comprehensive psychometric evaluation was conducted. Table 3.2 provides a psychometric summary for James. As can be observed in the table, a variety of different assessment procedures were used in the hope that a formal diagnosis could be assigned. Hartledge reports that there was a superiority of right hand function on both motor and sensory tasks and that this was beyond what might be usually explained by normal hand preference. Such information, according to the author, provided support for the notion of a cerebral organization discrepancy. The author suggests that this is important because the direction of the discrepency between hands and motor and sensory functions is consistent with other psychometric developmental behavioral and academic skill deficiencies. Based on this information, as well as other data gathered during the psycho-

Table 3.2. Psychometric Summary for James* (CA = 9½).

		WISC-R			
Verbal	*SS*	Performance	*SS*	Standard Scores	
Information	10	Picture Completion	10	VIQ	103
Similarities	12	Picture Arrangement	9	PIQ	88
Arithmetic	10	Block Design	8	FSIQ	96
Vocabulary	9	Object Assembly	8		
Comprehension	12	Coding	7		

Wide Range Achievement Test	Grade Level	Standard Scores
Reading	4.1	95
Spelling	3.7	91
Arithmetic	3.2	87
Constructional Praxis (Beery VMI)	**Age Level**	**Standard Score**
	8-7	89
Receptive Language (PPVT)	**Age Level**	**Standard Score**
	10-8	106
Motor (Rate of finger tapping)	**# taps/10 seconds**	
(Preferred hand) Right hand	39	
Left Hand	33	
Sensory (Recognition of numbers written on fingertips)		**# correct/20**
Right hand		17
Left Hand		15

*Hartledge, L.C. (1981). Clinical application of neuropsychological test data: A case study. *School Psychology Review, 10,* 362–366.

metric evaluation, the author suggests a fairly strong hypothesis of chronic functional superiority of left over right hemisphere functioning, and that while anterior and posterior portions of the right hemisphere are depressed when compared to the left, there might be slightly less impairment on posterior than anterior portions of the right hemisphere.

Although the evaluation was done for primarily psychometric evaluation and correct diagnosis of the child, the author did advance specific educational recommendations for the child, such as the use of (1) linguistic-phonic approaches to word attack skills because such a strategy utilizes the analytic sequential skills of the left hemisphere and deemphasizes visual/spatial cues which for James are less effective; (2) learning "rules" such as "i before e," which present spatial configuration material in the logic of language and are based on a left hemisphere approach; (3) encouraging James to read assignments twice because such studying would help develop information that is within the context of a meaningful sequential system; and (4) handling behavioral transgressions with an emphasis on verbal understanding of causes and consequences. The rationale for this is that verbal mediation is especially effective when used with children who have superior left hemispheres.

Thus, the psychometrically oriented case study could have implications for educational work; however, the point is that the assessment results were not translated into any interventions, but rather, resulted in a diagnosis. Other applications of assessment case studies could be documented (the interested reader should consult Part II of Davidson & Costello's [1969] book in which various applications of case study methods for assessment are outlined). These generally show that through various psychometric techniques and procedures, case study methods can be used to map various areas of functioning in cognitive and social domains. Nevertheless, in most of these investigations, there is no repeated measurement of the client for purposes of evaluating the effectiveness of some intervention.

Intervention Case Studies

By far the most common case study methods are those used within clinical and other areas of applied psychology to evaluate the effectiveness of treatment. The method by which this evaluation is done varies as a function of the type of case. This domain of case studies can generally be conceptualized within the context of the absence of experimental controls. As Kazdin (1980) notes:

> As traditionally conceived, the case study refers to investigating an individual or group of individuals in the absence of experimental controls. The lack of experimental control means that it is difficult to exclude many rival interpretations that could account for the client's behavior. Hence, the case study can

> be distinguished from experimental research where causal relationships can be drawn because the variables that influence behavior are manipulated directly and, with the inclusion of appropriate control conditions, can be accorded a causal role in behavior change. Of course, in some research, experimental manipulation of conditions is either not possible or not permissible due to practical or ethical constraints or because of the nature of the independent variable. In these situations, statistical techniques (e.g., correlational analyses) often can help rule out alternative interpretations. A case study omits experimental or statistical controls and hence provides information that must be interpreted with considerable ambiguity. (p. 12)

Pre-experimental Case Studies. As noted above, case studies can generally be considered pre-experimental because they do not rule out the usual threats to validity that more well-controlled experimental single-case time-series designs rule out. On the other hand, it is not reasonable to lump all types of case study investigations together and suggest that they are incapable of ruling out certain threats to validity. It is important to emphasize two features of drawing valid inferences in any type of experimental research. To begin with, whether the researcher is able to rule out certain threats to internal validity is always a matter of degree. Even in some well controlled experimental research it is not possible to address certain internal validity threats. Second, many of the threats to internal validity extend beyond experimental designs as traditionally conceived. In the past it has been customary to discuss internal validty as something that can be controlled through experimental design; yet this is only one method that can be used to rule out various sources of invalidity.

Uncontrolled case studies, as defined above, do not allow the researcher to draw totally valid conclusions. The primary reason for this is that various threats to internal validity are simply not ruled out. Nevertheless, the case study can be improved upon in a number of different ways. In order to do this, several different types of pre-experimental case study dimensions need to be addressed. In fact, these dimensions can be used to plan a case study to improve upon drawing valid inferences, or to examine published case studies in the field to improve upon interpretation from existing data. In this regard we expand upon the dimensions that Kazdin (1981) outlined in drawing valid inferences from case studies (see Figure 3.1).

Type of Data. One way in which case studies vary is the type of data that are gathered. At one extreme a researcher may provide subjective information on a client, including such things as self-report data or subjective evaluation (e.g., impressions) of change that may have occurred during treatment. On the other hand, a researcher may be in a position to gather more formal and objective data on the case. For example, repeated measures of frequen-

Characteristics	*Low Inference*	*High Inference*
Type of data	Subjective data	Objective data
Assessment occasions	Single point measurement	Repeated measurement
Planned vs. ex post facto	Ex post facto	Planned
Projections of performance	Acute problem	Chronic problem
Effect size	Small	Large
Effect impact	Delayed	Immediate
Number of subjects	$N=1$	$N<1$
Heterogeneity of subjects	Homogeneous	Heterogeneous
Standardization of treatment	Nonstandardized treatment	Standardized treatment
Integrity of treatment	No monitoring	Repeated monitoring
Impact of treatment	Impact on single measure	Impact on multiple measures
Generalization and follow-up assessment	No formal measures	Formal measures

FIG. 3.1. Dimensions of Case Study Investigations

cy counts or specific mechanical recordings of certain responses could be scheduled. Also, the researcher could use physiological equipment to help monitor the effects of treatment. Such direct measures usually have an advantage over more subjective descriptions typically used in conventional case study research. In addition, other types of data could be used including specific checklists and rating scales, and various types of global ratings. Nevertheless, none of these would be as valuable as direct measures of behavior. Again, it should be noted that these direct methods of assessment are independent of the experimental research design in the investigation.

Assessment Occasions. Another aspect of a case study that influences the degree to which valid inferences can be drawn is the number and timing of assessment occasions. At the minimum, assessment can occur at the beginning of treatment and again upon its termination. Ideally, however, assessment should occur repeatedly throughout the study. Such continuous assessment would allow one to rule out a greater number of threats to internal validity than would assessment that occurs only a limited number of times. Measures that lend themselves most readily to continuous assessment include direct observation of behavior and self-monitoring, while more traditional measures such as projective personality tests would be less adaptable to this method of assessment. Thus, when conducting a case study one must not only consider the desirability of continuous assessment but must choose measures that are capable of being used for this purpose as well (Hersen & Barlow, 1976).

Planned vs. Ex Post Facto Case Studies. An important distinction that must be made among various types of case studies relates to whether or not the researcher is able to manipulate some type of independent variable. Manipulation of the independent variable increases inference for concluding that this variable accounted for changes in the measures in the study. Ex post facto case studies are those in which the experimenter has no direct control over the independent variable, making it free to vary, or not vary, part of the usual experimental arrangements. For example, an investigator might reconstruct and examine possible factors that influence reductions in family arguments among husband, wife, and children. It might be determined that certain events, such as the visit of a mother-in-law, tend to be correlated with an increase in family arguments. However, since this type of intervention was not directly manipulated by the researcher (unless the researcher is a relative), one cannot draw valid inferences due to the lack of control over this variable. On the other hand, when the researcher has an opportunity to plan and manipulated an intervention, it is more likely that it could be responsible for an effect. In pre-experimental case study investigations the researcher is able to directly plan for the implementation of an intervention and to draw more valid inferences from the data (see Glass, Willson, & Gottman, 1975).

Projections of Performance. Distinctions among various types of case studies can be made on the basis of past and future projections of performance on client behavior. In some cases, a behavior problem or clinical disorder can be quite chronic. With an extended history of the disorder it is unlikely that, without some type of planned intervention, a change would occur. Thus, if the researcher can show that the disorder was chronic prior to implementation of the treatment, and that a dramatic change occurred once treatment was delivered, certain threats to validity might be ruled out. On the other hand, various problems that occur for brief periods of time and appear to be transient would typically not provide as strong an inference for the effect of treatment as those that are more chronic and resistant to treatment. Thus, the history of the problem takes on special significance in terms of drawing a valid inference from a case study.

There are at least two ways in which the researcher could determine whether or not the problem is chronic. First of all, one can examine the data on baseline, if available. The problem occurring over a period of several weeks or months may demonstrate that it does not improve with the simple passage of time. Second, it may be possible to examine the specific course of the disorder to determine when it began and the usual characteristics of the disorder over time (e.g., lack of change in client behavior, increasing seriousness of the problem). Finally, it may be possible to determine whether or not the problem is chronic by examining previous attempts to treat it. If there have been many previous and unsuccessful attempts to treat the problem with other interventions, it is likely that it is a more chronic and difficult one.

Effect Size. Another important characteristic of case studies that must be considered is the type of effect that occurs when the treatment is applied. Generally, an effect that is quite large will allow a greater degree of inference than one that is relatively small. Determining the nature of a large effect is subject to some debate in case study and single-subject research (see later discussion). Nevertheless, an effect that is clinically large (e.g., such as reducing disruptive behavior to near 0 rates accompanied by positive consumer evaluation of treatment) is likely to allow more inference that the treatment effect was responsible for change. Thus, the researcher can be more confident that the observed effects were due to the treatment and not to some uncontrolled variables in the study.

Effect Impact. Aside from the size of the effect, the impact of the treatment (i.e., whether or not the treatment effect was immediate or delayed) should be evaluated. Generally, an immediate impact of treatment will allow one to draw more valid inferences from case studies than a treatment that takes a longer period of time to show an effect. Again, the researcher must evaluate the immediacy of change within the context of other factors that could account for such a change in client behavior. Nevertheless, when the impact is considered along with the size of the effect when treatment is applied, greater inference is possible.

Number of Subjects. The number of subjects involved in a case study investigation can influence the degree of inference that can be drawn from the data. Although most case studies might involve only one subject, the researcher can have a greater degree of inference for the treatment effect when the treatment can be replicated across several cases. Generally, the more cases that show successful effects of the treatment, the more unlikely it is that certain extraneous events would be responsible for change. Thus, it is desirable for the researcher to replicate the treatment across a number of subjects whenever possible.

Heterogeneity of Subjects. In addition to replication across subjects, another dimension that the researcher could take into account is the diversity or heterogeneity of clients involved in the case study. Once successful replications occur across subjects of diverse characteristics (e.g., race, social class, age, type of problem, and so forth), the inferences drawn about treatment are generally stronger than if this diversity did not occur. Thus, the researcher can reduce various threats to internal validity when demonstrations across diverse cases can be scheduled as part of the research series.

Standardization of the Treatment. The standardization of treatment will also affect the degree to which valid inferences can be drawn from case studies. Whenever possible the treatment procedure should be standardized. First of all, a treatment needs to be explicitly defined and a protocol for its implementation developed. A protocol of this nature would not only allow the researcher to implement the treatments in a consistent manner, but would also allow for a post hoc determination of the fit between treatment description and its actual implementation. Second, standardization of procedures allows for replication of this same treatment across several different cases. Third, standardization of treatment would allow others in the scientific community to assess this information more easily once the successful treatment was developed. Such a successful standardized treatment could then be used in future well-controlled research by other investigators.

Integrity of Treatment. Aside from the standardization of treatment, some type of check on the integrity or accuracy of implementing the treatment should also be scheduled (Johnson & Pennypacker, 1980). It is important to emphasize that observation of the dependent variable as is usually done in behavior analysis research is insufficient to allow conclusions regarding the effects of a treatment on some target behavior. Thus, the researcher should schedule repeated checks on implementation of the independent variable to determine if there is a functional relation between the dependent target behavior and the independent treatment variable (Peterson, Homer, & Wonderlich, 1982). In addition, the researcher should emphasize a check on the integrity of the independent variable to determine whether or not it is actually occurring across various phases of the investigation.

At least two procedures might be used to check on the integrity of the independent variable. First of all, the researcher can use the same method by which the accuracy of the dependent variable is assessed, that is, by having multiple observers check on whether or not it is being implemented as specified. However, in many situations this might not be cost-effective. Nevertheless, in some instances the researcher can continually check on the accuracy of the independent variable by reviewing the protocol that has been standardized for implementation of the treatment. This type of process evaluation across various phases can help insure the integrity of the independent variable.

Impact of Treatment. The impact of treatment is often assessed on one primary dependent variable. This target behavior is usually chosen because it represents the major concern of the client and/or his/her careproviders. However, the credibility of case studies can usually be improved by gathering multiple measures of client behavior. Determining treatment impact on multiple measures is important for several reasons. First of all, several dimensions of client functioning might be influenced by a particular treatment. It is desirable to know how pervasive the treatment effects are in improving client functioning. Without this multiple measurement, important information might be lost. Second, choice of a target behavior is sometimes guided by the positive/negative effects that a particular treatment has. For example, Wahler, Sperling, Thomas, Teeter, and Luper (1970) treated two children who stuttered. However, these children also displayed oppositional and hyperactive behaviors. Reductions in the latter two behaviors were associated with decreases in stuttering. Thus, multiple impact assessment would allow an examination of potential improvements. Third, assessing treatment impact might even be indicated due to the nature of the problem on both theoretical and conceptual grounds. For example, fear has usually been regarded as a multidimensional construct consisting of behavioral, self-report, and psychophysiological domains (see Morris & Kratochwill, 1983, for an overview in the child fear literature). Whenever possible, researchers should employ measures across the three domains. Generally, case studies can be improved by multiple assessment of the treatment impact. Such assessment, coupled with the other dimensions discussed in this section, improve the inferences that can be drawn from the case report.

Generalization and Follow-up Assessment. Another dimension that would improve the validity and usefulness of case studies is the assessment of generalization and maintenance of behavior change. Although this issue has become increasingly recognized as a necessary ingredient of experimental studies (Stokes & Baer, 1977), there is no reason to exclude it as a consideration for case studies. Indeed, there is nothing about generalization and maintenance that restricts it to an experimental study alone. Generalization can be assessed across behaviors, settings, and subjects, as well as over time (i.e., follow-up). Generalization to other settings, for example, could easily be assessed when a clinician conducting a case study asks the client to collect data via self-monitoring on the number of positive self-statements that he or she makes outside the clinician's office. Thus, if the clinician has used positive self-statements during the therapy session as a basis for determining improvement, this self-monitoring data would provide a means of assessing generalization of improvement in the frequency of positive self-statements in other settings. Maintenance of these treatment effects could, in turn, be assessed by making a phone call to the client after the termination of treatment to determine how lasting the change in behavior was.

Measures of Social Validity. Related to the assessment of generalization and maintenance is the inclusion of measures of social validity. Although the validity of a case study can be improved by use of objective measures, this does not exclude subjective measures from consideration. Indeed, the desirability of using subjective measures of behavior change in addition to objective assessment is becoming increasingly recognized (Kazdin, 1977; Wolf, 1978). These measures would be particularly relevant to a clinical replication case study where the clinical effectiveness of a treatment is of interest. Without the assessment of social validity, a case study might yield significant results and yet not be recognized as being acceptable to the client and his or her care-providers. In addition, by assessing the social validity of a treatment, problems of implementing the treatment in a clinical setting could be revealed, thus allowing for treatment revision to occur if necessary. For example, social validity data may indicate that the treatment is aversive to parents. When this sort of information is obtained by a social validity measure, it would then be possible to revise the treatment to make it more acceptable and effective for parents to implement. A more detailed discussion of social validity is provided later in the chapter.

Analysis of Results. Another dimension that would allow for more valid inferences to be drawn from case studies is the manner in which the researcher analyzes results. This dimension must necessarily, however, be restricted to case studies that utilize objective and repeated assessment data. Thus, more subjective data that are gathered only in a pre/post fashion will likely not allow the type of analysis that is necessary to draw valid inferences from the investigation. But, assuming that a case study has utilized objective and repeated assessment data, and that it includes a baseline phase, validity of the study can be improved by examining the data through some type of formal analysis. For example, the magnitude of change as a result of treatment, and the rate of change, must be taken into account if the data are to be analyzed visually. If, for example, a behavior never occurs prior to baseline, and then suddenly occurs when treatment is implemented, the magnitude of change could be readily observable. In addition, if a behavior occurs at a stable low-frequency prior to treatment, and then begins to increase when treatment is implemented, a significant change of rate would have been demonstrated. However, if neither the change in magnitude nor rate is significant, the data interpretation must be approached with more caution. Although statistical analysis could be used under some conditions, it may not be required. Nevertheless, such statistical data analysis is possible and is discussed in more detail later in the chapter.

Example Case Studies

The aforementioned points demonstrate that there are many dimensions along which case studies can vary in terms of the inferences that can be drawn from them. Below we illustrate two different kinds of case study investigations and show how quite different conclusions can be reached based upon the manner in which the report provided various kinds of data.

Case Study 1. Bergman (1976) provided a case example of the effect of extinction on interpersonal closeness in the treatment of chronic schizophrenia. The case demonstrates how various clinical experiences serve to raise theoretical notions regarding how treatment might be implemented. The case illustration involved the treatment of a 25-year-old Caucasian male diagnosed as schizophrenic, chronic undifferentiated type (according to DSM-II standards). The client was hospitalized in a large state facility that specialized in long-term care. The client demonstrated intense perseveration and circularity in thinking and the author provided a demonstration of how this type of behavior was demonstrated during conversations. Typically, an attempt to relate to the client brought another question from him and the answer to the question brought him back to mentioning the facility to which he was transferred. Bergman first decided to modify this interactive style by relating through the use of extinction techniques while concomitantly establishing rapport with the client. After obtaining some baseline data, Bergman began to turn his head and remain silent for 60 seconds following any mention of the previous hospital by the client. He reports that initially the procedure decreased the rate slightly, but over time there was little change. This led him to conclude that the procedure was largely a failure. Subsequently, Bergman hypothesized that the client's style was to avoid contact. He reports the following:

> The tests of my hypothesis came over the next few meetings with Jim. As I was able to reestablish closeness with Jim, his symptomatic mode of relating evaporated. The maintenance of this contact was proven particularly useful in getting Jim to verbalize about a variety of things (e.g., sexual matters) that he had previously avoided. I believe that Jim could only open up (hence, trust) when I could demonstrate to him a consistent commitment of closeness. This was something he had never experienced from a male before, which he deeply desired. Here again the ward staff corroborated my impressions. They began using their own interpersonal closeness with Jim in order to facilitate his growth. (p. 396)

This case illustrates one of the most common forms of case study investigation. That is, a narrative account of therapeutic change of a client is presented through the therapist's subjective report. Although Bergman reports that he had gathered baseline data, there are none reported in his article. In addition, we have no evidence to suggest that assessment was continuous across the case. Essentially, based upon the criteria discussed previously in the chapter, there is little that can be gleaned from this case study, thus making it impossible to interpret. It represents the most basic form of case study investigation that a clinical researcher is likely to find in the professional literature. Nevertheless, case studies need not adhere to this format.

Case Study 2. Roberts and Gordon (1979) report the successful treatment of a 5-year-old girl who, subsequent to an accident in which she received burns over approximately 30% of her body, experienced nightmares and night terrors. These occurred 15–20 times each night. In addition, the authors report that she had developed a strong phobic reaction to a wide range of fire-related stimuli. The authors report rather extensive behavioral assessment of the case involving interview data, questionnaire data (e.g., The Louisville Behavior Checklist, The Walker Problem Behavior Identification Checklist, and The Locke-Wallace Marital Adjustment Inventory for the parents). The treatment procedure consisted of the following: First of all, the mother was instructed to stay in the daughter's room for the entire night after the child had fallen asleep. As soon as the first response in a chain of the night terrors occurred, the mother was instructed to disrupt the sequence by awakening her daughter. The mother would not talk to her daughter during this time and allowed the child to go back to sleep. During the baseline period the nightmare incident was defined as the last behavior in a chain. Screaming was defined as the first behavior in the chain (clutching the nightgown). The authors note that during subsequent treatment phases where the problem was ignored, the nightmare was defined again as the last behavior in the chain (screaming). Although this procedure changes the response definition across phases of the study, the authors argued that it was necessary to implement the clinical intervention.

Results reported in Figure 3.2 show that the wake-up procedure initially increased the frequency of the onset of nightmares. Nevertheless, this trend reversed; after a brief period of time there was no more than one nightmare per night after a week of treatment. Following this procedure the mother was instructed to no longer remain in the room and the nightmares were to be completely ignored by the parents. This was continued for almost four weeks until the child was readmitted to a hospital. The parents were then instructed to reinstitute the wakeup procedure for the following three nights. At this point, the parents also reported that the child's fears generalized. Specifically, the child became increasingly fearful of fire, the gas stove, lit cigarettes,

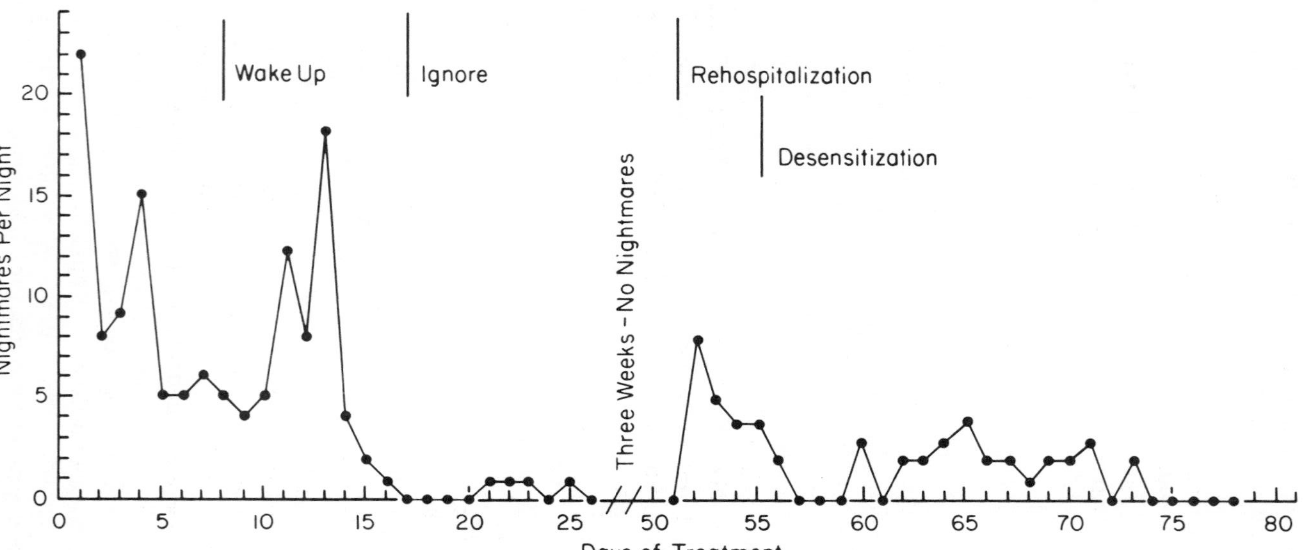

FIG. 3.2. Daily frequency of nightmare incidence across treatment conditions (Source: Roberts, R. N., & Gordon, S. B. (1979). Reducing childhood nightmares subsequent to a burn trauma. *Child Behavior Therapy, 1,* 373–381. Reproduced by permission).

and fires shown on television. It is at this point that the authors implemented a systematic desensitization treatment.

The desensitization procedure consisted of 10 magazine pictures of fires selected to represent a wide variety of settings. The child's mother was employed as a therapist to present the stimuli. As can be seen in the figure, nightmares decreased at this point, and the parents reported that the child no longer avoided them when they were smoking cigarettes or in the vicinity of the stove. The child generally did not exhibit any fearful reactions to fire-related stimuli. The 6-month follow-up indicated that there were no further problems.

This case study, while having some interpretive difficulties, demonstrates a great improvement over the previous case study described above. Specifically, it addresses some of the issues related to how case studies can be improved. First of all, it was demonstrated that the child did not improve over a period of several weeks after the incident occurred. Second, the authors were able to gather some baseline data prior to the interventions that were implemented. Moreover, the data were gathered in a continuous manner and follow-up was scheduled. Although the authors implemented several different treatments, and there is no reliability reported, this case represents a greater degree of inference for experimental control than those studies without these characteristics.

In summary, the researcher conducting a case study investigation faces a number of problems related to drawing valid inferences. In the typical case study, many threats to internal validity that are ruled out when more formal single-case experimental procedures are employed are not possible. Nevertheless, case studies can be distinguished by various characteristics that allow one to draw valid inferences. In this section we have discussed several specific procedures which can be used to draw such inferences. To the degree that the researcher is able to address these concerns in a case study investigation, more valid inferences can be drawn.

Case Studies as a Link between Research and Practice

In addition to the advantages of case studies described in the beginning of this chapter, therapeutic case studies, to the degree that they address the issues of drawing valid inferences, could potentially play an important role in linking clinical research and practice. At one end of the spectrum, therapeutic case studies can provide an impetus for controlled single-subject or group research on a particular disorder or therapeutic technique. Alternatively, case studies can provide an end-point for controlled research—i.e., they can serve as a vehicle for replication of experimental findings in clinical practice.

Case Studies as an Impetus for Research. Therapeutic case studies can provide a potential means for clinicians to publish information about techniques they utilize in their practice—i.e., techniques that have not yet been the subject of controlled research. This would serve at least two purposes. First, it would be a source of hypotheses for researchers interested in the technique or disorder described in the case study. While such hypothesis-generation is not limited to therapeutic case studies, such studies play a unique role in the development of treatments for various disorders. For example, a case study might describe the successful treatment of a disorder using a technique that had not yet been investigated. If the technique appeared to be a promising one, the treatment would then be scrutinized further via a single-subject design to determine its validity under well-controlled experimental conditions. Second, case studies can provide a way to keep research consistent with practice. While the link between research and practice is typically viewed as a situation in which research is the forerunner, this is not always the case. Indeed, in some instances, researchers have suggested a treatment technique or tactic which has already been used successfully in practice. An example of just such a situation comes from the social skills literature. Gresham (1981), in a review of the literature on social skills training with handicapped children, noted that, "To date, there is little, if any, research which has investigated the effects using social learning theory techniques such as modeling , coaching, role playing, and so forth, with nonhandicapped children to facilitate positive social interaction and peer acceptance of handicapped children" (p. 168). However, in a personal communication with one teacher, it was learned that she had frequently used training of this type in the past to facilitate the social acceptance of withdrawn third-grade children in her class. In yet another personal communication, a father related that his son, who has a harelip, was accepted by his peers to a much greater extent after his teacher had encouraged the other children to interact with him. These teachers probably never consulted the literature on social skills training; rather they utilized a technique that they thought might be useful, and were surprisingly successful. Information about these treatments never reached the literature, as it was not the product of a controlled experiment. If, however, these individuals had reported their findings in a case study, these techniques might have already been validated experimentally and be in use on a wider basis today. Thus, case studies can be viewed as a means of reporting clinical successes in order to keep researchers up-to-date on the progress being made by practitioners.

Case Studies as a Means for Testing Generalization. A major concern for both researchers and clinicians is the generalizability of research findings into the clinical setting. Generally, a treatment is constructed, evaluated and found effective in rigorous experimental conditions that are far removed from those existing in clinical settings. However, when this internally valid and effective treatment is disseminated into practice, it can "bomb." Valuable research time and money may be lost.

There are various reasons for the failure of treatment generalized from research to practice. Clinical research and practice differ in terms of therapist training, form of treatment (i.e., package or single component), use of specific instructions and consistent implementation procedures, as well as systematic monitoring and evaluation of results (Kazdin, 1982).

One way to bridge this gap between research and practice for more efficient knowledge building and clinical service is to employ more systematic procedures in clinical practice that resemble those of research (e.g., employing the use of written treatment manuals and evaluation forms). Another way to link research and practice is through clinical replications (Barlow, Hayes, & Nelson, 1984; Kazdin, 1982). Here a treatment found to be effective and internally valid in controlled experimental settings (i.e., analogue studies, group designs, and clinical trials) is tested in a clinical setting absent of such experimental controls, procedural regulations, and monitoring. The concern is to determine if what works in research actually does work in the clinical environment. Thus, the examiner can evaluate the client's responses to treatment and check for any discrepancy between this response and those found in controlled research.

Clinical replications combine the researcher's concerns for generalization and the clinician's concern for applicability and effectiveness. From clinical replication case studies researchers gain important information on the variables that contribute to external validity, effective methods of training, and on productive ways to disseminate treatment. Clinicians benefit from clinical replications because such research is more relevant to their immediate clinical problems and needs for treatment, and demonstrations that treatment is effective in their own setting. Also, a clinician can gain insights into the limits of practice and treatment ideas through clinical replications.

In order to achieve these benefits, clinical replications need to include some crucial facets (Kazdin, 1982). First, clinical replications must serve a purpose within the research continuum. This criterion is fulfilled by the clinical replication role of evaluating the end product of research. The treatment demonstrated to be internally valid and effective in controlled experiments is given a further test of external validity in clinical practice.

A second criterion is that clinical replications need to use standardized procedures that lend themselves to replication in a wide variety of clinical settings. This criterion can be met with the use of instructional manuals and loose monitoring of treatment implementation. Also, techniques for drawing valid inferences from case studies as described earlier in the chapter (e.g., number of assessment occasions, type of data, etc.) can strengthen validity.

Third, the client's response must be evaluated to determine whether the treatment effect in the clinical setting approximates that found in clinical research. Standard forms of evaluation may be included as part of the treatment package manual provided to clinicians in efforts to meet the second criterion mentioned above. Such evaluations may take the form of self-reports, interviews, or rating scales.

Some considerations must be taken into account when conducting and evaluating clinical replications. One concern in the clinical setting is that the priority is service and amelioration of the problem and not research. Therefore, occasionally the treatment must be altered to meet the individual's needs or therapist limitations. Another possible problem is the perceived value of case studies by both researcher and clinician. The former may envision traditional limitations of case studies with clinical replications, and the latter may see them as artificial in the clinical setting.

However, clinical replication case studies serve an important role for both researchers and practitioners. Serving as an end-point for controlled clinical research, clinical replications address the question of whether or not a treatment hypothesized, designed, and validated earlier in the research continuum can be implemented in clinical practice. Clinical replications also provide a "feedback loop" to clinical researchers and clinicians that may lead to further treatment enhancement by adding necessary components or eliminating ineffective ones. Clinical replication may even take the researcher and clinician back to the beginning point of research with a new treatment hypothesis.

EXPERIMENTAL SINGLE-CASE RESEARCH DESIGNS

Single-case experimental research designs generally represent an improvement over the pre-experimental case studies described in the previous section. With a formal single-case experimental design, it is possible to rule out threats to validity that might otherwise remain in the usual pre-experimental case study. Nevertheless, the same pre-experimental case study characteristics previously discussed can be used to increase inference in an experimental single-case design. For example, single-case research designs can generally be improved by monitoring the integrity of the independent variable. In the past this has not been a common characteristic of research using these designs, but when done, it improves inference for drawing a functional relation between the independent and dependent variables.

A major feature of single-case experiments is that a design is arranged to reduce threats to internal validity. The features of the designs are established so that it becomes much less likely that extraneous factors would explain the effects demonstrated on the dependent measures. Several characteristics of single-case experimental designs are necessary to draw valid inferences. First of all, a major feature of single-case experimental designs is that the dependent measures are repeatedly assessed across various phases of the experiment. Usually, data are collected prior to the intervention and represent a baseline.

Following this, a series of intervention phases are implemented. Nevertheless, an essential feature is that the client's behavior is measured repeatedly so that various trends in the data can be examined.

A second major feature related to repeated assessment refers to assessing client variability across time. As the target responses are repeatedly measured, variability will usually be apparent in the data. The level and trend of the target behavior have a bearing on the inferences that can be drawn about the future course of behavior. For example, if the performance during treatment departs greatly from that during baseline, the investigator will be able to draw stronger inferences for an intervention effect. Usually, some stable measures are considered essential during the baseline phases. Nevertheless, a researcher can still draw valid inferences if the trend is in the opposite direction of that anticipated during the intervention phase. Also, there are some designs (to be discussed below) that handle trends in the data that might emerge as problematic.

A third feature of single-case designs is the careful specification of the independent and dependent variables, setting, therapist, and client characteristics that occur during the experiment. It is important that the investigator holds certain variables constant during the intervention phase and that the therapeutic components are isolated so that a functional relation can be established between the independent and dependent variables. Also, specification of various conditions surrounding the experiment is deemed essential for the replication of findings and for establishing the external validity of the investigation.

Another characteristic of single-case research designs is the replication of effects. The various designs used in single-case research vary on how this is accomplished. Usually, internal validity is achieved by replication of effects across clients, client measures, settings, or within subject(s). The issue of determining the number of replications is a matter of some debate. Nevertheless, in most designs at least two and probably four replications are considered necessary to test the hypothesis that the independent variable is responsible for change in the dependent variable. Replication is also critical if results are to be generalized beyond the case being investigated.

Another important consideration in single-case research is the flexibility of the design in response to ongoing change in the dependent measures. Sometimes individual clients respond quite differently to treatment across phases. This was demonstrated in the previous investigation by Roberts and Gordon (1979) in which several different interventions were scheduled across the investigation. However, sometimes there is a tradeoff with this flexibility in establishing internal validity. When the researcher can establish withdrawal of treatment or return to baseline phases between various interventions, the inference for the intervention effect is usually increased. Specific issues relating to how this is accomplished are discussed later in this section. Nevertheless, the ability to change the design in response to certain features of client response to treatment is a unique feature of these designs that does not occur in most experimentation in clinical psychology.

Single-Case Research Designs: Applications

There are many variations of single-case research designs in the professional literature. Within the past few years a variety of unique design formats have been developed, but most single-case research designs can be broken down into some basic components (Hayes, 1981).

Within-Series Designs. Within-series designs evaluate change in client measures within various phases of the investigation. Typically, in these designs the most basic form is an A/B/A/B strategy in which A represents a baseline phase and B represents a treatment designed specifically for the subject. In this type of design, treatment effects are replicated during the second B phase. The tactic of replicating treatment effects can also be used in comparing different treatments. For example, a researcher can compare a B phase to a C in several replication attempts (e.g., B/C/B/C/B/C).

The A/B/A/B design format represents a relatively simple phase change strategy. A more complex phase change strategy can be scheduled in within-series designs. Essentially, these designs operate under the same logic, but the more complex phase change designs examine the effects of multiple intervention components. The strategy that the researcher adopts is one in which various combinations of treatments can be tested against their individual components. For example, in a two-phase option a researcher can compare one treatment, such as B, to a treatment package consisting of B + C + D components where B represents praise, C represents feedback, and D represents token reinforcement strategies. Essentially, the logic of the within-series complex phase change designs is the same as the simple phase change designs. That is, the researcher attempts to replicate the intervention package across various phases of the study (e.g., B/B + C + D/B/B + C + D/B/B + C + D/B).

In the more complex within-series strategy the researcher can manipulate two or more variables separately or in combination. In this strategy the treatment effects are often additive. That is, certain treatment components may contribute more to the therapeutic effects than other components. In this type of research it may be necessary for the investigator to tease apart the separate components, and certain strategies have been developed for carrying out this task (see Barrios, in press).

Jason and Liotta (1982) used a within-series single-case research design to evaluate a program designed to reduce cigarette smoking. The study was conducted in a university cafeteria and the target area was a "No Smoking" section containing 13 round tables. The dependent measures consisted of observers recording the number of individuals who smoked one or more cigarettes, and the number of seconds any smoking was occurring within the target area. The design consisted of an A/B/A/B/B + C/B/B + C/ and a follow-up assessment. The intervention, or B phase, consisted of mounting a tent-like sign on each table with the following words on it: "No Smoking Section for Health and Comfort of Patrons." Also four larger signs were placed on walls with the following words on them: "No Smoking Section. Please Don't Smoke in this Section." The B + C phase (or sign + verbal prompting) consisted of the sign intervention and the addition of a university student approaching smokers and saying: "I am concerned about keeping this section for non-smokers. Would you either stop smoking in this area or move to the smoking area?" After a 5-minute interval, if the smoker continued, the prompter again indicated, "I'd just like to once again remind you that this is a no-smoking section. Would you please not smoke here?" Three students served as prompters during this condition.

Results presented in Figure 3.3 demonstrate that during the two phases, cigarette smoke was emitted for an average of 39 out of an observed 50 minutes, and the average of 7.7 individuals were observed smoking in the target area per day. However, during the sign phases the average number of smokers was reduced to 5.3 per session, and cigarette smoke was observed for an average of 26 minutes. However, as can be observed in Figure 3.3, the sign-plus-prompting intervention condition resulted in an average of 1.6 smokers observed smoking an average of 6.2 minutes. This study demonstrated that the sign-plus-verbal-prompting was generally a more effective intervention condition than the simple sign prompting condition alone. However, there are some difficulties with the design. To begin with, it would have been desirable for the authors to schedule another baseline phase between the sign prompting (B) and the sign-plus-verbal-prompting (B + C) phases. Also, the study does not demonstrate that a sign-plus-verbal-prompting is effective independent of the order in which the interventions were introduced. That is, it is possible that the sign-plus-verbal-prompting would not have as great an effect if preceded by the sign prompting condition alone.

In the within-series designs it should be noted that the withdrawal of the intervention may not always result in an initial return to baseline levels, as was true in the current study. To some degree this compromises the integrity of the design and does not allow as great a degree of inference for an experimental effect. Obviously, there are also some measures that will simply not return to baseline levels as when certain learning occurs, or when contingencies in the environment serve to "catch" the behavior into naturally occurring reinforcement. Also, there are situations in which the withdrawal of treatment may simply be unacceptable from the standpoint of the client, careproviders, or even the experimenter. Obviously, there are certain legal and ethical issues that could be raised by withdrawing treatment for certain types of severe disorders. In the study mentioned above this is not a major issue.

Another type of within-series procedure is called the changing criterion de-

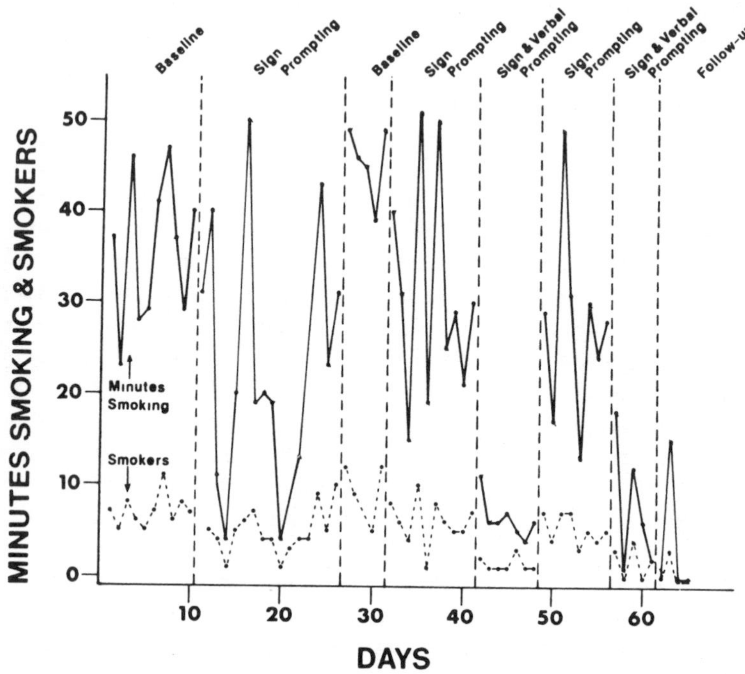

FIG. 3.3. Minutes smoking and number of smokers observed in the cafeteria's no smoking section across experimental conditions. (.-.-= minutes smoking; .---. = number of smokers). (Source: Jason, L.A. & Liotta, R.F. (1982). Reduction of cigarette smoking in a university cafeteria. *Journal of Applied Behavior Analysis, 15,* 573–577. Copyright, 1982 by the Society for the Experimental Analysis of Behavior, Inc. Reproduced by permission.)

sign. This design allows threats to internal validity to be ruled out by bringing the level of the dependent measure under the control of certain criteria that are modified during the study (Hall & Fox, 1977; Hartmann & Hall, 1976). In this strategy a baseline phase is usually scheduled followed by an intervention phase, which is implemented continuously for a period of time until criterion performance is achieved. However, at certain selected points during the treatment phase, the researcher schedules step-wise changes in the level of the performance on the dependent measure. Certain criteria are linked with treatment contingencies and if the dependent measure generally follows the step-wise change in the preset criteria, validity for the treatment effect is increased.

An example of the changing criterion design is found in a study by Foxx and Rubinoff (1979) designed to evaluate the behavioral treatment of caffeinism. The investigation focused on three habitual coffee drinkers who were interested in reducing their daily consumption of caffeine to more acceptable levels. The authors employed a changing criterion design to evaluate the effectiveness of a program consisting of self-monitoring and plotting daily intake of caffeine. In addition, subjects received monetary prizes for not exceeding the treatment phase criteria while forfeiting a portion of their prize when they did exceed the criteria. Results reported in Figure 3.4 for Subject Number #3 (a psychologist) showed that coffee drinking decreased from baseline over the treatment phases. Specifically, with this subject the criterion level for each treatment phase was 144 mg. of caffeine less than the previous treatment phase. The horizontal lines indicate the criterion level shifts for each phase, whereas the broken horizontal lines indicate the mean for each condition. As noted in the figure, there were days in which the client exceeded the phase criterion. As can be seen in Figure 3.4, the psychologist's consump-

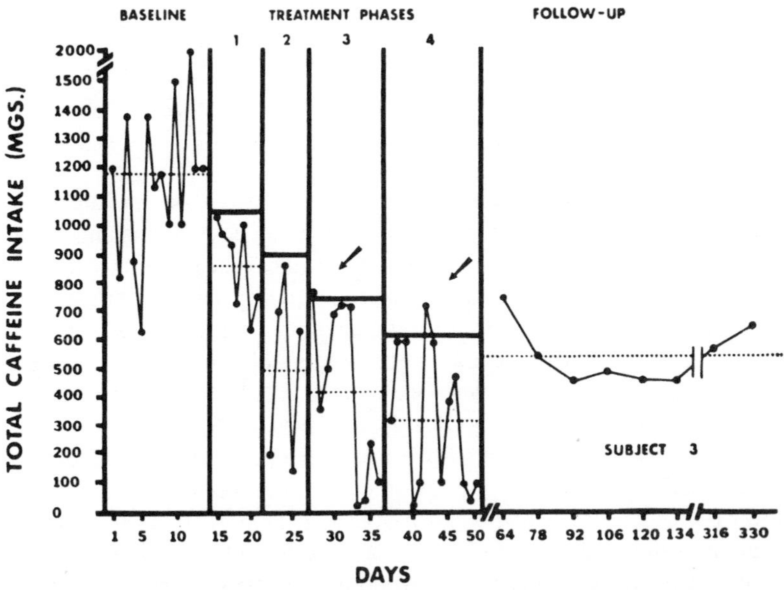

FIG. 3.4. Subject 3's daily caffeine intake (mg.) during baseline, treatment, and follow-up. The criterion level for each treatment phase was 144 mg. of caffeine less than the previous treatment phase. Solid horizontal lines indicate the criterion level for each phase. Broken horizontal lines indicate the mean for each condition. Arrows indicate days in which the treatment phase criterion was exceeded (Source: Foxx, R.M. & Rubinoff, A. (1979). Behavioral treatment of caffeinism: Reducing excessive coffee drinking. *Journal of Applied Behavior Analysis, 12,* 335–344. Copyright, 1979 by the Society for the Experimental Analysis of Behavior, Inc. Reproduced by permission).

tion of caffeine was eliminated or was reduced to more acceptable levels. In addition, the treatment effect was maintained during a 10-month follow-up. This program appeared to be quite effective in reducing the amount of caffeine consumed by the other two subjects in the experiment as well.

As noted in the Foxx and Rubinoff (1979) study, the changing criterion design requires a demonstration of changes in the dependent measure along with the criterion shifts over the treatment phase. In order to establish the internal validity of the design the researcher must demonstrate that each criterion shift results in a change in behavior. Moreover, it is important for the investigator to have the behavior stabilize in the within-phase series before proceeding to the next step-wise level. In addition, each step-wise criterion change must be large enough to distinguish it from variability occurring in the data. Procedures that can be used in the changing criterion design include randomly varying the length of the criterion, as well as the depth, and the direction of the criterion shifts (Hayes, 1981). These strategies can increase inference for experimental control because they serve to exaggerate the influence of the criterion shifts. Generally, the changing criterion design is useful in those investigations where shaping a behavior gradually over the treatment phase is needed. Where larger shifts in behavior are expected to occur, the researcher could probably use a different type of research design, because the changing criterion design appears most suited to gradual changes in behavior over time.

Between-Series Designs. There are two types of between-series single-case research designs: The Alternating Treatments Design (ATD) and the Simultaneous Treatment Design (STD). Both designs allow the researcher to compare two or more interventions across time. The comparisons that are made between the different interventions on the dependent measures take into account shifts in level and trend in data as the intervention is applied over time.

The ATD allows the researcher to expose the client to separate treatment conditions for equal time periods (Barlow & Hayes, 1979). In this design the investigator alternates treatments for a brief time period (e.g., treatment B is administered in one session and treatment C in another session). The investigator is able to establish alternation of treatment either by counterbalancing or by randomly assigning it across phases of the investigation. With the ATD the investigator is able to compare two or more treatments in a relatively brief period of time while avoiding some of the major disadvantages of withdrawal designs (e.g., withdrawal of treatment, stability of the data series, among other features).

Agras, Leitenberg, Barlcw, and Thomson (1969) evaluated the effects of social reinforcement on a 50-year-old woman who was claustrophobic. According to the authors, the client was unable to remain in a room with the door closed, go into such places as an elevator, movie theater, or church, or even drive her car for long distances. The authors measured the phobia by recording the time the woman was able to sit in a small windowless room before she felt uncomfortable. These data were collected four times over the day. The intervention consisted of two therapists working with the woman for two sessions each. Therapist 1 provided praise when the woman was able to increase the amount of time that she remained in the room during the trials. The second therapist simply maintained a pleasant relationship but did not provide any contingent praise. Essentially, the client was exposed to a multiple schedule over various phases of the study. Results of the investigation reported in Figure 3.5 indicate that the average amount of time that the woman spent in the small room was fairly low during baseline. However, at the beginning of the treatment the woman showed higher performance with the therapist who provided reinforcement than the one who did not. During the second intervention phase, the therapists alternated their roles so that the one who provided contingent praise stopped and the other one took over this treatment activity. As can be observed in this phase of the investigation, the client discriminated between treatments and began to perform better again with the praise condition. The conditions were again alternated during the third phase where they returned to their original roles. Generally, the results showed that the woman was able to remain in a small room for longer periods of time with a therapist who provided reinforcement.

This study represents an early example of what is currently called an ATD. This strategy was often called a multiple schedule during the early years of operant research as it was being applied to phobic clients. It can be observed that the ATD can be quite useful for comparing two distinct and independent treatments as can be noted by the Agras et al. (1969) study. Investigators were able to compare these treatments over three phases of the investigation while balancing therapists. This type of strategy usually provides a considerable savings in time over a within-series single-case research design.

In contrast to the ATD design, the STD presents treatments to the subjects simultaneously (Kazdin & Hartmann, 1978). Nevertheless, the simultaneous availability of the treatments does not necessarily insure that the client is exposed to all treatments equally. In fact, the STD really evaluates a client preference among treatments because the treatments are available at the same time in the same session. It is possible that the STD could provide the researcher with information on client responsiveness to treatments where definite preferences exist. However, there are few applications of the STD in the literature. Generally, the STD and ATD allow the investigator to compare two or more treatments. However, the designs are not limited to two treatments. The researcher can schedule more than one, but the logistical considerations in balancing all the features of the designs with three or more conditions becomes somewhat burdensome. Thus, for practical reasons the usual applications of these designs involve only two treatment comparisons.

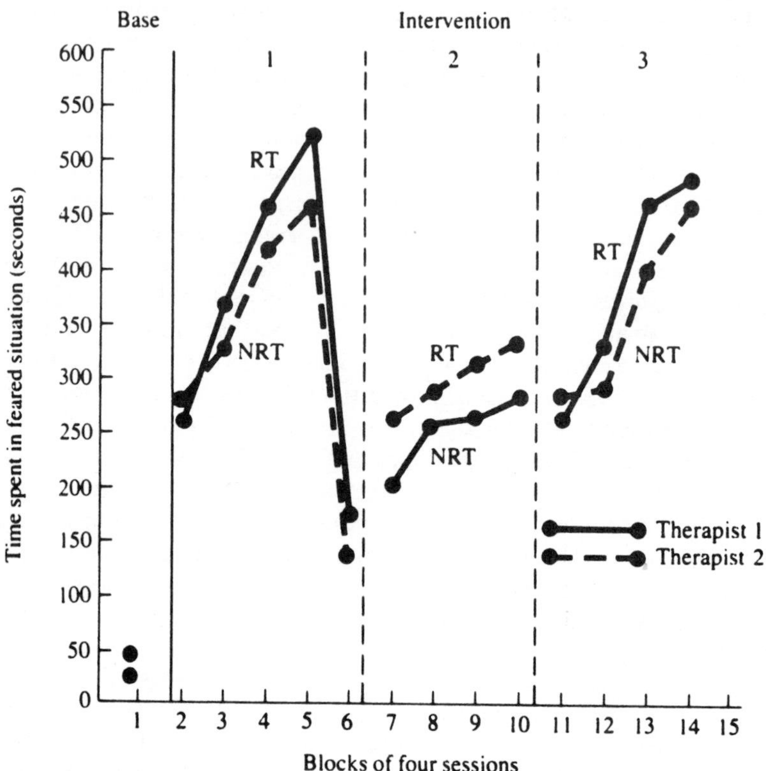

FIG. 3.5. The effects of reinforcing and non-reinforcing therapists on the modification of claustrophobic behavior. One therapist provided reinforcement (reinforcing therapist or RT) while the other did not (non-reinforcing therapist or NRT). The therapists eventually switched these contingencies. (Source: Agras, W.S., Leitenberg, H., Barlow, D.H. & Thomson, L.E. (1969). Instructions in reinforcement in the modification of neurotic behavior. *American Journal of Psychiatry, 125,* 1435–1439. Reproduced by permission.)

Combined Series Designs. In the combined series single-case design the researcher draws a comparison both within and between series. The multiple baseline design (MBD) represents the most common example of this strategy because it includes a simple within-phase element and replicates the treatment across either subjects, settings, or behaviors. The internal validity of the design is met through staggering the interventions across time. Once changes are observed in the first A/B series, the remaining series receive the intervention in sequential fashion. Each time a replication occurs across either subjects, settings, or behaviors, the researcher is more confident that there is a functional relation between the independent and dependent variable. These designs are most useful because the researcher has the option of implementing them across three different aspects of dependent measures. Also, the researcher can schedule further replications depending upon practical and ethical considerations. It is also possible that the MBD is more compatible with the usual practice of many applied researchers because it is not necessary to withdraw the treatment once it has been implemented. However, this is an option for the researcher if he/she desires to do so.

An example of the MBD will elucidate its utility in applied and clinical research. Bornstein, Bach, Heider, and Ernst (1981) employed an MBD to evaluate behavioral marital therapy for two couples. The couples reported several areas of conflict, including financial, social, and personal independence, as well as a multi-dimensional assessment format including self-report, and external observers' reports of marital interaction. The treatment program consisted of instructing the couples in appropriate forms of communication and problem solving. The specific therapy was based on the behavioral marital therapy of Jacobson and Martin (1976) and communications (Olson, 1976). Specifically, the authors intervened by helping the couples to be specific in describing their problems, developing effective listening skills, helping them to communicate directly with each other, and maintaining a positive problem-solving approach. Also, during a "couple generated" discussion a therapist would intervene whenever the oportunity arose to increase/decrease behavior under consideration. In such instances the therapist provided instructions, feedback, coaching, modeling, reinforcement, role reversal, and contracting.

Results of the investigation reported in Figure 3.6 show the laboratory-based data. The data on rate per minute of complaining, criticizing, agreement, and positive problem solving all appeared to improve as a function of the intervention. The treatment also appeared to be successful during a one-year follow up.

The Bornstein et al. (1981) study represents an example of how an MBD can be implemented across behaviors. An important consideration that is often raised in the design is whether or not generalization across the behaviors will occur once intervention is introduced to one specific behavior. For example, the researcher might be concerned that after the intervention package is implemented with complaining behaviors, criticisms would also decrease. However, it appears that this was not the case. Also, it can be demonstrated that once agreement was increased, positive problem solving did not increase until the intervention was introduced.

DATA ANALYSIS

An important consideration in case study and single-case research designs is determining whether or not the treatment was responsible for observed changes in the dependent variable. In order to examine this the researcher must deter-

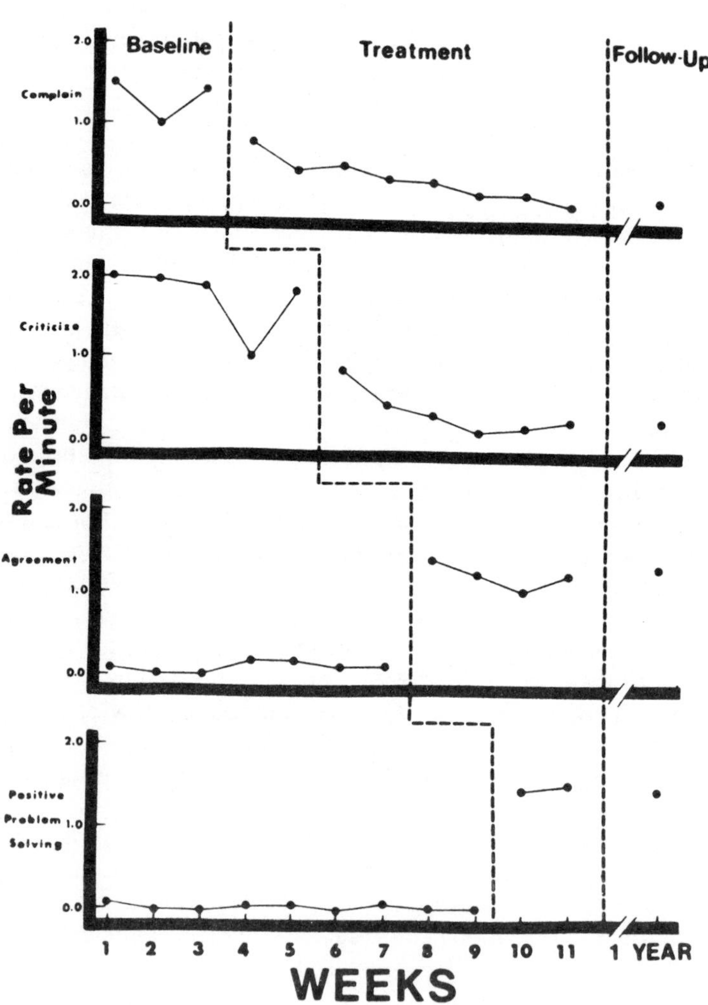

FIG. 3.6. Laboratory observational data for Couple 1 across baseline treatment and follow-up phases. (Source: Bornstein, P.H., Bach, P.J., Heider, J.F., & Ernst, J. (1981). Clinical treatment of marital dysfunction: A multiple baseline analysis. *Behavioral Assessment, 3,* 335–343. Copyright, 1981 by Association for Advancement of Behavior Therapy. Reproduced by permission).

mine whether and to what degree the treatment and dependent measures covary. In single-case research several different types of data evaluation strategies are employed to make this determination. These usually include visual analysis, statistical analysis, and certain clinical or therapeutic criteria.

As traditionally conceived, the choice of a particular data analysis strategy represents a statistical conclusion validity concern (Cook & Campbell, 1979). Various analytic methods used to assess the covariation can pose threats to validity and interpretation of the data and so represent an important validity concern in single-case research. In single-case research, a major controversy relates to the criteria that are used to draw inferences regarding covariation between independent and dependent variables. Issues surrounding these concerns are highlighted below. The interested reader should refer to several other volumes for more detailed discussion of these concerns (Kazdin, 1982; Kratochwill, 1978).

Visual Data Analysis

Visual analysis procedures represent the most common strategy for a data analysis in single-case research. To some extent this is true because many of the data analysis procedures grew out of the operant tradition, which infrequently uses any kind of statistic in single-case research. The emphasis on visual analysis is still prominent with certain individuals from the behavior analysis tradition who recommend these strategies to the exclusion of any statistical analytic technique (Johnson & Pennypacker, 1980).

Visual analysis procedures are generally easy to learn and apply. The primary justification for use of visual analysis is that such techniques act as a filter to eliminate small effects and hence promote large intervention effects in applied behavior analysis research (Baer, 1977; Parsonson & Baer, 1978). Generally, weak experimental effects that might be detected through statistical procedures are considered small, non-durable, less replicable, and less generalizable, and, overall, less meaningful than those produced by large experimental effects.

Visual analysis is usually appropriate when the observed effects of the intervention are large. However, determining what a large effect is can be debatable. In fact, a large effect is really a relative term, and often depends upon the subjective impression of the experimenter. What represents a large effect to one investigator is often not a large effect to other investigators or reviewers of the experimental research report. Perhaps the clearest use of visual analysis occurs under conditions where the data patterns are ideal for inspecting some type of treatment effect. This occurs when an intervention is implemented on a dependent measure that has not been previously present (Kazdin, 1982). For example, Piersel and Kratochwill (1981) evaluated the effects of a teacher-implemented contingency management package in the treatment of selective mutism. The contingency management package employing extinction and positive reinforcement was implemented in a multiple baseline fashion across two children who had a 0 level of verbalizations in a classroom setting. Figure 3.7 presents the data for both subjects over baseline and intervention phases. It can be observed that baseline verbalizations (number of words) for each subject was zero. In this case there is perfect stability over time and absence of trends and variability in the data. The intervention produces some change that is considered valuable and represents some demonstration that the intervention effect has occurred. In this instance, the usual statistical evaluation of the data is not needed to demonstrate some intervention effects (this does not preclude the possibility of the application of certain statistical tests such as time-series analysis to evaluate patterns of the data, such as variability during the intervention, seasonal effects, and so forth). Actually, there are many examples in the applied literature showing that baseline behavior is relatively stable, zero, or at very low rates. In such cases the intervention program provides a demonstration that some type of effect has occurred independent of whether or not one might consider the effects large.

Considerations. Visual analysis procedures have a number of considerations that must be addressed by the applied researcher. First of all, graphical analysis can be improved by employing a variety of technical aids developed for this purpose (e.g., standard deviation bands, regression lines to fit the data, mean lines: Parsonson & Baer, 1978). Second, a major assumption of visual analysis is that data be evaluated over time and that enought points be collected to discern various data patterns. Without continuous assessment of the dependent measure the researcher may not be able to draw appropriate inferences. A third concern relates to the actual patterns of data that occur. Such factors as baseline stability, variability, score overlap, number of data points, trend, changes in level, and analysis across phases must be considered. Especially important is a concern raised recently in the literature regarding auto-correlation (i.e., a statistical estimate of the present value of data as predicted from past values). This concern is important because it has been demonstrated that with certain patterns of data, statistical serial dependency may be present and render the data somewhat uninterpretable through visual analysis. For example, Jones, Weinrott, and Vaught (1978) noted that when serial dependency is present, agreement between statistical and visual analysis methods is reduced. Finally, use of visual analysis in applied behavioral analysis research has been premised on addressing therapeutic or clinical criteria. When clinical or therapeutic criteria are invoked it is often argued that statistical criteria may be redundant. This issue is examined next.

Clinical and Therapeutic Criteria. Clinical or therapeutic criteria are often used to complement visual analysis of data. Clinical and therapeutic criteria have usually been discussed within the context of social validation (Kazdin,

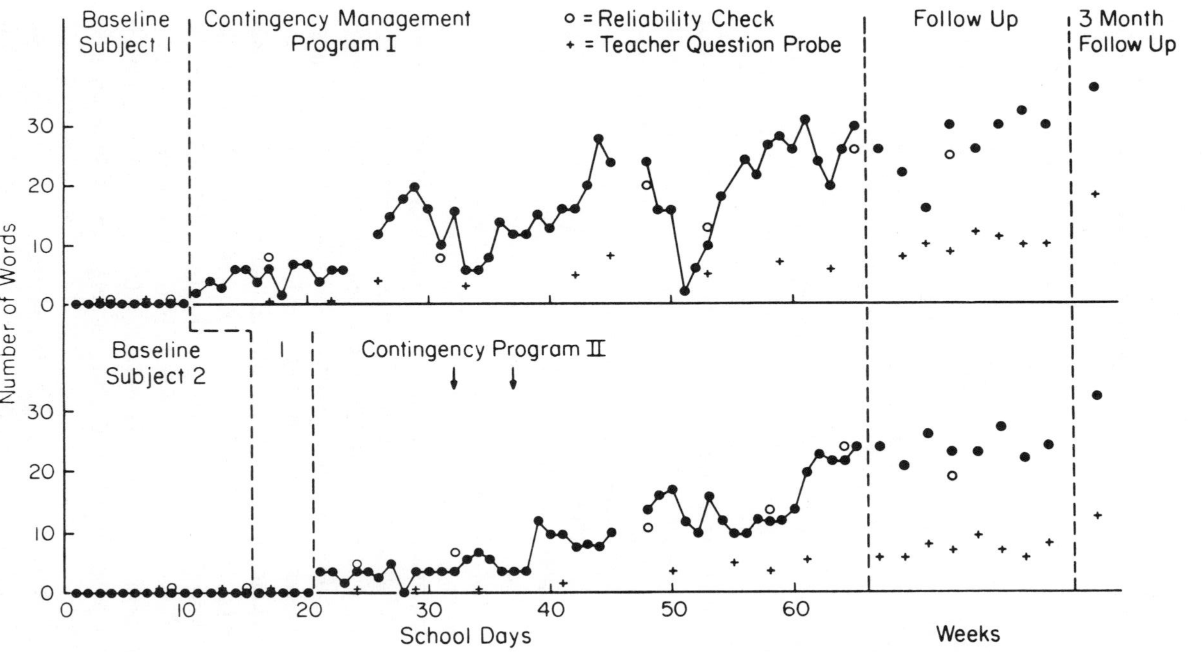

FIG. 3.7. The number of words spoken by Shannon (Subject 1) and Patrick (Subject 2) during baseline and treatment phases across all settings where behavior was observed. Open circles represent reliability checks. Stars indicate teacher probes in the generalization settings. Missing data refer to those days when the subjects were absent from school. Follow-up data were gathered in the classroom and generalization setting over 8 weeks and upon return to school the following fall. (Source: Piersel, W.C., & Kratochwill, T.R. (1981). A teacher-implemented contingency management package to assess and treat selective mutism. *Behavioral Assessment, 3,* 371–382. Copyright 1981 by Association for Advancement of Behavior Therapy. Reproduced by permission.)

1977; Wolf, 1978). For example, Wolf (1978) noted that social validation can be used to evaluate whether an intervention produces changes of clinical or therapeutic significance. Kazdin (1977) outlined two specific methods for evaluating the clinical or therapeutic effects produced in single-case and group research designs. These are referred to as the social comparison and subjective evaluation methods. In the social comparison method, behavior of the client is compared with that of others whose behavior has not been defined as problematic. Subjective evaluation refers to assessment of the client's performance as solicited by other individuals in the natural environment. Behaviors are usually regarded as clinically important if the treatment program brings a client's performance within the range of socially acceptable levels. The importance of these validation methods is that they can be used to complement visual inspection of the data and provide some type of formal criterion towards which interventions can be focused and against which program outcomes can be evaluated.

As an example of the use of social validation criteria in evaluating therapeutic effects, Matson (1982) conducted a study to assess treatment of the behavioral characteristics of depression in the mentally retarded. In the study, four mentally retarded adults in the mild-to-moderate range were treated in a multiple baseline fashion across behaviors typically associated with the depression construct. The intervention consisted of individual therapy sessions involving information, performance feedback, and token reinforcement. Specifically, treatment was provided for such behaviors as the number of words spoken, somatic complaints, irritability, grooming, negative self-statements, positive affect, eye contact, and speech latency. Social validation criteria were established by evaluating eight mentally retarded persons who did not meet the criteria for depression on the MMPI Self-rating Depression Scale, Beck Depression Inventory, and clinical judgments. The later clinical judgments served as the social validation criteria and consisted of twice rating each of the eight target behaviors on the subjects to establish a criterion level of performance. The treatment brought the subjects' performance within the range of the normative performance of the retarded nondepressed subjects. In the Matson study, the social comparison method of social validation was employed to evaluate the clinical importance of change. As noted above, in this strategy normative comparisons are developed through comparison with so-called "normal peers" as judged by individuals in the environment. Subjective evaluations can also involve asking certain judges to define criteria for good performance in areas of social functioning (e.g., social skills, creative behaviors).

Despite the positive characteristics of social validation, there are some considerations that must be taken into account in the use of this strategy. For example, it is possible that normative standards may be inappropriate to serve as a criterion to evaluate change. One might question use of mentally retarded peers as a criterion against which the effectiveness of depression treatment was evaluated as in the Matson (1982) study. It might be argued that the behavior of nonretarded individuals should serve as a criterion. Nevertheless, it can readily be seen that such issues are subject to debate. Also, individuals who conduct a subjective evaluation may not always establish consistent criteria and may disagree on what is an appropriate criterion for evaluating change. Moreover, certain scales or strategies used to establish the criterion in social validity outcome measures could be questioned on various psychometric grounds, as for example, lacking reliability and validity (see Kazdin, 1977). Thus, even though social validity can improve upon visual analysis, social validation still has a subjective component and leaves the level of performance needed for clinical change somewhat informal or unspecified. In this regard, it may not establish a reliable decision rule.

Social validation procedures are typically recommended within the context of clinical or therapeutic research. However, as noted at the beginning of this chapter, not all single-case research designs are used in this form of research. There are some cases where social validation strategies may not be deemed appropriate as a formal criterion for data analysis. For example, in certain types of program evaluation research, where large numbers of subjects are studied across time, social validation would appear to be inappropriate, as in the case of evaluating helicopter patrolling strategies and their influence on city crime rates (Kirschner, Schnelle, Domash, Larson, Carr, & McNees, 1980), disciplinary procedures in state prison inmates (Schnelle & Lee, 1974), as well as many other areas. Thus, the investigator must look to other areas to consider a more formal criterion for data analysis.

Statistical Data Analysis

Statistical analysis of single-case research data has been the subject of considerable debate in the clinical literature. Because statistical analysis is a relatively complex area only a brief overview of some of the more salient issues will be presented here. The interested reader is referred to several sources that provide a more detailed discussion of this area (Kazdin, 1982; Kratochwill, 1978).

Statistical analysis of single-case data requires that the researcher address several important features before embarking upon a statistical analysis. Usually, statistical analysis has been invoked under conditions where large effects are not found. However, use of statistical tests depends on the overall characteristics of the data that are employed. First of all, correlated data have been known to cause difficulty in interpretation through visual methods. It is possible that application of certain statistical tests will allow the investigator to deal with this problem and make a more reliable decision regarding the intervention effect. Also, variability and trend in the data often cause interpretive problems. It is the application of statistical tests that can deal with these kinds of components of the data.

Another major feature of statistical analysis is that it provides the researcher a formal and usually reliable criterion from which to base conclusions. Generally, statistical analysis can produce a reliable decision-rule, although in certain types of time-series analysis many data points (e.g., 50) are necessary in order for reliable model identification to occur (McCleary, Hay, Meidinger, & McDowell, 1980).

Another major advantage of statistical analysis is that it can be used to detect relatively small but reliable effects when certain therapeutic interventions are being evaluated. The importance of evaluating statistically significant but small effects can be seen as important within the context of integrating treatment approaches into a package to effect a larger change in behavior that might not be possible through any single component. It is also possible that variables which initially produce small effects could bring about large effects when replicated across different therapists, subjects, or disorders. Finally, statistical analysis of single-case data could be useful when an investigator is embarking upon a new area of research. In some cases planning intervention programs necessitates examining many different kinds of interventions with many different components. It is possible that application of statistical tests would allow detection of reliable treatment effects where visual analysis could have been equivocal.

An example of the way in which a statistical analysis can complement visual inspection of the data and can help conclusions about the outcome is in an investigation by Wolfe, St. Lawrence, Graves, Brehony, Bradlyn, and Kelly (1982). These authors evaluated the effects of an intensive behavioral parent-training program for a child-abusive mother. A "bug-in-the-ear" technique was used to reduce abusive-related behaviors in a relatively low functioning child-abusive mother. The mother displayed very high rates of aversive behavior towards her three children. Using a MBD, the investigators evaluated the effects of the intervention across hostile physical and verbal behaviors and positive verbal and physical behaviors. Figure 3.8 presents data for each of these target behaviors during compliance and cooperative interaction tasks. The solid circle represents the compliant task and the open triangle represents the cooperative task. Interpretation of the data in the top two series on hostile, physical, and verbal behaviors presents a few interpretive problems because there is little variability and virtually no trend once the intervention is introduced. With introduction of the training in positive behaviors, interpretation of the data is not at all straightforward through visual analysis. In order to determine changes in the positive data series in both the compliance and cooperative tasks, the investigators conducted a time-series analysis. Analysis of the data indicated that positive physical behaviors during the compliance task showed statistically significant changes in both level and slope. How-

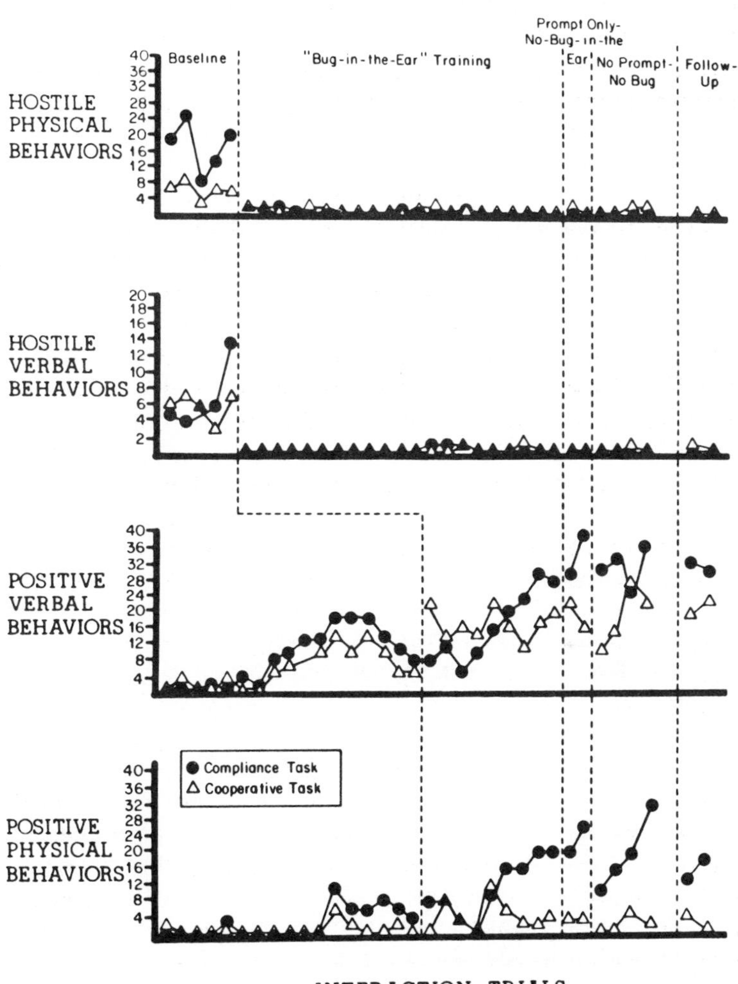

FIG. 3.8. Clinic observations of parent target behaviors across experimental conditions. Frequencies per 10-minute sample of parent hostile, physical and verbal behaviors (top two graphs) and parent positive verbal and physical behaviors (bottom two graphs) during compliance task and cooperative task are shown (Source: Wolfe, D.A., St. Lawrence, J., Graves, K., Brehong, K., Bradbyn, D., & Kelly, J.A. (1982). Intensive behavioral parent training for a child abusive mother. *Behavior Therapy, 13,* 438–451. Copyright, 1982 by Association for the Advancement of Behavior Therapy. Reproduced by permission.)

ever, during the cooperative task, increases in positive physical behavior were not significant for level or slope. Also, results of the analysis showed that the mother's use of positive verbal behavior was nonsignificant for both the cooperative and compliance task. In summary, this study demonstrates that statistical analysis can be used to draw inferences from the data which might otherwise not be possible through visual analysis alone.

Several considerations can be raised over the use of statistical tests in single-case research. To begin with, as noted in the above discussion, it may not always be necessary to employ statistical tests. This is so when baseline levels are at extremely stable and low rates or even nonexistent, or when the effects of the intervention are large, such as in modification of client behaviors that achieve rates well above normative criteria. Another concern is selection of a test that is appropriate for single-case data. Again, in this literature there is considerable debate regarding what is or is not an appropriate statistical test. Usually, conventional parametric tests (e.g., *t*-tests, analyses of variance, multiple regression) are not appropriate for most single-case research designs. The primary reason is that in the use of conventional parametric tests, inferences are made about unobserved samples of the subject under consideration; yet, non-random time frames from the experiment are usually selected. Thus, the generalization implicit in these tests is not met. Also, most traditional parametric procedures assume that estimates of "error" in the data are independent. Application of conventional parametric tests with autocorrelated data will result in an inflated Type I error rate. Nevertheless, when data do not display autocorrelated error, the researcher could use more traditional parametric procedures.

Another concern in applied and clinical research where single-case designs are used is the requirement that statistical tests usually impose on the investigator. In certain types of statistical analyses, baseline series must be included and they must usually be of a certain length. The applied investigator may not always have the luxury of including this kind of baseline phase in the study. In addition, certain types of statistical tests such as time-series analysis, require that the phases be long enough to identify models appropriate for the running of the statistical test. Also, tests, such as the R_n statistic (Revusky, 1967) require a certain number of baseline series in the design in order to be used. Various practical and ethical considerations could be paramount and require that the investigator not meet design and statistical requirements for use of these tests.

Once a decision has been made that a statistical test can be used, the investigator must select from a number of available procedures. Generally, two types of alternatives have been used, including non-parametric methods (e.g., Edgington, 1980; Levin, Marascuilo, & Hubert, 1978) and time-series analysis (McCleary et al., 1980). In randomization tests, random assignment is used as a basis for drawing inferences from the data. However, these types of tests, like their large-N-between-group design counterparts, typically do not use as much of the data and so the researcher may not obtain as much information in the analysis as in other methods.

Time-series analysis strategies can be used in typical single-case research designs where the data series is relatively long. These procedures address the issue of autocorrelated data by removing it through specification of an appropriate model for the analysis. After the model has been identified, the test can be applied and, depending on the type of program, the investigator can obtain an estimate of significant changes in level and slope as well as variability and seasonality in the data. These procedures usually require a computer program and a great deal of sophistication in mathematical statistics.

Even when statistical tests are used, another important consideration is that the investigator must take into account the overall series of phases in the design to draw inferences regarding an experimental effect (Kazdin, 1982). Thus, it is a pattern of data across all the phases that result in drawing valid inferences from the experiment. Statistical tests that are employed may not always be applied to all the phases, and hence, may be of limited usefulness.

EVALUATION OF TREATMENT OUTCOMES

A researcher can have a vast number of questions when he/she is evaluating a treatment. Yet, there is a priority list to the seemingly endless number of questions. Both applied and basic researchers are first and foremost concerned with whether or not a treatment makes a difference in the target behavior. Once an effect has been determined, refined questions can be addressed. These questions include how much effect is possible, under what conditions it occurs and for whom, what improvements can be made in it, and what are the final after-effects of the treatment. Recently, several dimensions of treatment evaluation strategies have been conceptualized and some can be used in single-case research (Kazdin, 1982).

Generally, a treatment is designed in response to a clinical need for ameliorating a problem. Since the main objective in clinical work is to provide service or care, the treatment usually is composed of several components, any or all of which the clinician believes might be effective. Determining whether such a treatment does indeed relieve the client's problem is called the *treatment package strategy*. The treatment is given in its entirety to see if desired changes occur. For example, to eliminate an adult phobia a graded in vivo exposure package of reinforced practice may be presented with all five components proposed by Leitenberg (1976). The components are: graded exposure to fear-eliciting stimuli, therapeutic instructions, client control of progress, performance feedback, and performance-contingent reinforcement. Since the need for treatment arises in the clinical setting, using a single subject time-series design is most cost-efficient and relevant for evaluating the treatment package, although group designs can also be used. At this point, the researcher is not concerned with why the treatment works, just that it does work.

Having found an effect, more specific questions can be asked, such as what components are necessary to bring about the positive change. These questions can be answered through a *dismantling treatment strategy*. Within this strategy individual components are isolated and systematically eliminated from the treatment in order to observe the influence each component has on the general treatment effect. Information of this sort is valuable for developing the treatment package into a more concise, cost-efficient program.

Although single-subject time-series designs can be implemented to address dismantling strategy questions, they tend to run into trouble when isolating and comparing different components due to sequence effects. For evaluating more specific questions dealing with comparisons of components and treatments, group designs tend to be the better choice. Using the previous example, the components of reinforced practice can be presented in various combinations to different homogeneous groups and compared across conditions for their individual effects in a group design. When a group design is impossible to implement for reasons of subject availability, a single-subject design in which components of the treatments are systematically withdrawn can be carried out.

Having determined the necessary components, the researcher may wonder what he/she can add to improve the treatment. The *constructive treatment strategy* addresses this question. It is the opposite of dismantling strategy; rather than systematically removing components from the treatment, components are added to make a qualitatively more effective treatment. However, the components added should be assessed for their independent effectiveness before combining them with the other components. In the example of reinforced practice, a component that has been tested for its additive effect in enhancing fear reduction is the therapist modeling of appropriate approach behaviors (Barlow, Agras, Leitenberg, & Wincze, 1975). Again, single-subject time-series designs may present unclear findings due to the sequence of treatment. Such concerns can be controlled in group designs.

The experimenter may also wonder how much exposure to the fear-inducing stimulus is needed for sufficient fear reduction in the client. Using a *parametric treatment strategy,* the experimenter can vary specific aspects of the treatment to check for the maximal amount of change possible. The variation of the components is usually done quantitatively, but qualitative variations can also be applied. Taking the exposure component found crucial in the dismantling strategy, the length of reinforced practice sessions can be varied across groups or single subjects. As an example, Stern and Marks (1973) found two continuous 2-hour sessions better than four half-hour sessions separated by 30-minute rest periods on the same day for agoraphobic clients. The optimal response can therefore be achieved on the average after two continuous 2-hour sessions, thus answering treatment cost questions.

Given that the researcher has used the four previous evaluation strategies to design a specific, concise, effective treatment, he/she may question if the treatment actually ameliorates the problems faster and better than another treatment. Through a *comparative treatment strategy*, the researcher can compare two or more treatments to determine which one is most effective. A problem with this strategy is that the different treatments may have different types of effects across the independent variables, and thus cannot be directly compared. Rather than ask which treatment is better, the question should be which treatment works best for the problem at hand. In the example, the package of reinforced practice was compared to imaginal flooding and systematic desensitization to assess which approach was more effective in reducing anxiety to certain stimuli (Crowe, Marks, Agras, & Leitenberg, 1972). Reinforced practice was found to be superior to both alternative treatments. Since both treatments are assessed on the same dependent variable, such a comparison is feasible.

Following the aforementioned sequence, the experimenter may conclude that he/she has a valid treatment. But what of external validity (i.e., To what client population can this treatment generalize? Does the type of therapist play a role in the generalizability?). Examining attributes of the client and therapist that might influence the applicability of the treatment is called the *client-therapist variation strategy*. Such client characteristics as age, sex, socioeconomic status, and education, as well as therapist characteristics such as sex, age, training, prestige, and personality traits, can be selected for manipulation to determine the boundaries of treatment application. For example, the experimenter may ask if there is an interaction between the client's age and the magnitude of fear reduction. Addressing this question, Agras, Chapin, and Oliveau (1972) reported that clients younger than 20 years of age improved 100% as compared to 43% of those older who improved. Here, single-subject designs run into problems since they are unable to detect interaction effects. Factorial designs are usually the preferred study for demonstrating main and interaction effects.

A final question a researcher may ask is what happens to the client at the end of treatment (e.g., Are there side effects? Do the effects generalize? Do they last?). Furthermore, the researcher may want to know how the results developed and what the process of change entailed. Evaluation of this type is called an *internal structure or process strategy* and requires continuous data collection before, during, and after treatment. This type of assessment is rare in group designs but is a common characteristic of single-subject designs. By employing these designs, process questions about trends, immediacy, and magnitude of effects, changes in behaviors not focused on, and the nature of behavior in follow-up can be addressed. Knowing the nature of the client's change in behavior after intervention has ceased helps strengthen inferences drawn from the treatment and points out covariations or events that can lead to new hypotheses, new studies, and new treatments.

In summary, single-subject designs play an active role in evaluating treatment outcome questions. Although they may have problems in providing unambiguous answers for some evaluation questions due to sequence effects and juxtaposition of treatments, they do address other questions that might be left unanswerable in group research alone.

SUMMARY AND CONCLUSIONS

Case study and single-case research designs have been used frequently in clinical and applied research in psychology. In this chapter we noted that, as traditionally conceived, case study investigation refers to relatively uncontrolled and subjectively described clinical cases. However, case studies need not be restricted to this form of methodology. Independent of some type of formal research design, case studies can be improved by taking into consideration such factors as the size and impact of the effect, as well as: (1) obtaining objective data, (2) utilizing repeated measurement, (3) noting the chronicity of the case, (4) monitoring the integrity of the independent variable, (5) employing some type of formal data analysis, and (6) by collecting information about the generalization and maintenance of treatment effects in addition to the social validity of the outcome.

In contrast to case-study investigation, single-case research designs usually employ some type of formal design structure in order to assist in drawing valid inferences from the data. These strategies have provided important options to both case-study and traditional large-*N*-between-groups designs in clinical research. The methods also have emphasized repeated assessment of client variables across time and have provided the potential for conducting research in a variety of applied areas where clinical psychologists function.

Several different types of single-case research designs were described including within-series designs, between-series designs (including alternating and simultaneous treatment), and combined-series designs, which usually involve MBDs across subjects, settings, or behaviors. Some special issues in the use of these designs as well as the analysis of the data were described.

Use of single-case research designs requires a number of important assumptions. These strategies represent an important methodological tool in the clinical psychologist's armamentarium for developing a sound empirical knowledge base in the field. They have a unique role to play in research and in developing treatments that will be used in the future practice of clinical and applied psychology.

REFERENCES

Agras, W.S., Chapin, N.H., & Oliveau, D.C. (1972). The natural history of phobias. *Archives of General Psychiatry, 26*, 315–317.

Agras, W.S., Leitenberg, H., Barlow, D.H., & Thomson, L.E. (1969). Instructions and reinforcement in the modification of neurotic behavior. *American Journal of Psychiatry, 125*, 1435–1439.

Barlow, D.H., Agras, W.S., Leitenberg, H., & Wincze, J.P. (1975). An experimental analysis of the effectiveness of "shaping" in reducing maladaptive avoidance behavior: An analysis study. *Behavioral Research & Therapy, 13*, 141–152.

Barlow, D.H., & Hayes, S.C. (1979). Alternating treatments design: One strategy for comparing the effects of two treatments in a single subject. *Journal of Applied Behavior Analysis, 12*, 199–210.

Barlow, D.H., Hayes, S.C., & Nelson, R.O. (1984). *The scientist practitioner: Research and accountability in clinical and educational settings.* New York: Pergamon.

Baer, D.M. (1977). Perhaps it would be better not to know everything. *Journal of Applied Behavior Analysis, 10*, 167–172.

Barrios, B. (in press). Single-subject strategies for examining joint effect: A critical evaluation. *Behavioral Assessment.*

Bergman, R.L. (1976). Extinction and interpersonal closeness treatment techniques in chronic schizophrenia: A serendipitous case study comparison. *Psychotherapy: Theory, Research and Practice, 13*, 395–396.

Bornstein, P.H., Bach, P.J., Heider, J.F., & Ernst, J. (1981). Clinical treatment of marital dysfunction: A multiple-baseline analysis. *Behavioral Assessment, 3,* 335–343.

Cook, T.D., & Campbell, D.T. (Eds.). (1979). *Quasi-experimentation: Design and analysis issues for field settings.* Chicago: Rand McNally.

Crowe, M.J., Marks, I.M., Agras, W.S., & Leitenberg, H. (1972). Time-limited desensitization, implosion, and shaping for phobic patients: A cross-over study. *Behavior Research and Therapy, 10*, 319–328.

Davidson, P.O., & Costello, C.G. (1969). N = 1: *Experimental studies of single cases.* New York: Van Nostrand-Reinhold.

Dukes, W.F. (1965). *N* = 1. *Psychological Bulletin, 64,* 74–79.

Ebbinghaus, H. (1886). *Uber das Gedachtnis: Untersachungen Zur experimentelen Psychologie.* Leipzig: Duncher and Humbolt.

Edgington, E.S. (1980). Random assignment and statistical tests for one subject experiments. *Behavioral Assessment, 2,* 19–28.

Foxx, R.M., & Robinoff, A. (1979). Behavioral treatment of caffeinism: Reducing excessive coffee drinking. *Journal of Applied Behavior Analysis, 12*, 335–344.

Glass, G.V., Willson, V.L., & Gottman, J.M. (1975). *Design and analysis of time-series experiments.* Boulder: University of Colorado Press.

Gresham, F.M. (1981). Assessment of children's social skills. *Journal of School Psychology, 19,* 120–133.

Hall, R.V., & Fox, R.G. (1977). Changing-criterion designs: An alternate applied behavior analysis procedure. In C.C. Etzel, J.M. LeBlanc, & D.M. Baer (Eds.), *New developments in behavioral research: Theory, method, and application.* Hillsdale, NJ: Lawrence Erlbaum Associates.

Hartmann, D.P., & Hall, R.V. (1976). A discussion of the changing criterion design. *Journal of Applied Behavioral Analysis, 9*, 527–532.

Hartledge, L.C. (1981). Clinical application of neuropsychological test data: A case study. *School Psychology Review, 10*, 362–366.

Hayes, S.C. (1981). Single case experimental design and empirical clinical practice. *Journal of Consulting and Clinical Psychology, 49,* 193–211.

Hersen, M., & Barlow, D.H. (1976). *Single case experimental designs: Strategies for studying behavior change.* New York: Pergamon Press.

Israelsohn, W.J. (1960). Description and modes of analysis of human growth. In J.M. Tanner (Ed.), *Human growth.* Oxford: Pergamon.

Jacobson, N.S., & Martin, B. (1976). Behavioral marriage therapy: Current status. *Psychological Bulletin, 83,* 540–556.

Jason, L.A., & Liotta, R.F. (1982). Reduction of cigarette smoking in a university cafeteria. *Journal of Applied Behavior Analysis, 15,* 573–577.

Johnson, J., & Pennypacker, H.S. (1980). *Strategies and tactics of human behavioral research.* Hillsdale, NJ: Erlbaum.

Jones, R.R., Weinrott, M.R., & Vaught, R.S. (1978). Effects of serial dependency on the agreement between visual and visual inference. *Journal of Applied Behavior Analysis, 11,* 277–283.

Kazdin, A.E. (1977). Assessing the clinical or applied significance of behavior change through social validation. *Behavior Modification, 1,* 427–452.

Kazdin, A.E. (1980). *Research design in clinical psychology.* New York: Harper & Row.

Kazdin, A.E. (1981). Drawing valid influences from cases studies. *Journal of Consulting and Clinical Psychology, 49,* 183–192.

Kazdin, A.E. (1982). *Single-case research designs: Methods for clinical and applied settings.* New York: Oxford Press.

Kazdin, A.E., & Hartmann, D.P. (1978). The simultaneous-treatment design. *Behavior Therapy, 8,* 682–693.

Kirschner, R.E., Schnelle, J.F., Domash, M., Larson, L., Carr, & McNees, M.P. (1980). The applicability of a helicopter patrol procedure to diverse areas: A cost-benefit evaluation. *Journal of Applied Behavior Analysis, 13,* 143–148.

Kratochwill, T.R. (Ed.) (1978). *Single-subject research: Strategies for evaluating change.* New York: Academic Press.

Kratochwill, T.R. (in press). *Time-series research.* New York: Academic Press.

Kratochwill, T.R., & Mace, F.C. (1983). Time-series research in psychotherapy. In M. Hersen, L. Michelson, & A.S. Bellack (Eds.), *Issues in psychotherapy research.* New York: Plenum.

Kratochwill, T.R., & Piersel, W.C. (1983). Time-series research: Contributions to empirical clinical practice. *Behavioral Assessment, 5,* 165–176.

Leitenberg, H. (1976). Behavioral approaches to treatment of neuroses. In H. Leitenberg (Ed.), *Handbook of behavior modification and behavior therapy.* Englewood Cliffs, NJ: Prentice-Hall.

Levin, J.R., Marascuilo, L.A., & Hubert, L.J. (1978). *N*-nonparametric randomization tests. In T.R. Kratochwill (Ed.), *Single subject research: Strategies for evaluating change.* New York: Academic Press.

Matson, J.L. (1982). The treatment of behavioral characteristics of depression in the mentally retarded. *Behavior Therapy, 13,* 209–218.

McCleary, R., Hay, R.A., Meidinger, E.E., & McDowell, D. (1980). *Applied time-series analysis for the social sciences.* Beverly Hills, CA: Sage.

Morris, R.J., & Kratochwill, T.R. (1983). *Treating children's fears and phobias.* New York: Pergamon.

Olson, D.H. (1976). *Treating relationships.* Lake Mills, IA: Graphic Publishing.
Parsonson, B.D., & Baer, D.M. (1978). The analysis and presentation of graphic data. In T.R. Kratochwill (Ed.), *Single subject research: Strategies for evaluating change.* New York: Academic Press.
Peterson, L., Homer, A.L., & Wonderlich, S.A. (1982). The integrity of independent variables in behavior analysis. *Journal of Applied Behavior Analysis, 15,* 477–492.
Piersel, W.C., & Kratochwill, T.R. (1981). A teacher-implemented contingency management package to assess and treat selective mutism. *Behavioral Assessment, 3,* 371–382.
Revusky, S.H. (1967). Some statistical treatments compatible with individual organism methodology. *Journal of the Experimental Analysis of Behavior, 19,* 319–330.
Roberts, R.N., & Gordon, S.B. (1979). Reducing childhood nightmares subsequent to a burn trauma. *Child Behavior Therapy, 1,* 373–381.
Ross, A.O. (1981). Of rigor and relevance. *Professional Psychology, 12,* 318–327.
Schnelle, J.F., & Lee, J.F. (1974). A quasi-experimental retrospective evaluation of a prison policy change. *Journal of Applied Behavior Analysis, 7,* 484–496.
Stern, R., & Marks, I.M. (1973). Brief and prolonged flooding: A comparison in agoraphobic patients. *Archives of General Psychiatry, 28,* 270–276.
Stokes, R.F., & Baer, D.M. (1977). An implicit technology of generalization. *Journal of Applied Behavior Analysis, 10,* 349–368.
Tanner, J.M. (1962). *Growth at adolescence* (2nd ed.). Oxford: Blackwell Scientific Publications; Philadelphia: Davis.
Tanner, J.M. (1970). Physical growth (3rd ed.). In P.H. Mussen (Ed.), *Carmichael's manual of child psychology.* New York: Wiley.
Wahler, R.G., Sperling, K.A., Thomas, M.R., Teeter, N.C., & Luper, H.L. (1970). The modification of childhood stuttering: Some response-response relationships. *Journal of Experimental Child Psychology, 9,* 411–428.
Wolf, M.M. (1978). Social validity: The case for subjective measurement, or how applied behavior analysis is finding its heart. *Journal of Applied Behavior Analysis, 11,* 203–214.
Wolfe, D.A., St. Lawrence, J., Graves, K., Brehong, K., Bradbyn, D., & Kelly, J.A. (1982). Intensive behavioral parent training for a child abusive mother. *Behavior Therapy, 13,* 438–451.
Woodworth, R.S., & Schlosberg, H. (1954). *Experimental psychology* (rev. ed.). New York: Holt, Rinehart, & Winston.

4

Group Comparison Designs

J. Gayle Beck
Frank Andrasik
John G. Arena

INTRODUCTION

Group comparison research is one of the hallmarks of clinical experimentation. While other experimental approaches (such as single case methodology) exist and play important roles in the science of clinical psychology, between-group designs provide a systematic framework for examining large-scale group differences, no matter whether they are used to explore treatment outcome, psychopathology, personality, or assessment questions. The types of experimental issues that group comparison research is capable of addressing center on probability statements about group differences: Does Treatment A produce sizably greater gains than Treatment B or no treatment in a specified group of patients? Is Group A statistically different on some personality index relative to Group B? Does Group A respond to experimental manipulation in a quantitatively different fashion than Group B? In approaching experimental questions such as these, a researcher employing a group comparison design seeks statistically-significant differences between samples, following the tradition of Fisher (1956, 1967). Ultimately, the hope of such an approach is to discover lawful relationships which follow a predictable pattern across individuals. The role of only one between-subjects (or group comparison) study is to make a small contribution to the broader-scale search for scientific knowledge.

The purpose of this chapter is to provide an overview of group comparison designs. In outlining the more common designs, a number of relevant issues will be discussed. These relate to internal and external validity concerns (see Chapter 2) in constructing and implementing a between-group project, such as selection of subjects and dependent measures. Additionally, topics such as ethics, approaches to data analysis, and interpretation of findings will be discussed briefly, especially as these topics relate to some of the criticisms that have been leveled against group comparison designs (e.g., Hersen & Barlow, 1976; Leitenberg, 1973; Sidman, 1960). The purpose of this review is not to discuss the relative merits of single case versus group designs, as alternative design strategies are discussed elsewhere. Rather, it is intended to provide an overview of the various group designs, including issues central to conducting this type of research.

BETWEEN-GROUP DESIGNS

Principles of Experimentation

"True" experimental designs differ from pre- or quasi-experimental designs (Campbell & Stanley, 1963) by their incorporation of random assignment of subjects to groups, and various control or comparison groups. Randomization can be accomplished in several fashions. The most straightforward involves using any procedure that ensures each subject an equal chance of group assignment. Towards this end, it is common to use a table of random numbers or a coin toss. Unfortunately, this does not necessarily ensure comparable groups, which may create problems for treatment-outcome research and assessment studies exploring the effects of various testing procedures (Campbell & Stanley, 1963). An alternative procedure is to match pairs of subjects on relevant dimensions (e.g., severity of symptoms, socioeconomic status, and age) and then randomly to assign each member of the pair to one of two groups. This approach is termed *randomized blocks assignment* or *stratified block randomization* and is frequently used in research requiring equivalent groups (e.g., treatment outcome studies: Kendall & Wilcox, 1980; experimental analysis of psychopathology: Chapman & Knowles, 1964). A third strategy termed *yoking* can be employed as well, which is a specialized type of randomized block design. In this approach, subjects are paired; one subject receives the experimental manipulation, while the other is exposed to equivalent aspects of this procedure minus one salient dimension. For example, many learned helplessness studies (e.g., Hiroto, 1974; Seligman & Maier, 1967) yoke the experimental subject with the control subject, ensuring the former an equal number of reinforcements minus the critical dimensions of control over reinforcement delivery (for a discussion of potential problems with yoking, see Church, 1964). A fourth approach to random assignment is the use of a *repeated measures design,* where every subject is exposed to each experimental condition in a counterbalanced fashion. Unfortunately, a researcher employing this approach must know in advance that the effects of each manipulation will not carry over into subsequent conditions; if this is not known, a threat to internal validity (i.e., testing) is introduced. Generally, repeated measures designs are recommended when subject recruitment is difficult (e.g., experiments with hard-to-reach populations such as rape victims) or the experimenter has sufficient experience with the manipulations to ensure the lack of carry-over effects. Of course, counterbalancing the order of presentation of experimental conditions can help to control for unknown carry-over effects. Generally, randomization strategies help to control for selection biases: a threat to the internal validity of any design.

A second experimental principle entails the use of control groups. The selection of an appropriate comparison group or control procedure is not as straightforward as randomization procedures and will be detailed in a later section. However, all between-groups designs entail the use of some type of control condition. This rules out potential threats to internal validity, such as history, maturation, and testing. Proper care is necessary to rule out confounding by statistical regression, as will be elaborated below.

These two experimental principles form the backbone of many between-subjects designs. Their existence enables the researcher to test causal hypotheses by controlling some of the factors relevant to internal validity. Other related factors, such as instrumentation, experimental mortality, and selection-maturation interactions are controlled by most true experimental designs, as well.

Specific Designs

This section will outline the different experimental designs that are common in clinical research. A summary of these appears in Table 4.1, along with relevant considerations for their use. The symbolic notation of Campbell and Stanley (1963) is adopted to provide a graphic display of each design. In this system, *O* stands for assessment or measurement process, and *X* indicates the exposure of a group to an experimental variable or event (randomization of subjects to groups is assumed, in light of the preceding discussion). Additionally, the symbol *Y* is used to indicate an attention-control condition and *Z* stands for a placebo control condition.

Pretest-Posttest Control Group Design. In this design, one group is given an experimental treatment with assessment preceding and following this event, while a second group receives only the two assessment occasions. This design is most widely used in treatment-outcome studies. The use of a pretest allows the investigator to rule out alternative explanations for the findings such as history effects, testing, and other threats to internal validity discussed in Chapter 2. An example of the use of this design is provided by Shipley and Fazio (1973). These authors compared a treatment oriented toward problem solving with a waiting-list control condition, employing depressed college students as subjects. Results indicate that this brief intervention strategy was significantly more effective, relative to no treatment, in alleviating self-reported depression.

One of the strengths of this design, aside from the control over threats to internal validity, is the use of a pretest. This observation period allows the investigator to match subjects on important dimensions (e.g., age, severity

Table 4.1. Common Group Comparison Designs

Design	Group		Strengths (+) and Weaknesses (−)
Pretest-posttest control group design	Group A:	$O\ X\ O$	+ adequately controls for threats to internal validity
	Group B:	$O\quad O$	+ pretest scores may be used for additional analyses
			− lack of control for pretest sensitization
Posttest only control group design	Group A:	$X\ O$	+ Adequately controls for threats to internal validity including pretest sensitization
	Group B:	O	− group differences are assumed, but not assessed
Solomon four group	Group A:	$O\ X\ O$	+ adequately controls for threats to internal validity, especially focusing on pretest sensitization
	Group B:	$O\quad O$	+ built-in replication of experimental manipulation
	Group C:	$X\ O$	− requires large number of subjects
	Group D:	O	− failure to control for effects of participating in experimentation
Attention and control group design	Group A:	$O\ X\ O$	+ increased control over effects of experimental participation
	Group B:	$O\quad O$	+ potential for partial replication of experimental manipulation
	Group C:	$X\ O$	+ suitable to clinical settings
	Group D:	O	− failure to control for subject expectancies
	Group E:	$O\ Y\ O$	− possibility of confounds in attention control group
	Group F:	$Y\ O$	− costly design, in its entirety
Placebo and control group design	Group A:	$O\ X\ O$	+ allows for separation of specific and nonspecific effects
	Group B:	$O\quad O$	+ controls for both participation and expectancy
	Group C:	$X\ O$	− placebo involves deception
	Group D:	O	− placebo may deter client from seeking needed treatment
	Group E:	$O\ Z\ O$	− placebo may have short conceptual lifespan
	Group F:	$Z\ O$	− costly design, in its entirety
Factorial design (e.g. 2×2)	Group A:	$O\ X_1\ O$	+ allow for investigation of interactive effects of two or more variables
	Group B:	$O\ X_2\ O$	+ economical in terms of subjects required
	Group C:	$O\ X_3\ O$	+ flexible type of design
	Group D:	$O\ X_4\ O$	− with multiple factors, interpretation can be difficult

Key: O indicates assessment.
X indicates exposure to an experimental manipulation (X_1, X_2, etc. indicate factorial variations in the experimental manipulation).
Y indicates attention control condition.
Z indicates placebo control condition.

of symptoms). This, in turn, can be included as a separate variable in the design, provided the number of subjects is large enough. Additionally, pretest measurement allows the investigator to make more definite statements about changes observed following the experimental manipulation. Without the use of this observation point, the design would yield only statements concerning group differences: a less refined experimental conclusion. Additionally, as pointed out by Kazdin (1980), when used for treatment-outcome research, this design allows the examination of pretest factors that predict dropping out of treatment. This can include a comparison of subjects who dropped versus those who did not, or given a large enough sample, classification and quantification of the various factors which predict attrition.

This design does have several shortcomings. The most notable is the lack of control for pretest sensitization, or the possibility that administration of a pretest "sensitized" the subjects to respond to the experimental manipulation in a specific fashion. This potential confound cannot be assessed with this design and can limit the generalizability of the findings. One solution to this is to separate the pretest and experimental manipulation in time and context. For example, in a treatment study, the pretest could be administered several weeks prior to intervention and in a non-clinical setting (e.g., the client's home, by mail). There are limits to this strategy, however, as the more removed the pretest is from the intervention, the greater the risk of other threats to internal validity, such as history.

Posttest Only Control Group Design. This design is similar to the previous one, minus the administration of a pretest. The posttest only design controls for the possibility of pretest sensitization and adequately addresses all of the possible threats to internal validity. Potential group differences are controlled hypothetically by randomization of subjects in group assignment, although this can never be assured or assessed. This is the major weakness of this design and probably accounts for its infrequent use in clinical research. Additionally, the types of refined analyses discussed above, such as exploration of factors that predict attrition, and blocking subjects by relevant characteristics, cannot be accomplished with a posttest only design. There are situations, however, where this design can be employed; for example, in research on testing procedures (i.e., studies examining the effects of different instructions upon performance), or research exploring the impact of social processes, such as persuasion, upon volunteering.

Solomon Four Group Design. As shown in Table 1, this design is a composite of the two designs discussed previously and is intended to examine the effects of pretesting upon the results of an experimental manipulation (Solomon, 1949). Four groups are included; only two receive pretesting (as in the pretest-posttest design). The other two groups resemble the posttest only design. As an example of the use of this design is provided by Mungas and Walters (1979). These investigators evaluated pretesting effects of self-report measures of assertion and a structured role-play task on the evaluation of social skills training with college students. The results indicate that both types of measures (self-report and role-play) showed significant pretest effects through treatment interactions, suggesting that pretest sensitization is an important confound with these outcome measures. As in this example, the design enables the researcher to explore interactions between testing and experimental manipulations. Additionally, a built-in replication of the manipulation is included, in the absence of assessment sensitization. Specifically, the two groups that receive the active manipulation can be compared, and pretest-posttest differences within each group explored. Overall, this design provides a strong method of examining the effect of any manipulation, addressing threats to internal validity. It also provides a controlled exploration of pretest sensitization effects and the potential for replication within a single study. However, the design's major drawback is the cost involved: Twice the number of subjects are required for use of the Solomon four group design, thus doubling the research effort required. While the role of pretest sensitization is generally not widely known in clinical research, reactive effects from a variety of assessment procedures have been well-documented. These include self-monitoring (e.g., Bellack, Rozensky, & Schwartz, 1974; Maletzky, 1974; Nelson, Lipinski, & Black, 1975), questionnaires (e.g., Kiecolt & McGrath, 1979; Rock, 1981), and structured assessments such as role-plays, behavior avoidance tests, and structured interactions between clients (e.g., Bernstein & Nietzel, 1974; Johnson & Brown, 1969). This suggests a need for increased use of Solomon four group designs in clinical research, albeit in a carefully chosen fashion. Additionally, this design does not control for the effects of participating in experimentation, a confound which is especially salient for treatment outcome studies.

Attention and Control Group Design. This design is employed primarily in treatment outcome research and is intended to control for the effects of contact with psychological services. Six experimental groups are included, encompassing the four groups in the Solomon design, plus two additional conditions; in one of these, subjects receive preassessment, followed by some form of contact or attention intended to control for experimental participation, and postassessment. The second group is identical, minus the preassessment observation point. A variety of attention controls have emerged in the literature. Perhaps the most common is the waiting-list control procedure, where prospective clients are told that treatment is not available to them at that point in time, but will be in a number of weeks. Following the completion of the wait-list interval, subjects are generally offered treatment. This strategy has several advantages over a no-treatment attention control (simply offering assessment), as waiting lists are not uncommon in clinical settings and clients are motivated to complete the postassessment by the prospect of treatment. Also, inclusion of a second treatment group, after the formal end of the project, provides an opportunity for partial replication of any treatment effects observed. Unfortunately, attrition from the waiting list can be problematic; this can occur in an obvious fashion (e.g., failure to return for postassessment) or in more subtle ways. For example, Frank (1973) reports that 50% of a group seeking psychotherapy had also sought help from nonprofessional sources (e.g., clergy, friends). Researchers using this attention control procedure need to be aware of such subtle confounds, especially in light of broader therapy outcome issues (e.g., spontaneous remission of symptomology: Bergin & Lambert, 1978).

One of the major strengths of this design comes from the increased experimental control over contact with psychological services. This concern is especially relevant as several reports have shown that wait-list control subjects often feel helped by a single assessment contact (e.g., Malan, Heath, Bacal, & Balfour, 1975; Sloane, Staples, Cristol, Yorkston, & Whipple, 1975). However, as pointed out by Mahoney (1978), this design does not control for subjects' expectancies concerning the experimental project and perceived demands of the situation (Orne, 1962). These effects can be pervasive, especially in treatment outcome evaluations. It is rare to see this design employed in its entirety. Rather, the clinical literature reveals several partial forms of the design to be particularly popular and useful. An example of the use of this design is provided by Blanchard, Theobald, Williamson, Silver, and Brown (1978). This study employed a waiting list control as a comparison for two treatment groups in examining relaxation and biofeedback training for migraineurs. Initial analyses showed both treatments to be superior to no treatment, but the two treatments did not differ. Six of 10 control subjects opted for treatment once the waiting list interval was over, which permitted a replication of the initial findings. It is not mentioned whether any of the wait-list subjects pursued treatment elsewhere in the interim, nor whether this may have accounted in part for the disinterest of four subjects to be treated.

Placebo and Control Group Design. This design is similar to the one previously described, except that a placebo control group is employed in place of a control for experimental attention alone. The use of a placebo control group allows the investigator to examine the specific effects of treatment above and beyond "nonspecific" effects (Paul, 1967). The latter include clients' expectancies for change, contact with and attention from a therapist, clients' responses to perceived experimental/therapeutic demand, and the provision of a therapeutic rationale. While cumulative research findings are mixed concerning the exact role of these "nonspecific" factors in producing behavior change (Kazdin & Wilcoxon, 1976; Shapiro & Morris, 1978; Wilkins, 1977), placebos have been shown to affect behavior, sometimes in a robust fashion (e.g., Bootzin, Herman, & Nicassio, 1976; Frank, 1961, 1968). Thus, this design is necessary in order to make an empirical statement about the specific effects of any given intervention.

O'Leary and Borkovec (1978) raise a number of critical issues involved in the use of placebo groups, with special reference to treatment research. From an ethical perspective, placebo groups are inherently deceptive, providing clients with a therapeutically inert experience (at least theoretically so) under the guise of a potentially helpful treatment. Additionally, use of a placebo control may deter the client from seeking help elsewhere, an especially salient problem in conducting research with severely distressed individuals. These clients may be impelled to consent to an experimental placebo, in light of their pressing need for intervention. In the long run, such an experience may diminish a client's expectancy for change and possibly create deterioration in functioning, both clinically undesirable outcomes. Methodologically, it is difficult to ensure that the therapists who are delivering the placebo are instilling the same degree of positive expectancy for change in their clients, a factor that creates a subtle confound as therapist expectancies can exert a powerful effect on clinical outcome (Wilkins, 1977). Additionally, placebos tend to have a short conceptual lifespan (O'Leary & Borkovec, 1978); if an "effective" placebo is discovered, active research is often begun to determine its relevant effects. Thus, what originally was construed as a placebo may be reconceptualized as desire to please the therapist or an instructional set. O'Leary and Borkovec recommend the conservative use of attention placebos, contingent upon the severity of the problem involved, length of the proposed placebo, and knowledge about the natural course of the specific disorder. These recommendations appear warranted, in light of the issues highlighted above.

An example of the use of a placebo control is provided by Paul (1966); in this oft-cited work, systematic desensitization was compared with brief insight therapy in treating speech anxious students. A placebo group was employed as one of the control conditions, where clients were given a complex procedure and a carefully detailed rationale concerning seemingly relevant factors maintaining their anxiety. Results indicate that the placebo control group showed gains equivalent to the sample receiving insight therapy, an effect that was maintained at 2-year follow-up. This study highlights an important aspect of placebos; given the strong results provided by Paul's procedure, it would appear that the rationale and methods involved generated adequate client expectancies for success. And, it was a credible manipulation. Both of these factors are important to control in the use of placebos, especially as a weak, uncredible placebo does little towards examining the specific effects of the active intervention. These dimensions need to be assessed when using a placebo-control, a task that can be accomplished with questionnaires such as Borkovec and Nau's (1972), or by having subjects simulate the perceived effects of the placebo treatment (e.g., Lick & Bootzin, 1970).

Wilkins (1979) argues that researchers need "to get specific" when designing tests of "nonspecific" effects, as the latter term is devoid of a conceptual or operational base. He advocates that researchers identify possible factors or procedures which may influence therapy outcome (in addition to those hypothesized as critical or specific to an approach) and study them accordingly. Andrasik and Holroyd (1980) illustrate one way to "pin-down" nonspecific effects within the confines of biofeedback treatment for tension headache. Four groups were compared: no-treatment control; standard, clinical biofeedback; and two biofeedback control procedures. Elements basic to all types of treatment, but not specific to this particular treatment, were identified and operationalized so that they could be included in the biofeedback control procedures. These consisted of:

(a) headache monitoring,
(b) muscle contraction explanation of headache,
(c) a treatment rationale stressing the application of biofeedback,
(d) specific suggestions and demands for improvement,
(e) verbal reinforcement for improvement (for both biofeedback task and headache improvement), [and]
(f) progressively shaped feedback to ensure sucess at learning the biofeedback task. (Andrasik & Holroyd, 1980, p. 57)

Credibility questionnaires were administered periodically to test for comparability of groups along the preceding dimensions. The only difference between the clinical biofeedback and biofeedback control procedures was the direction of learning of control of muscle tension. Results indicated that the hypothesized key ingredient of EMG (electromyographic) biofeedback had little to do with outcome, as all three biofeedback procedures led to similar outcomes. These findings were replicated in a 3-year follow-up investigation (Andrasik & Holroyd, 1983).

O'Leary and Borkovec (1978) have suggested a number of alternatives to placebo controls. These will be discussed in a later section, but are important variations on the central concern addressed by this design. As with the attention and control group design, it is rare to see the placebo and control group strategy used in its entirety (as outlined in Table 1). This most likely is due to the substantial increase in subjects and procedural effort involved.

Factorial Designs. Unlike the previous designs, factorials allow the investigation of two or more factors in a single experiment. In its simplest form, a factorial design would consist of two levels of two separate variables (see Table 4.1). For example, in a psychopathology study on depression, an examination of experiment-delivered outcomes (negative and positive) and social situations (home and work) would be explored in interaction to determine possible effects on depressed affect and negative thoughts, following the clinical observations of Beck, Lewinsohn, and others (Beck, 1972; Lewinsohn, 1975; Rehm, 1977). This design is portrayed in Figure 4.1.

Factorial designs can consist of multiple levels of several variables in their expanded use, and are best viewed as a research approach, rather than a specific design. Given that one of the strengths of this approach is the inclusion of interaction effects between two or more relevant factors, this type of design probably is best employed following careful examinations of each factor in isolation. In other words, the use of complex factorials is not recommended for preliminary empirical examinations.

Beck, Barlow, and Sakheim (1983) provide an example of a $2 \times 3 \times 2$ factorial design in investigating the effects of focus of attention and perceived partner arousal on sexual responding. Two subject groups were sampled: sexually functional men and men with chronic erectile difficulties. Thus, the design consisted of two levels of attentional focus (self versus partner focus), three levels of partner arousal (high, low, and ambiguous), and two levels of the grouping factor (functional and dysfunctional men). Results indicate that the two experimental factors affected responding in a complex fashion; for example, men with sexual problems showed higher arousal during ambiguous partner arousal when focusing upon the partner, while functional men showed more arousal when attending to their own responses in this condition. This example demonstrates use of a repeated measures approach, as discussed earlier, in a factorial design, as all subjects received the six experimental conditions.

One of the strengths of factorial designs is the opportunity to examine the combined effects of the independent variables. This is especially important, as interactions between factors help to provide a more refined analysis of the phenomena under study. Additionally, factorial designs allow greater econ-

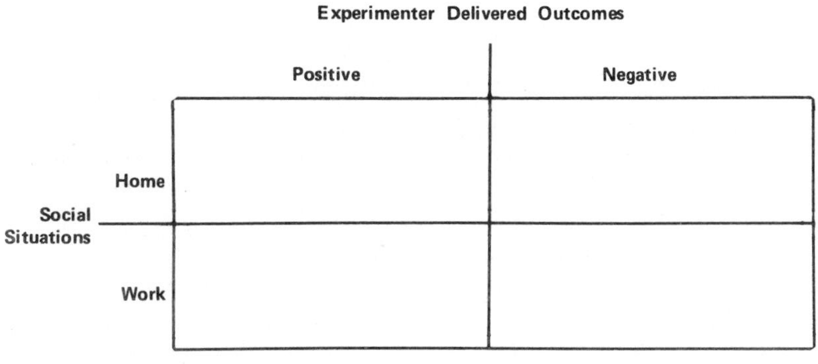

		Experimenter Delivered Outcomes	
		Positive	Negative
Social Situations	Home		
	Work		

FIG. 4.1. A hypothetical 2×2 factorial design

omy, as fewer subjects are required, relative to a series of individual studies exploring each variable in isolation. A number of variations in this design are available. For example, one of the randomization strategies discussed earlier can be combined with a factorial. Subjects can be grouped on some dimension (e.g., grade point average, scores on a pretest measure), and these groups or blocks are then assigned to various experimental conditions (one block in each group per condition). This variation, known as a randomized block or stratified design, as discussed earlier, provides one method of examining subject classification by treatment interactions, and exemplifies a variation on the usual factorial design. More detailed descriptions of this and other refinements in the factorial design are available in Keppel (1973) and Kirk (1968).

There are several limiting characteristics of factorial designs as well. In creating a study with this approach, the researcher can easily be tempted to build in too many factors. This quickly can lead to a mammoth project, requiring more subjects than are available to adequately fill each cell of the factorial. For example, with a four variable factorial design, where each variable has three levels ($3 \times 3 \times 3 \times 3$ design), if the investigator desired 10 subjects for each experimental cell, a total of 810 subjects would be required to complete the project. Additionally, it becomes exceedingly difficult to interpret complex interactions when multiple factors are involved. From a standpoint of exploring clinical phenomena, the hypothetical example outlined above provides an extreme example of "losing the phenomena" amidst an elegant experimental design. It becomes difficult to assess clinically meaningful patterns in individual clients when faced with such a quantity of data. This is related to a separate issue, clinical versus statistical significance, which will be discussed later.

General Considerations and Decision Rules

Each of the designs outlined above has both strengths and limitations. In approaching the prospect of conducting a group comparison study, the researcher needs to weigh these options. Certain designs are best suited for specific types of experimental questions, a situation that can guide the choice of a specific design. A decision tree is provided in Figure 4.2, detailing some of these considerations. While not exhaustive, the successive questions posed in Figure 4.2 help to determine which of the available research strategies may be most appropriate. Other considerations, such as availability of subjects, may be relevant factors in the choice of a design as well.

The above is intended to provide a review of available group designs. Many variations on these designs are possible, of course. For example, it is not unusual to see the attention and placebo designs employed with only three

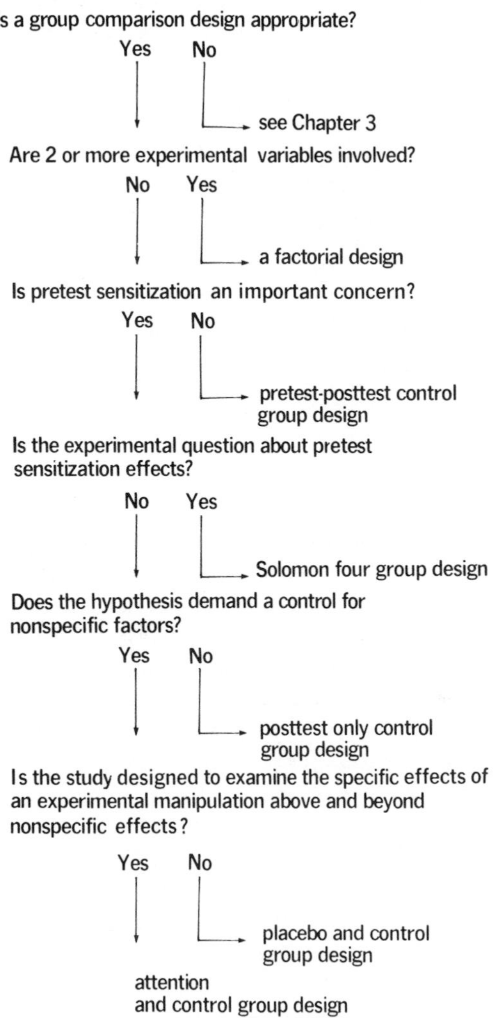
Is a group comparison design appropriate?
Yes No
see Chapter 3
Are 2 or more experimental variables involved?
No Yes
a factorial design
Is pretest sensitization an important concern?
Yes No
pretest-posttest control group design
Is the experimental question about pretest sensitization effects?
No Yes
Solomon four group design
Does the hypothesis demand a control for nonspecific factors?
Yes No
posttest only control group design
Is the study designed to examine the specific effects of an experimental manipulation above and beyond nonspecific effects?
Yes No
placebo and control group design
attention and control group design

FIG. 4.2. A decision tree for choosing among the available group comparison designs

groups: the experimental group, a condition that receives only pre- and post-assessment, and the attention or placebo conditions. In other words, the cells that were designed to assess pretest sensitization effects are commonly dropped from the design. The cost of this omission is the unknown effects of many of our assessment devices upon results obtained with experimental manipulations. However, flexibility is available in the use of these basic experimental designs.

RELATED CONCERNS IN EMPLOYING A GROUP COMPARISON DESIGN

After choosing a design, the investigator is confronted with a number of other research issues. These can be grouped into the following categories: methodological issues, including the selection of subjects, choice of control procedures, assessment strategies (operationalization of the independent variables); implementation concerns, such as ethical considerations and procedural reliability; data analysis, covering topics such as statistical control procedures and the multifaceted meaning of "significance"; and interpretation of findings. Each of these areas can influence the outcome of a research project, affecting the pattern of the results, the generality of the findings, and/or the implications of the data for future studies.

Methodological Issues

Subject Selection. Subject selection is one dimension of group research that establishes the degree of external and ecological validity. The characteristics of the individuals under study (including both demographic factors and diagnostic variables), manner of recruitment, selection and formation of groups, and motivation of subjects are all important concerns. A central issue in this regard is whether to employ "analogue" or "clinical" samples; more specifically, whether to test hypotheses with a sample of individuals who are not seeking psychological services and are recruited from a college campus or community survey (a non-clinical or analogue sample), or to employ a sample of individuals presenting for therapy obtained in a clinical setting. While the topics of analogue and clinical research are of larger scope, involving a variety of other dimensions such as choice of experimental setting, type of manipulation, etc. (e.g., Bernstein & Paul, 1971; Borkovec & O'Brien, 1976; Cooper, Furst, & Bridger, 1969; Kazdin, 1978, 1980; Levis, 1970), the dimension of interest for this discussion is subject characteristics. At one end of the continuum, college students can be employed for an analogue between-group study. These individuals are usually younger, better educated, of different socioeconomic status, and do not have psychiatric diagnoses, relative to a typical sample of clients presenting for outpatient care. Depending upon the experimental question, these differences may not be important. For example, if the investigator wishes to explore the effects of providing written instructions on subsequent test performance, it is probably most cost-efficient to employ a non-clinical sample. However, for therapy outcome questions, explorations of psychopathological processes, empirical examinations of various personality constructs, etc., the type of sample becomes a more salient aspect of the research. A good example of this is provided by Mathews (1978) in a review of recent research on behavioral fear-reduction techniques. Unlike earlier reviews, Mathews examined studies conducted with analogue and clinical populations separately, revealing important differences in responses to treatment between these two groups. Andrasik, Pallmeyer, Blanchard, and Attanasio (1983) report parallel findings in the headache literature, showing that clinic patients responded differently than college student volunteers when presented with the same biofeedback training schedules. Thus, while the analogue clinical distinction may be best regarded as a continuum (Kazdin, 1978), it would appear necessary to employ subjects drawn from clinical populations for the study of questions relating to therapy and psychopathology.

The selection of subjects should be accompanied by careful inclusion and exclusion criteria. If a clinical sample is used, this often involves psychiatric diagnoses. A number of diagnostic schemes exist (e.g., The Research Diagnostic Criteria: Spitzer, Endicott, & Robins, 1978; the third edition of the *Diagnostic and Statistical Manual* of the American Psychiatric Association [DSM III], 1980; the Feighner criteria: Feighner, Robins, Guze, Woodruff, Winokur, & Muñoz, 1972), which may be employed. While these possess some degree of overlap (e.g., Helzer, Brockington, & Kendell, 1981), use of any given diagnostic system is likely to result in a sample with characteristics specific to that system. This becomes important in making cross-study comparisons, as slightly varied samples may respond differently to experimental manipulations. While current diagnostic practices are more specific and symptom-oriented than their predecessors, there remain many problems in clinical diagnosis. As discussed by Garfield (1978), issues such as choice of adequate control groups, base rates, and lack of cross-validation continue to remain salient in this area. Thus, it is important for an investigator to rely upon more than psychiatric diagnosis in selecting a sample. A related concern is diagnostic reliability. While DSM-III represents a notable achievement in improved reliability (Spitzer, Williams, & Skodol, 1980), some of the newer diagnoses in this system do not possess high interrater reliability (e.g., somatoform disorders, personality disorders). Thus, if the experimental question concerns one of these diagnostic classes, the investigator needs to provide additional inclusion and exclusion criteria. The final research report should contain a careful description of the subjects, including details of the selection criteria and formal screening measures that were used.

Every research area has its own relevant subject characteristics that need to be considered in sampling. Copeland (1981), for example, has reviewed a number of these considerations for research on cognitive self-instructional programs for children. Relevant dimensions include age, cognitive ability, and attributional style. Other areas have different concerns. Experimental studies of male sexual dysfunction require examinations of potential organic factors such as diabetes and medication effects as exclusion criteria (Slag, Morley, Elson, Trence, Nelson, Nelson, Kinlaw, Beyer, Nuttall, & Shafer, 1983), while duration and severity of the problem are relevant inclusion criteria in light of population base rates (Frank, Anderson, & Rubinstein, 1978). Without highlighting every current research topic, it is important to note that careful selection criteria help to rule out alternative explanations for findings, as well as providing homogeneous groups, a critical element for replication.

While not directly related to subject characteristics, the researcher needs to consider how large a sample is required for the proposed project. In every research area, informal rules exist concerning adequate *N*s. These vary depending upon whether clinical subjects are required, the difficulty in reaching potential participants, amount of time needed to run a subject through the procedure, and type of dependent measures employed. Beyond informal guidelines, a statistical procedure known as a power analysis can be conducted. This determines the projected sample size required for statistically significant differences, in light of effect size and error variance (see Cohen, 1977, for details). A power analysis can tell the investigator exactly how many subjects are needed to obtain an experimental effect, provided close estimates of both types of variance are available. A careful balance needs to be struck, however, between finding statistically significant results and exploring clinically meaningful phenomena. With a large enough sample, very small group differences may achieve statistical significance, but this has little meaning for understanding clinical processes.

Another concern in subject selection is the manner of recruitment. Potential subjects can be solicited from media advertisements, drawn from outpatient and mental health clinics, or attracted to a specialized research clinic. Each of these recruitment strategies is likely to result in slightly different sample characteristics, differing on dimensions such as socioeconomic and educational status, demographic variables, and severity of presenting problems. Some reports of solicited versus unsolicited samples (e.g., Sallis, Lichstein, & McGlynn, 1980) have shown differences between these two, while others (e.g., Hersen, Bellack, & Himmelhoch, 1981) have not. Without considerably more data on the dimensions of difference of samples drawn with different recruitment strategies, it is difficult to establish the extent to which any given results can be generalized. Crucial factors, such as subject motivation, may exert profound effects upon the outcome of any study, especially treatment outcome research. Depending upon the experimental question involved, the issue of recruitment strategy may be especially salient for group comparison research.

A related issue in selection of subjects involves multiple treatment interference, a threat to external validity. This refers to a subject's prior exposure to experimental manipulations or treatments. An example can clarify this point. Chambless, Foa, Groves, and Goldstein (1982) conducted an examination of the efficacy of exposure and communications training in treating agoraphobic clients. While this design was fairly complex, one group received eight sessions of flooding, followed by 4 months of weekly psychotherapy. It is impossible to make a statement about the effects of psychotherapy on agoraphobia, from this report, given that this treatment was preceded by another therapeutic approach. With reference to subject selection, any potential subject who has previously participated in experimentation can confound the results of a study. This influence can be pervasive. For example, Brody (discussed in Reppucci & Clingempeel, 1978) attempted to manipulate the choice of delayed and immediate reward, employing an institutionalized delinquent sample. Unlike previous work, these findings revealed that subjects consistently chose delayed reward. In interviewing the subjects after completion of the investigation, Brody discovered that similar experimentation had been conducted recently in the institution, a factor to which he attributed his results. Most likely, past experience with experimentation influences a subject's participation to the extent that the present investigation resembles past exposure. In treatment outcome research, it is exceedingly difficult to locate a clinical sample that has not sought professional help previously. One solution to this potential confound, given its unavoidable nature, is to assess the extent and duration of prior therapies, possibly employing these characteristics as statistical covariates, an analytical procedure discussed below. Ultimately, the issue of multiple treatment interference needs to be addressed, in one fashion or another, in subject selection.

Depending on the type of study, a comparison or control group may be needed. There is an especially popular type of design, termed *contrasted groups*, for research in experimental psychopathology. In the selection of a comparison group, the first question confronting an investigator is whether to choose a group of normal (nondiagnosable) subjects or to contrast the group of interest with subjects bearing different psychiatric diagnoses. This choice is mandated by the experimental question. Preliminary studies may address whether the pathological group differs from normal controls on some dimension. Once this question has been given an affirmative answer, the research focus may shift to whether the observed differences are a function of specific pathological processes or are characteristic of general psychological impairment. The latter question then requires the use of subjects from different diagnostic categories. This type of study is "quasi-experimental," owing to the fact that other subject characteristics may be confounded with diagnostic groupings. For example, Chapman and Chapman (1977), in exploring a failure to replicate the results of a study on schizophrenic cognition, discuss the role of confounding factors such as degree of chronicity, severity of symptomology, and whether subjects are maintained on phenothiazines. A potential solution to this type of problem is to match individual clinical and control subjects on relevant dimensions. However, as discussed by Huesmann (1982), matching often introduces additional methodological problems. The use of a contrasted groups approach requires considerable skill and expertise on the part of the researcher, as many potential confounds can cloud the results of this type of study. Without knowledge of these confounds, the researcher can easily draw false conclusions from the data.

Another related subject selection strategy deserves mention; it is not unusual to see extreme groups selected from a given population, based on a pretest measure. These groups are then exposed to the same experimental manipulations. One of the dangers of this approach is regression to the mean, a statistical phenomenon that affects extreme scores and indicates error in measurement. Essentially, upon retesting, scores are likely to revert towards their group mean; this is especially true of extreme scores. Thus, selection of extreme groups may result in pre- to post-assessment differences, although this finding represents an interaction of treatment and statistical regression effects. Similarly, when matching subjects from two different populations, regression can affect the results if the two population means are different. A subject from the upper quartile of one population may be matched with one from the lower quartile of the second, resulting in significant posttest differences that are confounded by regression effects. While selection of extreme scores is commonly employed, it can create methodological problems for interpreting a group comparison design.

Selection and Specification of Independent Variables. Selecting and operationally defining independent variables is another important methodological concern for between-group research. Regardless of the nature of the experimental question, it is important that experimental variables first be clearly conceptualized and then precisely operationalized. Beyond this basic tenet, the specific concerns involved depend upon the type of research question. Two areas, experimental psychopathology and treatment outcome research, will be highlighted here as examples of relevant experimental topics.

Within the vast experimental psychopathology literature, a number of approaches to operationalizing independent variables have been used. One popular approach is to induce variations of the pathological state through physiological or environmental manipulations. For example, subjects can be asked to ingest alcohol, food, or nicotine, and subsequent effects on their behavior can be observed. A typical example of this type of research is a series of studies exploring the effects of alcohol upon sexual arousal (e.g., Briddell & Wilson, 1976; Lansky & Wilson, 1981; Wilson & Lawson, 1976, 1978). The control of subject expectancies has been particularly important in this line of investigation. For example, Wilson and Lawson (1976) manipulated subjects' expectancies of alcohol intake and actual alcohol consumption in a 2×2 factorial design. These data reveal that the expectation of having consumed alcohol produced significantly greater effects on sexual arousal, irrespective of blood alcohol levels. This is a good example of experimental control through the use of a factorial design and highlights the importance of incorporating carefully designed placebos. In this study, and others like it, drinks are flavored so that alcohol cannot be noticed by subjects, and elaborate procedures such as a medical assessment of presumed blood alcohol levels are used to build expectancies. Of course, careful posttest questioning is required to ensure the veracity of these manipulations. A related concern in operationalizing variables with physiological procedures is to ensure equivalent doses across subjects. Factors such as size, body weight, and metabolic rate appear relevant. Ideally, all subjects should receive equivalent amounts of the physiological substance, a dimension that can only be determined through precise biological assessment. An alternative solution is to use several dose levels and a subject sample that is homogeneous on relevant physical dimensions.

Environmental manipulations can be employed as well. This approach calls for exposing subjects to specific induction procedures designed to create analogues of the pathological process under investigation. A prototype of this type of work is seen in the learned helplessness literature (e.g., Hiroto, 1974). In this paradigm, a subject is placed in a situation where reinforcements are independent of his or her responding. Subsequent effects upon behavior, affect, motivation, and cognition are then observed, which seemingly mirror the impairments seen in clinical depression. An obvious concern is the degree of generalizability between the analogue manipulation and the clinical phenomena. Exposing normal volunteers to noncontingent reinforcement may have qualitatively different effects from relevant depressive processes. As discussed by Huesmann (1982), the similarity of analogue states to clinical phenomena does not firmly establish the analogue. However, this type of research does play a valuable role in experimental psychopathology, as it allows for true experimental control in the study of pathology. This type of study can then be augmented by other lines of evidence, to extend the generalizability of the results. Berkowitz and Donnerstein (1982) argue that the critical dimension for this type of study is the degree of *ecological validity*, which is not necessarily synonymous with external validity. According to these authors, the meaning that subjects attribute to experimental manipulations and the responses which they give determine in large part the extent to which parallels can be made between the laboratory and "real life." Granting the artificiality of the laboratory, the experimenter should strive for "experimental realism," attempting to explore empirical relationships which might otherwise be obscured by myriad social processes outside of the laboratory. This requires careful assessment of subjects' attributions about the experimental manipulations, and a willingness on the part of the investigator to consider more naturalistic data in reaching final conclusions.

Treatment outcome research poses a different set of issues in selecting and operationalizing independent variables. Implementation of a treatment study involves decisions about selection of therapists and administration of the intervention at its maximum strength. As Yeaton and Sechrest (1981) point out, however, the definition of "strong" psychotherapy is fuzzy, unlike its medical counterpart. These authors attempt to clarify the dimension of treatment strength, speculating that factors such as the length of intervention, adequacy of the theoretical rationale, existence of a detailed treatment protocol, and adequacy of therapist training are all involved. Ultimately, determining the strength of a given treatment will depend upon future conceptual advances. However, the odds of providing full-strength treatment are considerably higher with well-trained therapists. While the degree of therapist experience seemingly appears relevant, data on this issue are inconclusive (Parloff, Waskow, & Wolfe, 1978). Most likely, providing detailed treatment manuals and extensive training can assure therapist equality across clients and/or conditions, and can outweigh the nebulous effects of experience.

Therapist bias is a related concern; like most investigators, therapists often have investments in the outcome of therapy, sometimes favoring one approach over another. This type of confound can alter empirical results and has several possible solutions. If the investigator is interested in testing the strongest form of the treatment, expert therapists with open bias towards a particular approach can be employed. These individuals would then be nested within treatment conditions (or assigned to a single condition). DiLoreto (1971) provides an example of this approach, in his comparison of systematic desensitization, rational emotive therapy, and client-centered therapy. Therapists were chosen with strong commitments to one of these schools and only delivered that type of treatment. To use a nesting strategy, however, multiple therapists ideally should be employed for each treatment condition to minimize the effects of an aberrant therapist. A second approach to controlling for therapist bias is to cross therapists with conditions (i.e., each therapist sees equal numbers of clients in each condition). Paul (1966) used such an approach in comparing systematic desensitization with insight-oriented therapy. Crossing therapists potentially controls for a variety of nonspecific factors, such as interpersonal style and appearance. As discussed by Heimberg and Becker (in press), potential problems with crossing therapists include situations where specialized training is required (e.g., psychotherapy-drug comparisons) and inclusion of therapists with strong theoretical biases. The approach chosen ultimately depends upon availability of therapist, degree of theoretical bias, and whether the experimental question involves a "strong" test of two or more interventions.

A second methodological issue pertains to treatment administration. Relevant concerns include the duration of treatment, adherence of therapists to the treatment protocol, credibility of the therapeutic rationale(s) if two or more treatments are compared, and equation of important treatment parameters. In studies comparing one intervention to an attention or placebo control condition, the duration of the experimental conditions becomes important. As noted earlier, waiting-list control subjects may tend to seek treatment elsewhere, a possibility which increases the longer the wait-list interval. Similarly, the credibility of a placebo control may diminish over time, diluting the experimental control over expectancies achieved with this approach. These considerations need to be balanced against providing active intervention of sufficient length to produce gains. Determining duration will depend on the specific intervention under examination; for example, if one wished to examine Masters and Johnson's sex therapy (Masters & Johnson, 1970), a continuous 2-week interval would be required. The control group in this hypothetical examination would need to be equated on a host of other dimensions, however (e.g., day-long treatment sessions held in St. Louis with two therapists at a nationally renowned institute).

Adherence of therapists to treatment protocols ensures the veracity of the experimental manipulation. Ideally, this should not be assumed, but rather, periodic assessments of actual therapy sessions are needed. Adherence may change over time. DiLoreto (1971), for example, found that early sessions closely matched treatment protocols while some of the therapists deviated from treatment outlines in later sessions. A strategy could be used like that employed in behavioral assessment, wherein observers are provided with periodic spot-checks and feedback about their performance (Curran, Beck, Corriveau, & Monti, 1980; Johnson & Bolstad, 1973). This approach would provide both an assessment of adherence, as well as reducing therapist discrepancies from protocol. In assessing the content of treatment, audiotapes or unobtrusive observers could be employed, rather than therapist ratings, to guard against reporting bias.

The credibility of treatment rationales is another important dimension for operationalizing treatment manipulations. This concern has been discussed in the context of placebo control groups and is relevant to active therapy conditions as well. The provision of a credible rationale and generation of positive client expectancies need to be assessed in order to make definitive statements about the specificity of treatment effects. The importance of this cannot be overstated. For example, the efficacy of systematic desensitization, one of the more established behavioral techniques, has been established only against control conditions with less credibility (Kazdin & Wilcoxon, 1976). As discussed by Heimberg and Becker (in press), this issue is not a large concern when outcome is the main experimental focus. When questions of the processes by which interventions work are asked, this issue is paramount.

Studies that compare two or more treatment approaches have additional concerns in operationally defining the experimental manipulations. Treatments should be equated on dimensions such as length of intervention, spacing of sessions, and credibility. While this sounds repetitious, achieving this type of experimental control in practice can be difficult. For example, certain therapeutic approaches may require a longer time frame to reach equivalent levels of strength, relative to others. Similarly, some interventions may require spacing of sessions to allow for practice in the natural environment (e.g., relaxation training), whereas others conceptually call for intensive exposure to the therapeutic situation (e.g., insight-oriented therapy). To compare only two types of treatment, the requirements of each approach (both conceptual and technical) need to be considered in specifying treatment parameters and salient aspects need to be matched across interventions.

Selection of Experimental Control Strategy. Two of the designs outlined earlier call for specific control procedures and relevant concerns for their implementation have been raised. Given the existence of conceptual and methodological problems with placebo control strategies (O'Leary & Borkovec, 1978), the investigator needs to consider whether alternative research strategies might serve as well. O'Leary and Borkovec have outlined a number of alternatives to placebos. None of these strategies controls for therapist attention, however. The first alternative design controls for subject expectancy and therapist demand by providing counterdemand instructions. In this approach, the therapist advises clients not to expect positive gains until some specified amount of time has passed (e.g., after five treatment sessions). This within-subject control procedure may be contrasted with a second group that receives positive demand instructions during this interval. In using this design, the researcher needs to assess client expectancies closely to ensure that this brief control procedure is operative. This type of manipulation has been employed in research on sleep disturbance, effectively controlling for demand, suggestion, and expectancy effects (e.g., Borkovec, Kaloupek, & Slama, 1975). Potential problems with this approach include: (1) necessary knowledge of the time course of a given intervention, for the counterdemand instruction will lose its effectiveness if extended beyond the time when intervention actually begins to produce significant gains, and (2) similarly, a relatively short interval must be chosen and careful documentation of expectancies is needed, a methodological task that requires procedural attention.

Another alternative control procedure is the component control strategy proposed by Stuart (1973). This can involve the administration of one aspect of an intervention (e.g., instructions on problem solving for comparison with complete behavioral marital therapy, involving problem solving, communications training, and practice) or the administration of treatment components in theoretically inert combinations (e.g., imaginal exposure followed by relaxation, as a control for systematic desensitization). All clients can be provided with the same treatment rationale, providing increased experimental control. Assessment of client expectancies is needed to ensure equivalence across groups. One of the strengths of this approach is the potential to address theoretical questions as well to provide experimental control over nonspecific factors.

A third alternative to placebo controls is the use of the best-available treatment as a comparison group. This approach seems most fitting when introducing a new treatment procedure and when questions of efficiency as well as efficacy are involved. Both treatments need to be equated for duration, client expectancies, therapeutic demand, and other related factors. But this is not an easy task. Additionally, the question of whether to use crossed or nested therapists is important, as discussed earlier. The advantages of this approach are that it avoids the ethical and methodological problems involved in providing an "inert" placebo. However, equation of client expectancies can be a problem for this design. In selecting the best available treatment for use in this design, the researcher needs to consider what constitutes a fair comparison. Selection of a treatment that targets a completely separate aspect of functioning is likely to result in findings which tell us little about the specific effects of the experimental treatment. For example, within the literature on treatment of depression, several comparisons of drugs versus psychotherapy have been conducted. The predominant findings reveal that drugs affect symptomatology while psychotherapy has more profound effects on social functioning (cf. Weissman, 1979). While this is valuable information, if these were the only empirical examinations of the treatments, little could be said about their specific operation apart from nonspecific effects. (Fortunately, a number of other studies have been conducted in this literature using placebo and waiting list controls.) From the standpoint of choosing the "best available" treatment, this points to the need for careful definition of the experimental question as a conceptual guide for determining a fair "best available" treatment comparison.

A final alternative to placebo controls is the use of a neutral expectancy condition. Within the context of the traditional attention and control group design, Borkovec (1973) has proposed providing half of the clients in both groups with positive expectancy statements concerning the procedure, while the remaining clients are given a neutral expectancy set. This set entails providing a description of the procedures without any reference to therapy or treatment. This approach is especially suited for examining expectancy effects upon attrition and for exploring demand effects. However, there are several ethical problems involved in this approach, the most serious of which is providing treatment to subjects without their consent. That is, half of the subjects receive a neutral set that contains no references to therapy; the ethics involved in providing treatment to clients without their knowledge are questionable. This approach is not recommended for lengthy treatment trials or serious clinical problems and requires careful phrasing of consent statements with analogue populations. Optimally, the investigator can find an approach other than this to test nonspecific effects in treatment outcome studies.

Assessment Procedures. The topic of assessment issues, or choice of dependent variables, could easily have an entire chapter devoted to it. (For an extended discussion of this topic, the reader is referred to relevant chapters in Barlow, Hayes, and Nelson, 1984.) The research area where this concern is most salient is treatment outcome examinations. Therefore, relevant concerns will be raised in this context. The issues involved can be broken into several categories: what to measure, who provides the data, how often to sample and over what time span, and the choice of measurement approach.

It is almost axiomatic within treatment outcome studies to include multiple measures of change. This can include measures across multiple response domains (e.g., behavioral, cognitive/self-report, and physiological/affective) as well as more broad-band assessment of areas of functioning not directly targeted by treatment (e.g., vocational, educational, social). The first concern, multiple response measurement, generally addresses specified target complaints. For example, in treatment of anxiety disorders, it is becoming increasingly important to assess autonomic arousal, behavioral avoidance, and cognitive self-statements, following the recognition that anxiety is not necessarily a unified construct (Lang, 1968) and evidence that responding in these domains may not change in a synchronous fashion (e.g., Barlow, Mavissakalian, & Schofield, 1980; Grey, Rachman, & Sartory, 1981). This approach can be applied to most disorders and has the potential to advance our understanding of behavior change processes and the nature of pathological behavior. The second concern, assessment of functioning not directly targeted by treatment, entails determining the "breadth of change" (Kazdin & Wilson, 1978). While treatment efficacy is best determined by alterations in the presenting problem, improvements commonly generalize to other areas of clients' lives. Conversely, negative side effects of treatment can be detected with a broad-band assessment strategy. For example, Ayllon, Layman, and Kandel (1975), in a comparison of reinforcement and Ritalin for suppressing hyperactive behavior in children, report that while both approaches were equally effective, Ritalin suppressed academic achievement as well, thus rendering it a less desirable treatment.

With respect to who provides the data, multiple sources need to be assessed. This can include reports by the client, therapist, significant others (parents, spouses), uninvolved observers, independent ratings by professionals, etc. Strupp and Hadley (1977) have provided a conceptual frame within which to organize these multiple data sources. In this perspective, someone should be assessed from the viewpoint of society, the individual, and the mental health profession. This view recognizes the multiple goals of treatment and can provide a wider angled perspective on the radiating impact of treatment. The need for multiple sources is also based upon reactivity of measures and reporting biases of clients and therapists.

Frequency of measurement is another important concern. Within reasonable limits, it is often instructional to include mid-treatment assessments, especially if the investigator wishes to explore potential mechanisms through which the intervention produces change. To examine durability of treatment effects, follow-up assessment is needed. While a recent review

(Nicholson & Berman, 1983) concludes that information obtained at follow-up often adds little to that obtained post-treatment, this report did not include studies involving psychotic disorders, personality disturbances, or addictive problems. This review suggests more conservative use of follow-up, in light of limited time and resources available. If the investigator chooses to include a follow-up, given an experimental focus on a diagnosis with a high relapse rate or specific focus upon treatment durability, several details are important. The interval employed for follow-up depends, in part, on the nature of the problem under examination. For example, marked deterioration of treatment effects has consistently been found for weight reduction (Brownell, 1982) and smoking cessation (Lichtenstein, 1982) for the first year following treatment. Here the importance of lengthy follow-up (perhaps 1-year and beyond) is clearly established. Additionally, it is important to assess relevant dimensions, such as help-seeking at other agencies and differential attrition across groups. While difficult, it is necessary for clients to complete the same assessment battery or follow-up as employed throughout the treatment phase. A phone call or letter does not provide the same quality data necessary for drawing meaningful conclusions at follow-up. Some investigators often use monetary incentives for completion of follow-up as a way to increase compliance. The effects of this strategy have been little studied, unfortunately; unintended experimenter demand may be an important, undetected confound of this approach.

A final assessment issue concerns the use of unobtrusive measures (Webb, Campbell, Schwartz, & Sechrest, 1966). The advantages of measuring outcome unobtrusively are that the researcher can avoid potential reactivity effects and that subjects can be followed-up without concerns about compliance. Available techniques include archival records, such as school grades, and admission and discharge data from institutions, physical traces like contents of trash, and observation. In practice, use of unobtrusive measurement can be difficult, as records are often incomplete or suffer from inexact, changing criteria; physical traces are often anonymous; and observation may require hundreds of hours before the behavior of interest is finally displayed. The use of unobtrusive measures, however, can extend the external validity of findings and is a recommended approach, when possible.

Implementation Issues

Ethical Considerations. Ethical concerns obviously deserve mention with regard to the implementation of any between-group study. Often, deception is involved in experimental psychopathology and treatment outcome research. This can take the form of inducing an emotional state, such as anxiety, anger, or embarrassment; offering clients an inert treatment; or failure to inform subjects fully of all possible experimental manipulations. Any time deception is considered, the researcher needs to ask if the possible scientific gains outweigh potential risks to subjects. This is a difficult question, and one that is often impossible to answer prior to conducting a study. Another way to frame this issue is to ask if alternative approaches that do not involve deception are available for studying the experimental question. Several alternatives to placebo controls have been outlined earlier to address concerns over deception in treatment outcome research. When deception is unavoidable, the researcher needs to weigh available options and choose the least aversive deception with the lowest possibility for harm to subjects. For example, if the experimental question calls for invoking anxiety in subjects, a number of paradigms can be used: electrical shock and providing false feedback to subjects are two. Relevant literature should be examined for possible side effects and the expected range of individual variation in response to deception in making such a decision.

Debriefing necessarily follows use of deception and is intended to provide post-hoc consent and to minimize any unintended consequences. While a number of potential problems are not addressed by debriefing (e.g., subsequent mistrust of experimental participation, lowered self-esteem), the experimenter can minimize these by use of a carefully constructed debriefing interview, assessing all foreseen possible consequences. The long-term effects of deception can be followed-up after debriefing, via phone calls to subjects. Unfortunately, this is rarely done. As Kazdin (1980) discusses, whether subjects are debriefed should refer to the state in which they leave the laboratory, not merely the administration of an interview. Any particular deception-debriefing procedure thus demands pilot work and/or empirical grounding.

One of the fundamental ethical principles set out by the American Psychological Association (APA) is the provision of informed consent by subjects. This entails providing a detailed explanation of the procedure involved, which allows the individual to make a reasoned decision whether or not to participate, free of coercion (this procedure covers the elements of competence, knowledge, and volition, according to a legal analysis provided by Martin, 1975). In practice, this is accomplished by providing a written consent statement which details specific procedural steps and outlines potential benefits and risks to the subject. Included in this statement is a phrase indicating that the subject may withdraw participation at any time. Prior to participation, the subject is asked to read and sign this statement after all questions have been raised. When testing new treatment approaches, the experimental nature of the intervention needs to be detailed in the consent statement. This can pose problems, if it lowers expectancies for treatment success. This may be avoided by providing a statement of expected therapeutic benefits. When using a placebo comparison group, the issue of informed consent becomes intertwined with deception. This is an unavoidable dilemma, given the definition of a placebo group, and one that can only be avoided through the use of an alternative control strategy, as discussed earlier.

The ethics involved in withholding treatment are complex as well, especially in conducting research with fairly severe clients. Depending upon the context in which the research is being conducted, waiting lists may be common practice, thus lessening the problems in using this type of design. In any case, clients should be informed at the outset that there is a possibility of delaying treatments for a specified time. Only those who consent then can be randomly assigned to either active treatment or the attention control condition. If postponing treatment threatens to endanger clinical concerns, such as subsequent effectiveness of therapy or the well-being of the client during the waiting-list interval, another experimental design or a different subject sample should be chosen.

The above is intended to highlight some of the more pressing ethical concerns involved in implementing a group comparison study. Certainly, all of the ethical principles outlined by APA are relevant, as they are in any type of research. The crux of the above discussion is intended to alert the reader to the complex balance that must be struck between clinical and empirical concerns. In practice, most organizations regularly convene a panel of peers and community members to examine research proposals prior to implementation. This type of review is exceedingly helpful for the researcher contemplating a project involving deception or other risks.

Procedural Reliability. A second implementation concern is procedural reliability (Baer, Wolf, & Risley, 1968; Billingsley, White, & Munson, 1980). This refers to the degree to which all relevant variables (either independent variables or those which should remain constant) occur in accordance with the planned procedure. While it is assumed that experimental procedures are applied consistently, this is often not the case, as the previous discussion on therapist adherence to treatment protocol attests. Billingsley et al. (1980) present a system to assess procedural reliability, using an example from their work that involved exploring the impact of various components of classroom evaluation systems on the performance of handicapped students. This system consists of the use of classroom observers to code whether teachers consistently apply behavioral plans. While not directly applicable to work in other areas, this example highlights the importance of assessing what most often is assumed in research. The lack of procedural reliability threatens both the internal and external validity of a study and can obscure the types of functional relationships most sought. Hopefully, empirical reports will begin to include more assessments of the veracity with which procedural plans are followed; an inclusion that will heighten the believability of data and intervention procedures.

Data Analysis Issues

Statistical Procedures. A number of statistical procedures can be employed in analyzing data from a between-groups study (for specific details regarding statistical analyses, the reader is referred to Keppel, 1973, and Kirk, 1968). This section will highlight principles involved in statistical data analysis, as well as discuss the integration of statistical and clinical significance.

Despite a researcher's best efforts, treatment groups sometimes differ markedly prior to intervention, which may complicate subsequent data analysis and interpretation. Alternatively, the investigator may find other related factors are operative which are not included as independent variables. One commonly employed statistical procedure for controlling for such pretest differences among subjects is the analysis of covariance. Provided that subjects vary along a dimension that is not correlated with the dependent variables, scores obtained during the experiment can be adjusted statistically to obtain a "purer" examination of the experimental effects. This amounts to adjusting statistically for chance differences on the covariate (or the variable being controlled statistically) within each group and between groups. A visual example of this statistical approach is presented in Figure 4.3. The left panel presents the data prior to the analysis of covariance. As can be seen, the three groups differ at pretreatment and no apparent intervention effects are demonstrated. By statistically removing the pretreatment variance associated with

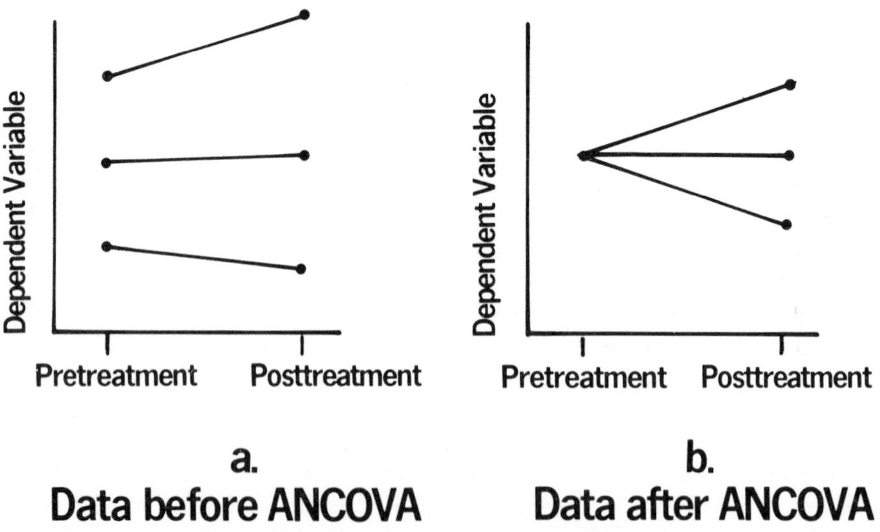

FIG. 4.3. Hypothetical data demonstrating statistical adjustment of pretreatment group differences with the analysis of covariance (ANCOVA)

an extraneous covariate, cell means are equated at pretreatment and experimental effects are shown (right panel).

A critical point in the use of the analysis of covariance is the independence of the covariate from the dependent measures; ideally, a measure taken before the experimental manipulation should be used to guard against unknown testing by treatment interactions. While the analysis of covariance is employed often enough to warrant mention here, it is important to note that this statistical procedure should never be used as a "rescue" strategy when the more routine analysis of variance fails to show significant effects. Rather, this procedure provides a statistical approach to removing extraneous intra-subject differences that may cloud clear interpretation of experimental findings. It also provides the experimenter with an alternative to experimentally grouping subjects along another dimension, thus reducing the number of variables employed and permitting a more direct examination of relevant factors.

A number of correlational procedures are also available which can help the investigator to refine data analysis and increase understanding of the experimental phenomena. Stepwise discriminant analysis, for example, can be used to determine factors that separate groups (Cooley & Lohnes, 1971; Dixon & Brown, 1979). This analysis computes linear functions for each variable involved and identifies those variables on which groups statistically differ. For example, Blanchard, Andrasik, Neff, Arena, Ahles, Jurish, Pallmeyer, Saunders, Teders, Barron, and Rodichok (1982) illustrate the utility of discriminant analysis procedures for identifying variables associated with treatment outcome. Following behavioral treatment, headache patients were termed "success" or "failure" based upon change in symptomatology. Scores from key psychological tests administered during baseline were able to correctly classify from 73.3 to 85.7% of all patients, taking into account type of headache and type of treatment. This approach to data analysis has the potential for uncovering important dimensions of difference between groups and can be used in a number of ways (e.g., to search for unsuspected dimensions of difference between clinical and nonclinical samples in experimental psychopathology studies, or to examine subject characteristics that differentiate treatment successes and failures as in the treatment outcome study discussed above). Use of this statistical tool has the potential to provide clinically meaningful data, as relevant subject characteristics are examined in interaction with group membership, response to treatment or whatever experimental focus is involved in the group-comparison design. Provided a large enough sample is employed in the study, discriminant function analysis can be used as a corollary analysis to univariate statistics such as the analysis of variance. A discriminant function approach provides more clinically meaningful information, relative to other regression analyses, as subject grouping forms the dimension to which regression is applied. Discrete group differences are maintained while linear equations are computed for dependent measures to determine what predicts group membership. This approach has many uses in clinical research and may, in time, reveal previously unsuspected information about clinical phenomena.

A related regression technique that has a different purpose is path analysis. This approach can be used to explore, in a correlational fashion, causal models. An example can clarify this procedure. Foa, Grayson, Steketee, Doppelt, Turner, and Latimer (1983) explored factors that predict success and failure in the treatment of obsessive compulsives. Results revealed that several variables were related to treatment outcome: pretreatment levels of depression and anxiety, reactivity to most feared stimuli, habituation of anxiety both within and between sessions, and age at onset of the disorder. These authors, drawing upon theories on the nature of anxiety and treatment processes, constructed a model utilizing these factors. The model was then tested by path analyses, which involves a series of multiple regression equations exploring the direct and indirect effects of experimental factors. While the data from this particular analysis are not strong, this example highlights the potential for path analysis in testing a causal model. This procedure enables the researcher to forge a link between conceptual issues and clinical data, a bridge which can only make our empirical data more meaningful and help to critically examine existing theoretical accounts.

Clinical versus Statistical Significance. A discussion of statistical procedures in the analysis of between-group studies would be incomplete without mention of the difference between clinical and statistical significance. A number of authors (e.g., Barlow, 1981; Chassan, 1960; Hersen & Barlow, 1976; Kazdin, 1980; Kazdin & Wilson, 1978) have discussed the differences between findings that are statistically significant and those which reveal clinically important phenomena. As any experienced researcher knows, statistically significant results can be obtained when actual group differences on the dependent measure are relatively small, provided the sample is large enough. This type of finding does little to advance our understanding of psychopathology, active treatment processes, personality constructs, and so on. What is needed, beyond statistical significance, is some assessment of clinically meaningful effects. This is different from assessing the percentage of variance accounted for, as would be done via a statistic like omega squared (e.g., Hays, 1973), for this type of index assesses affect size, not the clinical relevance of the effects. Kazdin and Wilson (1978) discuss a number of criteria which can be used in the treatment outcome research to address clinical effects. For example, data can be reported as the proportion of clients who improve significantly (according to well-defined criteria), a strategy that provides a more individual emphasis in data analysis. Alternatively, treatment failures and outliers from the group mean can be identified and relevant contributing factors explored, possibly through use of discriminant function analysis (as mentioned above).

An important dimension for examining clinical effects is the existence of normative standards with which to contrast clinical groups, as an index of the importance of change. Wolf (1978) introduced the concept of social validity or social acceptability of treatment effects. This refers to the acceptability of both treatment procedures and treatment results. Kazdin (1977) has offered two approaches to assessing the importance of treatment outcome, termed social comparison and subjective evaluation. Social comparison refers to using a "nondeviant" peer group's behavior as a standard for judging posttreatment gains. For example, Patterson (1974) compared posttreatment gains of conduct-disordered children with non-problem children. Home observations of behavior were made for both groups, matched on relevant dimensions (e.g., socioeconomic status, number of siblings). Pretreatment comparisons revealed the conduct problem children as more deviant than their peers, while comparisons at posttreatment showed that the clinical sample fell within the normative range of their nondeviant peers. While providing an example of social comparison, this report also provides an instance of clinically significant behavior change, as clients' behavior was brought within normative limits as a result of intervention.

A second approach to social validation discussed by Kazdin is subjective evaluation, which refers to assessing how the client is viewed by others. Significant others can be questioned to determine if specific treatment gains are detected, if global evaluations of the client have changed following treatment, and/or if the degree to which appropriate behavior is perceived has changed. Both of these social validation procedures suffer from potential problems (see Kazdin, 1980), the most notable of which is that norms may not be a desired goal for treatment, especially for certain behaviors such as cigarette smoking or drug consumption. This point addresses a philosophical problem as well, namely the multifaceted definition of "normal" behavior. While social validation procedures are not inherently problem-free, they do help the researcher address the clinical relevance of experimental effects and provide a more sensitive measure of clinical change relative to statistical significance.

Issues Concerning Interpretation of Results

Generalization. The final step in any between-group design involves interpretation of results. While each data set poses its own unique questions to the investigator, certain principles are common across studies. The first consideration in interpreting findings is the extent to which results can be generalized. Recognizing that it is impossible to sample all relevant dimensions of generalization, the researcher needs to address the extent to which critical dimensions were handled by the design. This includes the choice of the design proper, sample and measures chosen, procedural details, and so on. If innovative procedures were employed, the degree of generalization may be limited by their unknown effects upon the data. This can include all of the methodology and implementation concerns discussed earlier. In discussing implications of the results, limitations upon generalizing the findings need to be stated. Given that between-group research is grounded upon the search for probability-based statements about group differences, any one study does not provide a strong empirical statement, even given adequate sampling across all relevant dimensions of generalization. Thus the investigator is astute to point out limitations of the findings, experimental confounds that may hinder replication, and alternative designs that could be employed for subsequent examinations. Ultimately, generalization of findings can be determined only by replication, which often provides important qualifications and refinements in understanding clinical phenomena.

Negative Effects. The assumption has been made throughout this discussion that statistically significant differences were found; this often is not the case in research. *Negative effects* (or the lack of statistically significant findings) often are attributed to methodological weaknesses of the project or other sources of experimental bias, factors that possibly would be overlooked if statistical effects were obtained. Negative effects are published infrequently, owing to restrictions in journal space and editorial policies. This is unfortunate, as the conceptualization and methodology of a study are often more accurate determinants of its value. Some authors (e.g., Greenwald, 1975) have argued that the results of a study should have little bearing on publication decisions; rather, methodological and conceptual adequacy of the project should be used as primary criteria. Unfortunately, there is not full consensus in clinical psychology of what should constitute these criteria.

Additionally, negative effects can have many explanations, including a lack of relationship between the independent and dependent variables, choice of intensity or level of the independent variable (e.g., choosing two levels of an experimental variable that are close in intensity may not reveal differences), choice of assessment devices, and existence of a number of unassessed moderating variables. The careful investigator needs to consider these and other options when confronted with negative results. If the study entails an attempted replication of previous work, negative results may indicate unsuspected artifacts in the original study, especially if a number of investigators are unable to replicate it. Thus, negative effects, rather than being the researcher's bane, can play an important role in empirical clinical psychology, providing design and methodology concerns have been met adequately.

Replication. Replication lies at the heart of between-group research, as mentioned throughout this chapter. This can take the form of a direct replication wherein the experiment is repeated exactly, or systematic replication, which varies the experiment along at least one dimension (Sidman, 1960). Both types of replication play important roles in establishing the generality of findings and extending our understanding of clinical phenomena. Without replication, probability statements concerning group differences have little or no meaning, as any number of explanations for the findings can be accurate.

SUMMARY

The various concerns discussed above generally need to be addressed in conducting a group comparison study. Table 4.2 outlines these issues and provides a guide for the beginning researcher who is contemplating a between-groups study. The large number of details involved can seem overwhelming, yet careful attention to all aspects of methodology and implementation results in a more direct examination by allowing the investigator to rule out alternative explanations and experimental confounds.

This chapter has described commonly employed designs and relevant concerns in methodology, implementation, data analysis, and interpretation of

Table 4.2. A Checklist of Relevant Concerns in Conducting a Group Comparison Study

A. Methodological Concerns

Subject Selection:

- Is an analogue or clinical sample to be employed?
- Are inclusion and exclusion criteria carefully defined?
- Has the literature been examined for relevant subject characteristics that may interact with experimental manipulations?
- Is a large enough sample available?
- How are subjects to be recruited? Will this affect the experimental results?
- Have subjects been exposed to previous experimentation and/or treatment?
- What type of experimental control group is most appropriate?
- Are extreme groups to be used? If yes, have appropriate safeguards been devised to protect against statistical regression?

Selecting and operationally defining independent variables:

- If an experimental induction procedure is to be used, are relevant concerns (e.g., subject expectancies, dosage levels) adequately addressed?
- If an environmental manipulation is to be used, has the ecological validity been ascertained?
- If treatment is involved:
    - Is the intervention delivered at its maximum strength?
    - Are therapists to be employed with strong theoretical biases?
    - Are therapists to be crossed or nested?
    - How long will the intervention phase last?
    - Are treatment sessions to be monitored to ensure adherence to protocol?
    - If two treatments are compared, are the interventions equated on relevant parameters?
- Have alternatives to attention and placebo control groups been considered?

(continued)

Table 4.2. ***(continued)***

Assessment:
- Which dependent measures are to be employed?
- Who will provide the data (e.g., subject, therapist)?
- How often and over what time span will samples be taken?
- Will dependent measures be obtrusive?

B. Implementation Concerns

Ethics:
- Is deception to be employed? Have relative benefits and risks been weighed and non-deceptive alternatives not available?
- How will subjects be debriefed?
- How will informed consent be obtained?
- If treatment if to be withheld, is this appropriate to the sample involved?

Procedural Reliability:
- Is a system available to assess consistent application of experimental variables?

C. Data Analysis Concerns

- Have relevant parametric and correlational procedures been considered?
- How will clinical significance be assessed?
- Will social validation of behavior change be involved?

D. Concerns in Interpreting Results

- How far can the findings be generalized?
- If negative effects are achieved, are they a result of any methodological issues?
- What considerations are relevant for subsequent replication and extension of findings?

findings. Undertaking such a research project requires considerable skill, planning, and dedication, but the ultimate gain in knowledge from a well-designed study is not to be understated. Clinical psychology has witnessed a boom of research activity over the past several decades, a trend that has strengthened the field and aided our understanding of clinical processes. As this trend continues into the future, more refinements in our empirical inquiry process will occur. At the heart of between group research (past, present, or future) lies the search for scientific understanding of human behavior and lawful relationships. This principle will surely endure and guide our research endeavors.

REFERENCES

Andrasik, F., & Holroyd, K.A. (1980). A test of specific and nonspecific effects in the biofeedback treatment of tension headache. *Journal of Consulting and Clinical Psychology, 48,* 575–586.

Andrasik, F., & Holroyd, K.A. (1983). Specific and nonspecific effects in the treatment of tension headache: 3-year follow-up. *Journal of Consulting and Clinical Psychology, 51,* 634–636.

Andrasik, F., Pallmeyer, T.P., Blanchard, E.B., & Attanasio, V. (1983). *Continuous vs. interrupted schedules of thermal biofeedback: An explanatory analysis with clinical subjects.* Manuscript submitted for publication.

American Psychiatric Association (1980). *Diagnostic and statistical manual of mental disorders.* (3rd ed.). Washington, DC: Author.

Ayllon, T., Layman, D., & Kandel, H.J. (1975). A behavioral-educational alternative to drug control of hyperactive children. *Journal of Applied Behavior Analysis, 8,* 137–146.

Baer, D.M., Wolf, M.M., & Risley, T.R. (1968). Some current dimensions of applied behavior analysis. *Journal of Applied Behavior Analysis, 1,* 91–97.

Barlow, D.H. (1981). On the relation of clinical research to clinical practice: Current issues, new directions. *Journal of Consulting and Clinical Psychology, 49,* 147–156.

Barlow, D.H., Hayes, S.C., & Nelson, R.O. (in press). *The scientist-practitioner: Research and accountability in clinical and educational settings.* New York: Pergamon Press.

Barlow, D.H., Mavissakalian, M.R., & Schofield, L.D. (1980). Patterns of desynchrony in agoraphobia: A preliminary report. *Behaviour Research and Therapy, 18,* 441–448.

Beck, A.T. (1972). *Depression: Causes and treatment.* Philadelphia: University of Pennsylvania Press.

Beck, J.G., Barlow, D.H., & Sakheim, D.K. (1983). The effects of attentional focus and partner arousal on sexual responding in functional and dysfunctional men. *Behaviour Research and Therapy, 21,* 1–8.

Bellack, A.S., Rozensky, R., & Schwartz, J. (1974). A comparison of two forms of self-monitoring in a behavioral weight reduction program. *Behavior Therapy, 5,* 523–530.

Bergin, A.E., & Lambert, M.J. (1978). The evaluation of therapeutic outcomes. In S.L. Garfield and A.E. Bergin (Eds.), *Handbook of psychotherapy and behavior change.* (2nd ed.). New York: John Wiley & Sons.

Berkowitz, L., & Donnerstein, E. (1982). External validity is more than skin deep: Some answers to criticism of laboratory experiments. *American Psychologist, 37,* 245–257.

Bernstein, D.A., & Nietzel, M.T. (1974). Behavioral avoidance tests: The effects of demand characteristics and repeated measures on two types of subjects. *Behavior Therapy, 5,* 183–192.

Bernstein, D.A., & Paul, G.L. (1971). Some comments on therapy analogue research with small animal "phobias." *Journal of Behavior Therapy and Experimental Psychiatry, 2,* 225–237.

Billingsley, F., White, O.R., & Munson, R. (1980). Procedural reliability: A rationale and an example. *Behavioral Assessment, 2,* 229–241.

Blanchard, E.B., Andrasik, F., Neff, D.F., Arena, J.G., Ahles, T.A., Jurish, S.E., Pallmeyer, T.P., Saunders, N.L., Teders, S.J., Barron, K.D., & Rodichok, L.D. (1982). Biofeedback and relaxation training with three kinds of headache: Treatment effects and their prediction. *Journal of Consulting and Clinical Psychology, 50,* 562–575.

Blanchard, E.B., Theobald, D.E., Williamson, D.A., Silver, B.V., & Brown, D.A. (1978). Temperature biofeedback in the treatment of migraine headaches: A controlled evaluation. *Archives of General Psychiatry, 35,* 581–588.

Bootzin, R.R., Herman, P.C., & Nicassio, P. (1976). The power of suggestion: Another examination of misattribution and insomnia. *Journal of Personality and Social Psychology, 34,* 673–679.

Borkovec, T.D. (1973). The role of expectancy and physiological feedback in fear research: A review with special reference to subject characteristics. *Behavior Therapy, 4,* 491–505.

Borkovec, T.D., Kaloupek, D.G., & Slama, K. (1975). The facilitative effect of muscle tension-release in the relaxation treatment of sleep disturbance. *Behavior Therapy, 6,* 301–309.

Borkovec, T.D., & Nau, S.D. (1972). Credibility of analogue therapy rationales. *Journal of Behavior Therapy and Experimental Psychiatry, 3,* 257–260.

Borkovec, T.D., & O'Brien, G.T. (1976). Methodological and target behavior issues in analogue therapy outcome research. In M. Hersen, R.M. Eisler, and P.M. Miller (Eds.), *Progress in Behavior Modification* Vol. 3. New York: Academic Press.

Briddell, D.W., & Wilson, G.T. (1976). Effects of alcohol and expectancy set on male sexual arousal. *Journal of Abnormal Psychology, 85,* 225–234.

Brownell, K.D. (1982). Obesity: Understanding and treating a serious, prevalent, and refractory disorder. *Journal of Consulting and Clinical Psychology, 50,* 820–840.

Campbell, D.T., & Stanley, J.C. (1963). *Experimental and quasi-experimental designs for research.* Chicago: Rand McNally.

Chambless, D.L., Foa, E.B., Groves, G.A., & Goldstein, A.J. (1982). Exposure and communications training in the treatment of agoraphobia. *Behaviour Research and Therapy, 20,* 219–231.

Chapman, L.J., & Chapman, J.P. (1977). Selection of subjects in studies of schizophrenic cognition. *Journal of Abnormal Psychology, 86,* 10–15.

Chapman, L.J., & Knowles, R.R. (1964). The effects of phenothiazine on disordered thought in schizophrenia. *Journal of Consulting Psychology, 28,* 165–169.

Chassan, J.B. (1960). Statistical inference and the single case in clinical design. *Psychiatry, 23,* 173–184.

Church, R.M. (1969). Systematic effect of random error in the yoked control design. *Psychological Bulletin, 62,* 122–131.

Cohen, J. (1977). *Statistical power analysis for the behavioral sciences* (rev. ed.). New York: Academic Press.

Cooley, W.W., & Lohnes, P.R. (1971). *Multivariate data analysis.* New York: John Wiley & Sons.

Cooper, A., Furst, J.B., & Bridger, W.H. (1969). A brief commentary on the usefulness of studying fears of snakes. *Journal of Abnormal Psychology, 74,* 413–414.

Copeland, A.P. (1981). The relevance of subject variables in cognitive self-instructional programs for impulsive children. *Behavior Therapy, 12,* 520–529.

Curran, J.P., Beck, J.G., Corriveau, D.P., & Monti, P.M. (1980). Recalibration of raters to criterion: A methodological note for social skills research. *Behavioral Assessment, 2,* 261–266.

DiLoreto, A.O. (1971). *Comparative psychotherapy: An experimental analysis.* Chicago: Adline-Atherton.

Dixon, W.J., & Brown, M.B. (Eds.) (1979). *Biomedical computer programs—P series.* Berkeley: University of California Press.

Feighner, J.P., Robins, E., Guze, S.B., Woodruff, R.A., Winokur, G., & Munoz, R. (1972). Diagnostic criteria for use in psychiatric research. *Archives of General Psychiatry, 26,* 57–63.

Fisher, R.A. (1956). *Statistical methods and scientific inference.* Edinburgh, Scotland: Oliver & Boyd.

Fisher, R.A. (1967). *Statistical methods for research workers* (13th ed.). Edinburgh, Scotland: Oliver & Boyd.

Foa, E.B., Grayson, J.B., Steketee, G.S., Doppelt, H.G., Turner, R.M., & Latimer, P.R. (1983). Success and failure in the behavioral treatment of obsessive compulsives. *Journal of Consulting and Clinical Psychology, 51,* 287–297.

Frank, E., Anderson, D., & Rubinstein, D. (1978). Frequency of sexual dysfunction in "normal" couples. *New England Journal of Medicine, 299,* 111–115.

Frank, J.D. (1961). *Persuasion and healing.* Baltimore: Johns Hopkins University Press.

Frank, J.D. (1968). The role of hope in psychotherapy. *International Journal of Psychiatry, 5,* 383–395.

Frank, J.D. (1973). *Persuasion and healing.* (2nd ed.). Baltimore: Johns Hopkins University Press.

Garfield, S.L. (1978). Research problems in clinical diagnosis. *Journal of Consulting and Clinical Psychology, 46,* 596–607.

Greenwald, A.G. (1975). Consequences of prejudice against the null hypothesis. *Psychological Bulletin, 82,* 1–20.

Grey, S.J., Rachman, S., & Sartory, G. (1981). Return of fear: The role of inhibition. *Behaviour Research and Therapy, 19,* 135–143.

Hays, W.L. (1973). *Statistics for the social sciences* (2nd ed.). New York: Holt, Rinehart, & Winston.

Heimberg, R.G., & Becker, R.E. (in press). Comparative outcome research. In M. Hersen, L. Michelson, & A.S. Bellack (Eds.), *Issues in Psychotherapy Research.* New York: Plenum Press.

Helzer, J.E., Brockington, I.F., & Kendell, R.E. (1981). Predictive validity of DSM-III, and Feighner definitions of schizophrenia: A comparison with research diagnostic criteria and CATEGO. *Archives of General Psychiatry, 38,* 791–797.

Hersen, M., & Barlow, D.H. (1976). Single case experimental designs: Strategies for studying behavior change. New York: Pergamon Press.

Hersen, M., Bellack, A.S, & Himmelhoch, J.M. (1981). A comparison of solicited and nonsolicited female unipolar depressives for treatment outcome research. *Journal of Consulting and Clinical Psychology, 49,* 611–613.

Hiroto, D.S. (1974). Locus of control and learned helplessness. *Journal of Experimental Psychology, 102,* 187–193.

Huesmann, L.R. (1982). Experimental methods in research in psychopathology. In P.C. Kendall & J.N. Butcher (Eds.), *Handbook of research methods in clinical psychology.* New York: John Wiley & Sons.

Johnson, S.M., & Bolstad, O.D. (1973). Methodological issues in naturalistic observation: Some problems and solutions for field research. In L.A. Hamerlynck, L.C. Handy & E.J. Mash (Eds.), *Behavior Change: Methodology, concepts, and practice.* Champaign, IL: Research Press.

Johnson, S.M., & Brown, R. (1969). Producing behavior change in parents of disturbed children. *Journal of Child Psychology and Psychiatry, 10,* 107–121.

Kazdin, A.E. (1977). Assessing the clinical or applied significance of behavior change through social validation. *Behavior Modification, 1,* 427–452.

Kazdin, A.E. (1978). Evaluating the generality of findings in analogue therapy research. *Journal of Consulting and Clinical Psychology, 46,* 673–686.

Kazdin, A.E. (1980). *Research design in clinical psychology,* New York: Harper & Row.

Kazdin, A.E., & Wilcoxon, L.A. (1976). Systematic desensitization and nonspecific treatment effects: A methodological evaluation. *Psychological Bulletin, 83,* 729–758.

Kazdin, A.E., & Wilson, G.T. (1978). Criteria for evaluating psychotherapy. *Archives of General Psychiatry, 35,* 407–416.

Kendall, P.C., & Wilcox, L.E. (1980). A cognitive behavioral treatment for impulsivity: Concrete versus conceptual training with non-self-controlled problem children. *Journal of Consulting and Clinical Psychology, 48,* 80–91.

Keppel, G. (1973). *Design and analysis: A researcher's handbook.* Englewood Cliffs, NJ: Prentice Hall.

Kiecolt, J., & McGrath, E. (1979). Social desirability responding in the measurement of assertive behavior. *Journal of Consulting and Clinical Psychology, 47,* 640–642.

Kirk, R.E. (1968). *Experimental design: Procedures for the behavioral sciences.* Monterey, CA: Brooks/Cole.

Lang, P.J. (1968). Fear reduction and fear behavior: Problems in treating a construct. In J.M. Shlien (Ed.), *Research in psychotherapy* (Vol. 3). Washington, DC: American Psychological Association.

Lansky, D., & Wilson, G.T. (1981). Alcohol, expectations, and sexual arousal in males: An information processing analysis. *Journal of Abnormal Psychology, 90,* 35–45.

Leitenberg, H. (1973). The use of single-case methodology in psychotherapy research. *Journal of Abnormal Psychology, 82,* 87–101.

Levis, D.J. (1970). The case of performing research on nonpatient populations with fears of small animals: A reply to Cooper, Furst, and Bridger. *Journal of Abnormal Psychology, 76,* 36–38.

Lewinsohn, P.M. (1975). The behavioral study and treatment of depression. In M. Hersen, R.M. Eisler & P.M. Miller (Eds.), *Progress in Behavior Modification* (Vol. 1). New York, Academic Press.

Lichtenstein, E. (1982). The smoking problem: A behavioral perspective. *Journal of Consulting and Clinical Psychology, 50,* 804–819.

Lick, J.R., & Bootzin, R.R. (1970). Expectancy, demand characteristics, and contact desensitization in behavior change. *Behavior Therapy, 1,* 176–183.

Mahoney, M.J. (1978). Experimental methods and outcome evaluation. *Journal of Consulting and Clinical Psychology, 46,* 660–672.

Malan, D.H., Heath, E.S., Bacal, H.A., & Balfour, F.H.G. (1975). Psychodynamic changes in untreated neurotic patients—II. Apparently genuine improvements. *Archives of General Psychiatry, 32,* 110–126.

Maletzky, B.M. (1974). "Assisted" covert sensitization in the treatment of exhibitionism. *Journal of Consulting and Clinical Psychology, 42,* 34–40.

Martin, R. (1975). *Legal challenges to behavior modification: Trends in schools, corrections, and mental health.* Champaign, IL: Research Press.

Masters, W.H., & Johnson, V.E. (1970). *Human sexual inadequacy.* Boston: Little, Brown.

Mathews, A. (1978). Fear-reduction research and clinical phobias. *Psychological Bulletin, 85,* 390–404.

Mungas, D.M., & Walters, H.A. (1979). Pretesting effects in the evaluation of social skills training. *Journal of Consulting and Clinical Psychology, 47,* 216–218.

Nelson, R.O., Lipinski, D.P., & Black, J.L. (1975). The effects of expectancy on the reactivity of self-recording. *Behavior Therapy, 6,* 237–249.

Nicholson, R.A., & Berman, J.S. (1983). Is follow-up necessary in evaluating psychotherapy? *Psychological Bulletin, 93,* 261–278.

O'Leary, K.D., & Borkovec, T.D. (1978). Conceptual, methodological, and ethical problems of placebo groups in psychotherapy research. *American Psychologist, 33,* 821–830.

Orne, M.T. (1962). On the social psychology of the psychological experiment: With particular reference to demand characteristics and their implications. *American Psychologist, 17,* 776–783.

Parloff, M.B., Waskow, I.E., & Wolfe, B.E. (1978). Research on therapist variables in relation to process and outcome. In S.L. Garfield & A.E. Bergin (Eds.), *Handbook of psychotherapy and behavior change* (2nd Ed.). New York: John Wiley & Sons.

Patterson, G.R. (1974). Interventions for boys with conduct problems: Multiple settings, treatments, and criteria. *Journal of Consulting and Clinical Psychology, 42,* 471–481.

Paul, G.L. (1966). *Insight vs. desensitization in psychotherapy: An experiment in anxiety reduction.* Stanford, CA: Stanford University Press.

Paul, G.L. (1967). Strategy of outcome research in psychotherapy. *Journal of Consulting Psychology, 31,* 109–119.

Rehm, L. (1977). A self-control model of depression. *Behavior Therapy, 8,* 787–804.

Reppucci, N.D., & Clingempeel, W.G. (1978). Methodological issues in research with correctional populations. *Journal of Consulting and Clinical Psychology, 46,* 727–746.

Rock, D.L. (1981). The confounding of two self-report assertion measures with the tendency to give socially desirable responses in self-description. *Journal of Consulting and Clinical Psychology, 49,* 743–744.

Sallis, J.F., Lichstein, K.L., & McGlynn, F.D. (1980). Anxiety response patterns: A comparison of clinical and analogue populations. *Journal of Behavior Therapy and Experimental Psychiatry, 11,* 179–183.

Seligman, M.E.P., & Maier, S.F. (1967). Failure to escape traumatic shock. *Journal of Experimental Psychology, 74, 1–9.*

Shapiro, A.K., & Morris, L.A. (1978). Placebo effects in medical and psychological therapies. In S.L. Garfield & A.E. Bergin (Eds.), *Handbook of psychotherapy and behavior change* (2nd Ed.). New York: John Wiley & Sons.

Shipley, C.R., & Fazio, A.F. (1973). Pilot study of a treatment for psychological depression. *Journal of Abnormal Psychology, 82,* 372–376.

Sidman, M. (1960). *Tactics of scientific research: Evaluating experimental data in psychology.* New York: Basic Books.

Slag, M.F., Morley, J.E., Elson, M.K., Trence, D.L., Nelson, C.J., Nelson, A.E., Kinlaw, W.B., Beyer, S., Nuttall, R.Q., & Shafer, R.B. (1983). Impotence in medical clinic outpatients. *Journal of the American Medical Association, 249,* 1736–1740.

Sloane, R.B., Staples, F.R., Cristol, A.H., Yorkston, N.J., & Whipple, K. (1975). *Short-term analytically oriented psychotherapy vs. behavior therapy.* Cambridge, MA: Harvard University Press.

Solomon, R.L. (1949). An extension of control group design. *Psychological Bulletin, 46,* 137–150.

Spitzer, R.L., Endicott, J., & Robins, E. (1978). *Research diagnostic criteria (RDC) for a selected group of functional disorders.* New York: Biometrics Research, New York State Psychiatric Institute.

Spitzer, R.L., Williams, J.B.W., & Skodol, A.E. (1980). DSM III: The major achievements and an overview. *American Journal of Psychiatry, 137,* 151–164.

Strupp, H.H., & Hadley, S.W. (1977). A tripartite model of mental health and therapeutic outcomes: With special reference to the negative effects of psychotherapy. *American Psychologist, 32,* 187–196.

Stuart, R.B. (1973). Notes on the ethics of behavior research and intervention. In L.A. Hamerlynck, L.C. Hardy, & E.J. Mash (Eds.), *Behavior change: Methodology, concepts, and practice.* Champaign, IL: Research Press.

Webb, E.J., Campbell, D.T., Schwartz, R.C., & Sechrest, L. (1966). *Unobtrusive measures: Nonreactive research in the social sciences.* Chicago: Rand McNally.

Weissman, M.M. (1979). The psychological treatment of depression. *Archives of General Psychiatry, 36,* 1261–1269.

Wilkins, W. (1977). Expectancies in applied settings. In A. Gurman & A. Razin (Eds.), *Effective psychotherapy: A handbook of research.* New York: Pergamon Press.

Wilkins, W. (1979). Getting specific about nonspecifics. *Cognitive Therapy and Research, 3,* 319–329.

Wilson, G.T., & Lawson, D.M. (1976). Expectancies, alcohol, and sexual arousal in male social drinkers. *Journal of Abnormal Psychology, 85,* 587–594.

Wilson, G.T., & Lawson, D.M. (1978). Expectancies, alcohol, and sexual arousal in women. *Journal of Abnormal Psychology, 87,* 358–367.

Wolf, M.M. (1978). Social validity: The case of subjective measurement or how applied behavior analysis is finding its heart. *Journal of Applied Behavior Analysis, 11,* 203–214.

Yeaton, W.H., & Sechrest, L. (1981). Critical dimensions in the choice and maintenance of successful treatments: Strength, integrity, and effectiveness. *Journal of Consulting and Clinical Psychology, 49,* 156–167.

5
Correlational Methods in Clinical Research

Harvey A. Skinner

INTRODUCTION

Correlational methods are ubiquitous in clinical research. Study designs can range from the computation of a correlation coefficient between two measures based on a small sample ($n = 20$), to the complex and time consuming analyses involved in the statistical testing of causal models with a large sample ($n = 500$). Most research problems warrant methods somewhere between these two extremes. Although many excellent textbooks are available on correlational methods, they often focus more on computational details and statistical theory and may provide less insight on how to handle certain perplexing problems, such as having too many variables of potential interest, having a restricted or preselected sample, having missing data, or having concerns about the metric quality of measures. These issues are a central focus of this chapter.

The widespread availability of computer software packages (e.g., SPSS, SAS, BMDP) presents an almost irresistible temptation to use the most sophisticated multivariate techniques. Even though multivariate correlational methods have distinct advantages in allowing the simultaneous consideration of relationships among multiple measures, their use demands a corresponding level of expertise. Numerous pitfalls await the inexperienced researcher. In many respects, the advent of computer-based statistical packages has opened a Pandora's box. The control language required to use a powerful statistical procedure such as factor analysis is barely more complicated than that needed to compute a simple frequency distribution. In the precomputer era, one would not contemplate conducting a factor analysis without adequate knowledge of the tedious computational steps involved. Gulliksen (1974) recalls supervising 20 clerical workers for about 1 year during the 1930s in order to factor analyze 50 tests in Thurstone's first study of primary mental abilities. This technical difficulty forced the investigator to focus on a small

The author thanks Reinhard Schuller and Hau Lei for their statistical advice and assistance in the preparation of this chapter.

number of important measures. Thus, the computer revolution in data analysis is not without its drawbacks.

In reading various journal articles, one may suspect that sophisticated multivariate techniques are sometimes used in an attempt to obscure a lack of knowledge by sending up a "methodological smoke screen." It is ironic that simple linear models often work as well as or better than complex models with respect to statistical robustness and replicability (Dawes, 1979; Green, 1977). Moreover, when using a simple model one can generally convey what actually was accomplished. From painful experiences, I have learned that if you cannot effectively communicate to a wider audience what you have achieved in a study, then you might as well not have conducted the study in the first place (Skinner & Blashfield, 1982).

In this chapter, a number of broad issues are discussed in the use of correlational methods in clinical research. These issues have been stimulated by discussions with various colleagues about their research and by experience gained from reviewing manuscripts for clinical journals. A final section of the chapter will examine the revolution in quasi-experimental research due to the recent development of causal modeling techniques (Bentler, 1980). There is danger that in using sophisticated computer programs for causal modeling, investigators may be lulled into the same pitfalls of univariate correlational methods. Since the ultimate building block for a causal model is the correlation (covariance) coefficient, factors which influence this index are equally germane to univariate and multivariate studies.

PITFALLS IN THE USE OF CORRELATIONAL METHODS

Doing Research the Hard Way

All too often, analysis of variance (ANOVA) procedures are misapplied to a research problem that is basically correlational in design. For instance, a measure of individual differences, such as locus of control (Rotter, 1966), may be dichotomized at the sample median to produce two groups (internals and externals). Another example is the use of cutoff scores on a continuous measure such as the Beck Depression Inventory (Beck, 1972) to identify subgroups of individuals who are designated as either "depressed" or "not depressed." Then, these groups are compared on various "dependent" variables, which are often continuous measures (e.g., activity level, stressful life events, expectations of future behavior). In an illuminating article, Humphreys (1978) argues that this misapplication is "doing research the hard way," since a more powerful statistical test of hypotheses can be obtained from the correlation of the "dependent" and "independent" variables. Reliable information is lost when a continuous measure is categorized in order to create (artificially) an independent variable for ANOVA procedures. The product-moment correlation obtained after dichotomizing one variable at the median is reduced by approximately 20% to 40% of the underlying population value (Bollen & Barb, 1981).

Aside from a loss in statistical power when using ANOVA (or *t*-test) procedures in place of a correlational design, results from the study may be misinterpreted. Since subjects have not been assigned at random to different levels of the independent measure, experimental control over other stimulus and situational variables has not been achieved. When an individual difference measure is categorized and treated as an independent variable, the ANOVA procedures only yield an uncontrolled correlation between two or more categories and a continuous dependent variable, since no experimental manipulation of the "independent" variable has occurred. In addition, controversies often occur on criteria used for forming the various categories (see Hatzenbuehler, Parpal, & Matthews, 1983, for a discussion of classifying college students as depressed or nondepressed using the Beck Depression Inventory).

Another illustration of "doing research the hard way" is when a treatment outcome measure is categorized. In the alcoholism treatment literature, it is typical to see an outcome measure of drinking status (e.g., abstinent, light, moderate, heavy drinking) formed from inherently continuous measures of drinking frequency and quantity of alcohol consumed. Aside from arguments over threshold values in moving from one category to another (e.g., "moderate" to "heavy" drinking), this categorization results in a loss of information and statistical power. Bollen and Barb (1981) investigated the effect upon the correlation coefficient when two continuous measures are collapsed into a smaller number of categories. The greatest loss of information occurs when the continuous variables' correlation is low and only a few categories are used for the collapsed measures. For instance, an original correlation of $r = .20$ is reduced by 58% to $r = .12$ when the continuous variables are dichotomized. When more categories are used to approximate the continuous variables, the differences in correlation coefficients are smaller (Table 5.1).

Because of the difficulty involved in conducting a well designed treatment outcome study, one must question why researchers would make life even more difficult for themselves by discarding valuable information when a continuous outcome measure is categorized. This problem can masquerade in various guises in both univariate and multivariate analyses. For example, criterion groups denoting various "categories" of treatment success may be formed from a continuous measure, and subsequently a multiple discriminant analysis or multivariate analysis of variance (MANOVA) conducted to determine which client background and treatment process variables are most predictive of outcome. A more powerful statistical analysis would be to employ the continuous outcome measure as the *criterion*, and the client background and

Table 5.1. Correlation Coefficient for Original and Collapsed Variables*

Original Correlation	Reduced Correlation with Collapsed Variables			
	Number of Categories			
	2	3	4	5
.20	.12	.15	.17	.18
.40	.26	.30	.34	.36
.60	.41	.45	.50	.53
.80	.58	.62	.67	.71
.90	.72	.73	.77	.81

*Adapted from Bollen and Barb (1981) based on a simulation study with 50 samples of 500 observations each.

treatment process variables as *predictors* in a multiple regression analysis. It should be recognized that multiple discriminant analysis with two groups and multiple regression with a dichotomous criterion (group membership) are mathematically equivalent (Tatsuoka, 1971).

Being Misled by Empirical Data

Another basic pitfall is the interpretation of correlational results at face value. Unless careful consideration is given to factors in the study that may have affected the correlation coefficient (McNemar, 1969), there is danger of being "deceived" by the empirical data. For instance, a study must have adequate statistical power (Cohen, 1977), which refers to the probability of detecting a significant treatment effect (that is, reject the null hypothesis) when indeed a real effect exists in the population. Unless one has a reasonable chance (say 90%) of demonstrating empirically that a treatment has been successful, one must seriously question the merits of conducting the study in the first place. Otherwise, one may *falsely* conclude that a particular treatment has not been successful.

Consider a study designed to evaluate the usefulness of a measure of "social stability" in predicting outcome from treatment for alcoholism. Research has found social stability to be a consistent predictor of outcome (Ogborne, 1978). Assume that the "true" validity of a social stability index (e.g., Skinner, 1981) for predicting drinking status at 1-year follow up is 0.35. Under ideal conditions (i.e., the reliability of the outcome criterion is perfect, and there was no preselection of clients who entered the treatment program), a sample size of 65 clients is needed in order to have a 90% chance of empirically demonstrating a statistically significant correlation (Table 5.2). With more realistic conditions (i.e., criterion reliability of .80 and 50% preselection of clients), a sample size of at least 222 would be needed for good (90%) statistical power. Thus, the effect of criterion unreliability and subject preselection is to increase the necessary sample size required to detect a statistically significant correlation (Table 5.2). The sample sizes needed for adequate statistical power are much larger than has typically been assumed (Schmidt, Hunter, & Urry, 1976).

The parameters of sample size, selection ratio (preselection of clients), predictor reliability, and criterion reliability alone may account for inconsistent and inconclusive results in the search for prognostic indicators of treatment outcome. Schmidt and Hunter (1977) have provided an ingenious demonstration of this issue in their examination of validity outcomes across similar jobs in personnel settings. Although wide variation was observed in validation results from study to study, Schmidt and Hunter (1977) accounted for this distribution by a model that considered differences only in sample sizes, selection ratio, predictor reliability, and criterion reliability. The model assumed an identical correlation between the predictor and criterion in each study.

Another way of being "deceived" by empirical data is to fail to recognize that the measurement properties of a test may be altered if the new setting is appreciably different from the original context in which the measure was validated. For example, the reliability of a test that was developed in a heterogeneous sample of psychiatric patients may be substantially lower in a more homogeneous sample of patients with major depressive disorders. This at-

Table 5.2. Sample Sizes *(N)* Required for Power of .50 and .90 for Varying Criterion Reliability and Subject Preselection when True Validity = 0.35 ($\alpha = .05$, one-tailed)*

Degree of Preselection (Selection Ratio)	Criterion Reliability		
	1.00	.80	.60
1.00			
N (power = .90)	65	86	112
N (power = .50)	23	29	37
.70			
N (power = .90)	130	166	225
N (power = .50)	43	54	73
.50			
N (power = .90)	174	222	301
N (power = .50)	57	72	97
.30			
N (power = .90)	236	302	411
N (power = .50)	77	97	132

*Adapted from Schmidt, Hunter, and Urry (1976).

Table 5.3. Influence of Restriction of Range (Subject Preselection) on the Correlation Coefficient*

Degree of Preselection *(sd/SD)*	Original Correlation Coefficient		
	.30	.50	.70
.90	.27	.46	.66
.80	.24	.42	.62
.70	.21	.37	.57
.60	.19	.33	.51
.50	.15	.28	.44

*Adapted from McNemar (1969).
SD = standard deviation in original sample.
sd = standard deviation in restricted sample.

tenuation in reliability may be expected because of restriction of range in observed scores on the measure (McNemar, 1969). That is, if a broader range of subjects is studied the correlation will increase, and if a narrower range of subjects is examined the correlation will tend to decrease. Table 5.3 shows the influence on a correlation coefficient of varying levels of subject preselection. Restriction of range can occur when criteria for entrance to a treatment program restrict the range of scores on a test for the selected group.

Also, the predictive validity of an instrument may be dramatically altered by changes in the base rate. Consider a measure, such as the Social Stability Index (Skinner, 1981), that is being used to predict treatment outcome in an outpatient clinic for alcoholics. The intervention under study may be a traditional form of individual therapy or counseling. Socially stable clients scoring above a certain cutoff point on the Index are predicted to be "successful" in the treatment, whereas clients who are lower in social stability (below the cutoff) are predicted to be treatment "failures." Assume that a reasonably accurate outcome measure is available, which may be a composite of several variables, including alcohol consumption, work record, and family functioning. After a sample of clients ($N = 100$) has been treated and outcome data are collected, one may compare the *predicted* successes/failures from the Social Stability Index with the *actual* number of treatment successes/failures.

Figure 5.1 summarizes the four possible outcomes. Valid Positives *(VP)* occur when treatment success is predicted and success is obtained, whereas Valid Negatives *(VN)* occur when failure is predicted and it is obtained. False Positives *(FP)* take place when success is predicted but treatment failure occurs. False Negatives *(FN)* occur when treatment failure is predicted but success is obtained. The proportion of actual treatment successes $(VP + FN)$ is termed the Base Rate *(BR)*. The proportion of clients actually assigned to the treatment *(VP+FP)* is called the Selection Ratio *(SR)*. A key point is that the Base Rate *(BR)* and Selection Ratio *(SR)* constrain the degree of association that can exist between the predictor and criterion measures (Wiggins, 1973). For example, the effects of Base Rate and Selection Ratio upon test validity are illustrated in Figure 5.2. In his review of alcoholism treatment, Blane (1977) found that when outcomes are adjusted for dropouts during treatment, overall success rates are in the 25–50% range. Thus, a conservative estimate of 30% successes ($BR = 0.30$) is used in our example. When the Base Rate and Selection Ratio are equal ($BR = SR = 0.30$), the correlation coefficient (Φ) between the Social Stability Index and the outcome criterion has a theoretical limit of unity ($\Phi = 1.00$).

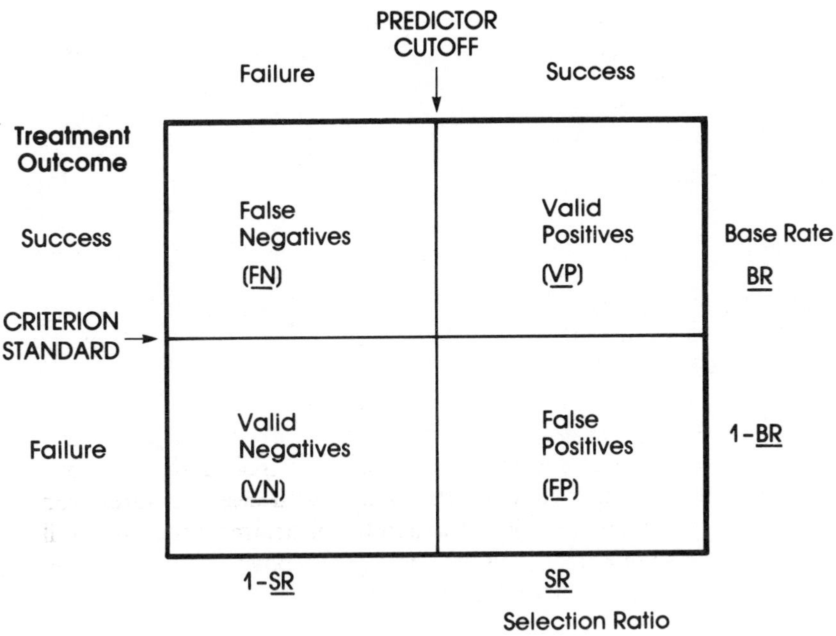

FIG. 5.1. Test Predictions and Treatment Outcomes.

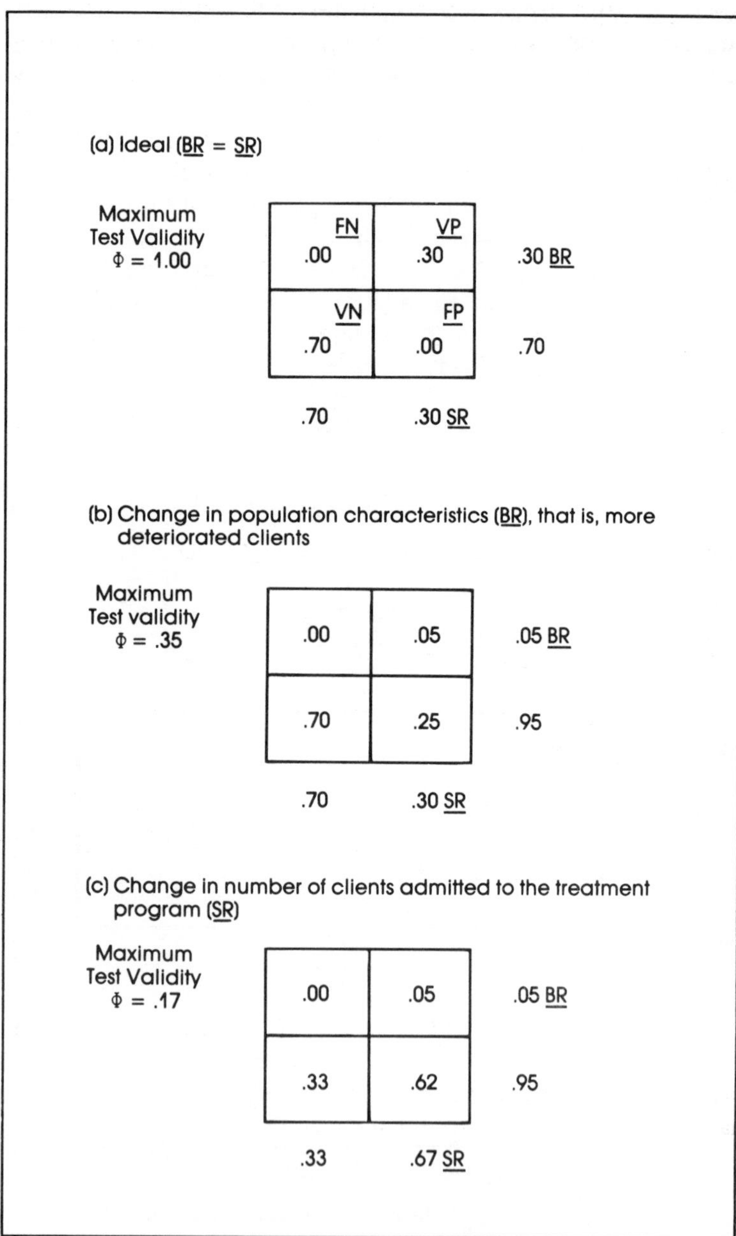

FIG. 5.2. Effect of Base Rate (BR) and Selection Ratio (SR) Upon Test Validity.

However, what if the client population were to shift over time such that more deteriorated clients presented for help at the clinic? These clients would have a poor prognosis and the Base Rate for successful treatment might be only 5% (*BR* = 0.05). As depicted in condition (b) of Figure 5.2, the maximum validity of the Social Stability Index would drop to 0.35 solely due to a change in the client population. Similarly, consider a situation where economic constraints have produced an administrative policy that requires a higher proportion of clients to be treated in this outpatient therapy. Perhaps a more costly inpatient program had to be closed, which resulted in the outpatient clinic having to assume care of more deteriorated clients. Consequently, two-thirds of the clients (*SR* = 0.67) are assigned to outpatient therapy. These administrative changes in the Selection Ratio result in a maximum validity coefficient of only 0.17. Thus, a measure with perfect prediction in one content can have its correlation with the outcome measure markedly decreased simply by changes in client characteristic *(BR)* or by alterations to the proportion of clients assigned to intervention *(SR)*. The message is clear: Whenever a test is used in a different context or circumstances change within a particular setting, appropriate reliability and validity checks must be made.

Too Many Variables/Not Enough Subjects

How often have you found yourself in the situation where you have a fairly large number of variables, but have data available from only a small number of subjects? This situation can be particularly treacherous if you are planning to use a multivariate technique, such as multiple regression analysis, where the expected value of the multiple correlation is not zero but is a function of the ratio of predictor variables to sample size (Cohen & Cohen, 1975). When examining a table of correlations, the probability of making at least one Type I error increases rapidly as the number of significance tests increases. Although procedures are available for guarding against this error rate (Larzelere & Mulaik, 1977), a careful reading of Paul Meehl's (1978) classic article on "tabular asterisks" is strongly recommended before the investigator compiles a large table of correlations.

Several approaches may be taken in order to reduce the number of variables to a manageable size. I would argue that the single most powerful data analytic technique is a "rational mind." Hence, the investigator should be able to select a small number of important variables based on theory and previous research. At the other extreme, I would recommend avoiding the use of entirely empirical procedures for variable selection, such as stepwise multiple regression or discriminant analysis. On a statistical basis, stepwise procedures are more likely to capitalize on chance and fail to replicate upon cross validation. A trivial difference may result in one variable entering the equation over another variable, even though the two measures may be equally important predictors of the criterion. Why should the investigator relegate his responsibility to the computer for selecting variables? It is rare that a study would be so exploratory that the investigator would not have some "hunches" regarding which measures are most important. The variables could be entered in a hierarchical fashion according to their (hypothesized) causal priority, and the statistical significance tested of increments to the multiple correlation. Cohen and Cohen (1975) provide full details on this powerful data analytic strategy.

Another strategy is to use a data reduction technique, such as principal components analysis (Gorsuch, 1974) or scaling procedures for data of rank order and categorical scale (Nishisato, 1980). Then, the "reduced" data set could be employed in subsequent analyses (Skinner, 1978a). For example, principal components analysis may be used to identify a parsimonious set of dimensions (factors) that reproduce reliable covariance among the variables of interest. The resulting factors may be interpreted as a descriptive model of relationships among variables; they may be used as a data-reduction technique for the generation of a small number of factor scales (scores) that may be explored in further analyses (e.g., as predictors in a multiple regression equation), and they may provide a basis for generating hypotheses that can be tested in future studies. Variables that are salient on a given factor could be combined to yield a simple index score. This strategy is useful for upgrading the metric quality of data since the composite score will be more normally distributed and conform more closely to an interval scale of measurement than the original variables (Gleason & Staelin, 1973). Also, the index score will be more reliable than any single variable in the linear combination (Nunnally, 1978).

A related problem is the issue of missing data, especially with respect to outcome measures. If the data may be assumed to be missing at random, then one may use various regression procedures to estimate the missing values (Frane, 1976). However, in clinical research there are often systematic reasons why one has failed to collect data on certain subjects. This is especially true with respect to treatment follow-up information, where it may be extremely difficult or impossible to locate subjects for whom the treatment has been less successful. Cohen and Cohen (1975) provide an excellent chapter on missing data and suggest the use of new variables (missing data dichotomies) to represent the absence of data. That is, a set of dummy variables are created that record either the presence (1) or absence (0) of data, and the missing data entries are filled with any constant. Then, the "missing data variable" is included as either part of the predictor or criterion sets of measures in subsequent analyses. This approach allows one to determine if there are systematic (nonrandom) factors that would account for missing data with specific subjects.

Misinterpretations of a Correlation Coefficient

Although correlational methods are taught in virtually every introductory statistics course, it is disquieting how often this simple index can be misinterpreted. The product-moment correlation coefficient *(r)* is sensitive only to *linear* relationships concerning the *relative ranking* of individuals on the two variables. Consider the following formula:

$$r_{xy} = \frac{\Sigma Z_x Z_y}{N}.$$

Basically, the correlation coefficient equals the average cross-product of standardized scores on the two variables (x and y). In moving from the original data to standard scores *(Z)*, the effect of level (variable mean) is removed and scatter (standard deviation) is set equal to 1.0 (Nunnally, 1978; Skinner, 1978b). Thus, one should always scrutinize the means and standard deviations for the original data when interpreting r. The distribution properties (skewness and kurtosis) and presence of outliers should be examined, since r can be adversely influenced by one or two outlying observations (Thissen, Baker, & Wainer, 1981; Wainer & Thissen, 1976).

For example, a relatively high correlation coefficient (e.g., 0.75) between subjects' and collaterals' reporting of an outcome measure such as alcohol use, would indicate only that the subjects and collaterals provided consistent rankings of which individuals drank low, moderate, and heavy amounts. This correlation does not provide any information about whether there may be a systematic difference in the actual level of alcohol consumption reported, nor does the index provide information on whether the data from one source may have considerably more variability or scatter.

A second source of misinterpretation is the failure to realize that one may have the same correlation coefficient (e.g., $r = .50$) but have different regression equations for the original data. Consider the linear regression equation for predicting $\hat{y}$ from x:

$$\hat{y} = ax + b,$$

where a is the slope and b is the intercept. The slope of the equation may be rewritten as:

$$a = \frac{S_y}{S_x} r_{xy},$$

where large S_x and S_y are the standard deviations for variables x and y, respectively. The slope of the original regression equation is influenced by the correlation coefficient as well as the scatter of each measure (Ehrenberg, 1978). The slope *a* measures the size of change in *y* that can be predicted for a unit change in *x*. With data in standardized form (*z* scores), the slope and correlation coefficient are identical (since $S_y = S_x = 1.0$). Thus, it is instructive to examine bivariate plots for both the original and standardized format. These plots (and an examination of residuals) may also indicate the presence of *non-linear* relationships that should be further explored.

Another major source of misinterpretation is the effect of sample size upon estimating the correlation coefficient. Table 5.4 summarizes the minimum correlation necessary for statistical significance at different sample sizes. With small samples that are characteristic of many clinical studies, a very large correlation coefficient is needed in order to achieve statistical significance. For example, with a sample size = 10 a correlation coefficient of 0.63 would be needed for significance at the .05 level. On the other hand, with large sample sizes that are characteristic in epidemiological studies, a very small correlation coefficient may achieve "statistical" significance but be of very small magnitude and have possibly limited "practical" significance.

Table 5.5 provides 95% confidence intervals for the correlation coefficient with varying sample sizes. As the sample becomes larger, there is a corresponding increase in the precision of estimating the underlying population correlation. With small samples that are common in clinical research, the sample *r* provides a rather poor estimate of the population parameter. Indeed, the confidence interval for the sample correlation coefficient is quite "flabby." For instance, with 30 subjects and an observed correlation of 0.50, the 95% confidence interval for this coefficient ranges between 0.17 to 0.73. In

Table 5.4. Minimum Correlation Necessary for Significance (2 tailed)* at Different Sample Sizes

Sample Size	Significance Level	
	.05	.01
10	.63	.77
20	.44	.56
30	.36	.46
40	.31	.40
50	.28	.36
100	.20	.26
200	.14	.18
500	.09	.11

*Adapted from Cohen (1977).

Table 5.5. Effect of Sample Size on 95% Confidence Intervals for the Correlation Coefficient

	Observed Correlation		
Sample Size	.30	.50	.70
10	−.41 to .78	−.19 to .86	.13 to .92
20	−.16 to .66	.07 to .77	.37 to .87
30	−.07 to .60	.17 to .73	.45 to .85
40	−.01 to .56	.22 to .70	.50 to .83
50	.02 to .53	.26 to .68	.52 to .82
100	.11 to .47	.34 to .63	.58 to .79
200	.17 to .42	.39 to .60	.62 to .76
500	.22 to .38	.43 to .56	.65 to .74

*Computational details are given by Cohen and Cohen (1975, pp. 56–58).

other words, one may conclude that the correlation coefficient is significantly greater than zero, but the underlying population correlation may range between the broad interval of 0.17 to 0.73 (the percentage of variance accounted for could range from 3% to 53%). You should pause and consider how often you have read a clinical study based on a small sample in which the investigator has drawn important conclusions from an observed correlation coefficient.

CAUSAL MODELING

Causal modeling techniques involve a generalized methodology for testing hypotheses with nonexperimental data. This methodology presents a marriage between factor analysis and path analysis traditions. A causal model consists of two elements. First, a *measurement model* specifies relationships between observed measures and latent variables or constructs as in factor analysis. For instance, a latent construct such as the trait anxiety may be measured by different techniques (self-report scales, behavioral ratings, physiological responses), where the factor loadings represent different relationships between the observed measures and the underlying construct. The use of factor analysis techniques has a long tradition in the study of intelligence and personality. Second, a *structural relations model* specifies the hypothesized pattern of causal influence among latent variables as a set of regression equations similar to path analysis. Although path analysis techniques have been widely used in sociological research (Duncan, 1966), this methodology has received less attention by psychologists until quite recently (Werts & Linn, 1970).

A good illustration of causal modeling is given in a recent article by Aneshensel and Huba (1983). They collected longitudinal data at four time periods in order to study relationships among depression, alcohol use and smoking. A simplified version of their causal model is given in Figure 5.3. The latent construct of depression was measured using four instruments, alcohol use was measured by two variables (quantity and frequency), and smoking was measured by the quantity of cigarettes consumed. The measurement aspect of the causal model in Figure 1 is depicted by the unidirectional arrows between the latent variable (circle) and the observed measures (boxes). The structural relations aspect of the causal model is shown as unidirectional arrows originating at one latent variable and pointing at another latent variable. The complete model is estimated simultaneously using maximum-likelihood procedures. Different models may be tested by examining the increments in goodness-of-fit of more restricted models (Bentler & Bonett, 1980). Aneshensel and Huba (1983) found that current levels of depression are dependent upon depression levels at all previously measured times. Alcohol use may lead to decreased levels of depression in the short time period. However, over longer periods of time alcohol use leads to a slightly heightened depression level. This study suggests that the immediate effect of alcohol use is to decrease levels of depression, whereas the long term impact of alcohol use is a further heightening of depression levels.

The statistician, Karl Joreskog, is generally recognized as the principal developer of causal modeling techniques by his work on statistical theory (Joreskog, 1978; Joreskog & Sorbom, 1979) and by his development of computer software programs, especially LISREL (Joreskog & Sorbom, 1978). An excellent introduction and review of causal modeling is given by Bentler (1980). The development of rigorous and generalized methods for causal modeling is a statistical revolution that may parallel the adoption of analysis of variance procedures in the 1940s (Rucci & Tweney, 1980). However, causal modeling techniques are still quite new, expensive and time-consuming to use. Technical difficulties remain to be solved regarding parameter estimation, and much needs to be learned about practical strategies for using the methodology effectively.

There is a real danger of being awed by this methodology. Cliff (1983) cautions that "somehow the use of one of these computer programs lends an air of unchallengable sanctity to conclusions that would otherwise be subjected to the most intense scrutiny" (p. 116). Cliff's (1983) article is "must" reading for any prospective user of causal modeling techniques. He discusses four well-established principles of scientific inference that may be obscured in the over-zealous rush to use sophisticated causal modeling techniques:

1. Data do not confirm a model, they only fail to disconfirm it because of the possible influence of variables that are not observed,

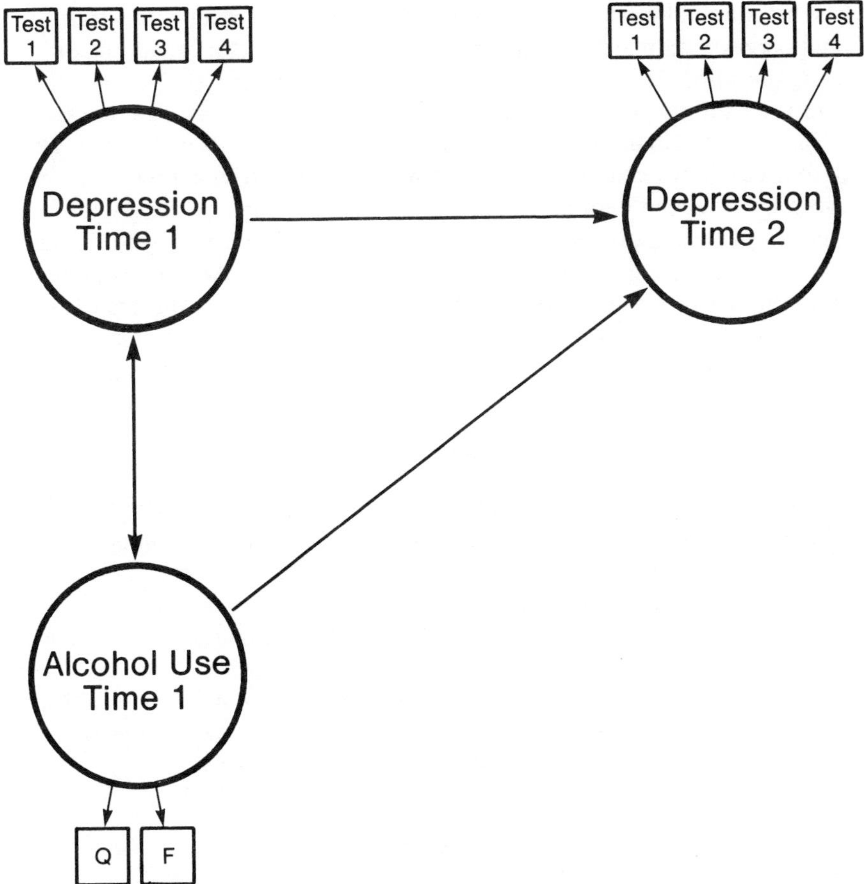

FIG. 5.3. Simplified Version of the Causal Model of Depression and Alcohol Use Evaluated by Aneshensel and Huba (1983). The construct Depression was assessed by four tests (1. CES-D, 2. hopelessness, 3. well-being, 4. death ideation), and the construct Alcohol Use was assessed by drinking Frequency *(F)* and Quantity *(Q)* consumed during the past 2 Months.

2. Correlation does not imply causation even when variables are separated in time,
3. Just because we name something (propose a structural model) does not mean that we have a scientific understanding of the processes involved, and
4. Ex post facto explanations are untrustworthy.

Paths between latent variables in the model are regression coefficients (beta weights), and all of the cautions learned about interpreting beta weights in multiple regression analysis should be observed. For instance, adding or deleting one variable from the model can dramatically alter the beta weights. Another issue concerns the use of the chi square statistic as a goodness-of-fit index. With small samples, a number of models may provide a plausible fit to the data, whereas in very large samples the most trivial discrepancy between a model and data may result in the model being rejected by the chi-square test. Bentler and Bonett (1980) have suggested alternative indices, and also recommend a step-up procedure for model testing. Another concern is the extent to which causal modeling procedures may capitalize on chance associations in the data. Further work is needed on the development of cross-validation strategies.

SUMMARY

In conclusion, this chapter has reviewed common problems in the use of correlational methods and has provided a commentary on causal modeling techniques, which appear to be the next revolution in data analysis in the social sciences. Even simple correlational methods are open to various misinterpretations and abuses. One should be well versed on these issues before embarking on the use of more sophisticated multivariate techniques. Although many excellent textbooks are available, there is no substitute for practical experience with these techniques. Data analysis is an "art" which involves considerable skills beyond the cookbook application of statistical methods.

REFERENCES

Aneshensel, C.S., & Huba, G.J. (1983). Depression, alcohol use, and smoking over one year: A four-wave longitudinal causal model. *Journal of Abnormal Psychology, 92,* 134–150.

Beck, A.T. (1972). *Depression: Causes and treatment.* Philadelphia: University of Philadelphia Press.

Bentler, P.M. (1980). Multivariate analysis with latent variables: Causal modelling. *Annual Review of Psychology, 31,* 419–456.

Bentler, P.M., & Bonett, D.G. (1980). Significance tests and goodness-of-fit in the analyses of covariance structures. *Psychological Bulletin, 88,* 588–606.

Blane, H.T. (1977). Issues in the evaluation of alcoholism treatment. *Professional Psychology, 8,* 593–608.

Bollen, K.A., & Barb, K.H. (1981). Pearson's *r* and coarsely categorized measures. *American Sociological Review, 46,* 232–239.

Cliff, N. (1983). Some cautions concerning the application of causal modelling methods. *Multivariate Behavioral Research, 18,* 115–126.

Cohen, J. (1977). *Statistical power analysis for the behavioral sciences* (rev. ed.). New York: Academic Press.

Cohen, J., & Cohen, P. (1975). *Applied multiple regression/correlation analysis for the behavioral sciences.* Hillsdale, NJ: Lawrence Erlbaum.

Dawes, R.M. (1979). The robust beauty of improper linear models in decision making. *American Psychologist, 34,* 571-582.

Duncan, O.D. (1966). Path analysis: Sociological examples. *American Journal of Sociology, 72,* 1-16.

Ehrenberg, A.S.C. (1978). *Data reduction: Analyzing and interpreting statistical data.* New York: Wiley.

Frane, J.W. (1976). Some simple procedures for handing missing data in multivariate analysis. *Psychometrika, 41,* 409-415.

Gleason, T.C., & Staelin, R. (1973). Improving the metric quality of questionnaire data. *Psychometrika, 38,* 393-410.

Gorsuch, R.L. (1974). *Factor analysis.* Philadelphia: Saunders.

Green, B.F. (1977). Parameter sensitivity in multivariate methods. *Multivariate Behavioral Research, 12,* 263-288.

Gulliksen, H. (1974). Looking back and ahead in psychometrics. *American Psychologist, 29,* 251-261.

Hatzenbuehler, L.C., Parpal, M., & Matthews, L. (1983). Classifying college students as depressed or nondepressed using the Beck Depression Inventory: An empirical analysis. *Journal of Consulting and Clinical Psychology, 51,* 360-366.

Humphreys, L.G. (1978). Doing research the hard way: Substituting analysis of variance for a problem in correlational analysis. *Journal of Educational Psychology, 70,* 873-876.

Joreskog, K.G. (1978). Structural analysis of covariance and correlation matrices. *Psychometrika, 43,* 443-477.

Joreskog, K.G., & Sorbom, D. (1978). *LISREL IV: Analysis of linear structural relationships by the method of maximum likelihood.* Chicago: National Educational Resources.

Joreskog, K.G., & Sorbom, D. (1979). *Advances in factor analysis and structural equation models.* Cambridge, MA: Abt Books.

Larzelere, R.E., & Mulaik, S.A. (1977). Single-sample tests for many correlations. *Psychological Bulletin, 84,* 557-569.

McNemar, Q. (1969). *Psychological statistics* (4th ed.). New York: Wiley.

Meehl, P.E. (1978). Theoretical risks and tabular asterisks: Sir Karl, Sir Ronald, and the slow progress of soft psychology. *Journal of Consulting and Clinical Psychology, 46,* 806-834.

Nishisato, S. (1980). *Analysis of categorical data: Dual scaling and application.* Toronto: University of Toronto Press.

Nunnally, J.C. (1978). *Psychometric theory* (2nd ed.). New York: McGraw-Hill.

Ogborne, A.C. (1978). Patient characteristics as predictors of treatment outcomes for alcohol and drug abuse. In Y. Israel, F.B. Glaser, H. Kalant, R.E. Popham, W. Schmidt & R.G. Smart (Eds.), *Research advances in alcohol and drug problems* (Vol. 4). New York: Plenum.

Rotter, J.B. (1966). Generalized expectancies for internal versus external control of reinforcement. *Psychological Monographs, 80*(1), (Whole No. 609).

Rucci, A.J., & Tweney, R.D. (1980). Analysis of variance and the "second" discipline of scientific psychology: A historical account. *Psychological Bulletin, 87,* 166–184.

Schmidt, F.L., & Hunter, J.E. (1977). Development of a general solution to the problem of validity generalization. *Journal of Applied Psychology, 62,* 529–540.

Schmidt, F.L., Hunter, J.E., & Urry, V.W. (1976). Statistical power in criterion-related validation studies. *Journal of Applied Psychology, 61,* 473–485.

Skinner, H.A. (1981). Assessment of alcohol problems: Basic principles, critical issues and future trends. In Y. Israel, F.B. Glaser, H. Kalant, R.E. Popham, W. Schmidt & R.G. Smart (Eds.), *Research advances in alcohol and drug problems* (Vol. 6). New York: Plenum.

Skinner, H.A. (1978a). The art of exploring predictor-criterion relationships. *Psychological Bulletin, 85,* 327–337.

Skinner, H.A. (1978b). Differentiating the contribution of elevation, scatter and shape in profile similarity. *Educational and Psychological Measurement, 38,* 297–308.

Skinner, H.A., & Blashfield, R.K. (1982). Increasing the impact of cluster analysis research: The case of psychiatric classification. *Journal of Consulting and Clinical Psychology, 50,* 727–735.

Tatsuoka, M.M. (1971). *Multivariate analysis.* New York: Wiley.

Thissen, D., Baker, L., & Wainer, H. (1981). Insolence-enhanced scatter plots. *Psychological Bulletin, 90,* 179–184.

Wainer, H., & Thissen, D. (1976). Three steps toward robust regression. *Psychometrika, 41,* 9–34.

Werts, C.E., & Linn, R.L. (1970). Path analysis: Psychological examples. *Psychological Bulletin, 74,* 193–212.

Wiggins, J.S. (1973). *Personality and prediction: Principles of personality assessment.* Reading, MA: Addison-Wesley.

Part 3
RESEARCH TOPICS

6
Personality

William Ickes

INTRODUCTION

Research in personality involves two major phases. The first phase, *assessment*, is concerned with the development of a valid and reliable means of measuring the personality trait or disposition of interest to the researcher. This phase includes, but is not necessarily limited to, such activities as the construction of an appropriate personality measure (e.g., paper-and-pencil test, structured interview), the psychometric refinement of the measure (e.g., to ensure a reasonably high level of internal consistency and reliability), and the discriminant and convergent validation of the measure (e.g., through its intercorrelation with other measures that are assumed to be conceptually similar versus distinct). This assessment phase of personality research is characterized by a fairly high level of methodological sophistication. However, because the methodological issues relating to personality assessment and test construction are considered in some detail in Chapter 10, they will not be discussed here.

The second major phase of research in personality incorporates everything not included in the assessment phase. This second phase, which might be called *application*, provides the focus of this chapter. A variety of research activities are included in this phase. These range from construct validation studies designed to determine whether or not the personality measure predicts its criterial behaviors (i.e., Does it appear to measure the trait it is supposed to measure?) through deductive (theory-testing) and inductive (theory-building) studies, to studies designed simply to answer some practical question (e.g., Does the personality measure predict which type of clients will respond better to a self-administered versus therapist-administered treatment program?)

Given the constraints on the length of this chapter, it would be difficult to discuss the range of methodological issues implicated in these various research activities if each type of application were considered separately. For-

Acknowledgements: Much of the material in this chapter appeared in earlier papers by Ickes (1981, 1982) and by Snyder & Ickes (in press). The author would like to thank Mark Snyder for his comments on the manuscript.

tunately, however, the most important methodological concerns are common to all of the applications described above. The reason for this commonality is that all of these research applications, in one way or another, force the researcher to deal with the problem of the degree of *correspondence* between personality traits and their criterial behaviors.

The correspondence problem is central in that it implicates most, if not all, of the important methodological issues encountered in the application phase of personality research. For this reason, the first section of the chapter provides a brief discussion of the correspondence problem and then describes how various researchers, in their attempts to come to grips with this problem, have provided the theoretical and methodological foundations for an alternative approach (i.e., the *moderating variable approach*) to the study of personality. In the second section, the insights of the moderating variable approach are translated into some general methodological prescriptions for clinical research in personality. In the third section, a personality study conducted by the author is reviewed and evaluated in terms of the methodological considerations discussed throughout the chapter.

THE CORRESPONDENCE PROBLEM AND THE MODERATING VARIABLE SOLUTION

For most of this century, theory and research in personality has been guided by the assumptions of a dispositional or trait approach. This approach seeks to understand consistencies in behavior "in terms of relatively stable traits, enduring dispositions and other propensities that are thought to reside 'within' individuals," (Snyder & Ickes, in press). When used effectively in personality research, the application of the dispositional approach typically constitutes a two-stage "bootstrapping" process. In the first stage of this process, contrasting personality types are identified who presumably differ in the regularity and consistency with which they display criterial behaviors of particular interest to the researcher. Work conducted during this stage concerns the development of an assessment instrument or measurement procedure, the psychometric refinement of such a measure, and subsequent attempts to establish its reliability and validity through appropriate empirical tests.

If the work conducted during this assessment and validation stage is successful, a second, "bootstrapping" stage begins in which the newly validated measure is now used to expand the researcher's conception of the particular clinical or social psychological phenomenon that the measure was designed to address. In this bootstrapping stage, researchers are not content with merely validating their personality measure in terms of criterial behaviors that have been specified a priori. Instead, they explore a range of previously unexamined behaviors in order: (a) to determine the boundary conditions for the clinical or social psychological phenomenon of interest, or (b) to examine the processes underlying the phenomenon at a level of detail not permitted by the relatively simplistic conception that guided the researchers' earlier validation work.

Although the application of the dispositional approach can be quite impressive when the two-stage process described above is successfully realized, a number of problems with the approach have nonetheless been noted (Snyder & Ickes, in press). From a conceptual standpoint, the approach tends to be relatively atheoretical almost by definition. The researcher who adopts this approach need not start with a theory of the phenomenon of interest and then proceed to test it directly. Instead, often in a virtual admission of ignorance, the researcher may begin by simply trying to identify individuals who, by their own self-reports or those of others, frequently manifest the phenomenon in their own behavior. Although the researcher's successful identification and subsequent study of such individuals (and their contrasting counterparts) may indeed lead to the inductive development of a well-articulated theory regarding the phenomenon of interest, it is important to note that such theory typically is the endpoint of the application of the dispositional approach and *not* its starting point. Moreover, to the extent that researchers' intuitions fail to generate profitable leads during the bootstrapping stage, the application of the dispositional approach will fail to provide much insight into the clinical or social psychological phenomenon of interest.

Other criticisms of the dispositional approach have questioned its central assumption that measures of traits and disposition are really useful in predicting behavior. A rather general criticism is that the approach gives too much emphasis to dispositional factors and not enough emphasis to situational ones (e.g., Alker, 1972; Bem, 1972; Bowers, 1973; Mischel, 1968). A more specific criticism is that the approach fails to specify in operational terms exactly how the hypothesized "consistency" or "correspondence" between traits and their criterial behaviors should be defined (e.g., Block, 1968; Magnusson & Endler, 1977). A third, and perhaps more damning, criticism is that dispositions traditionally have accounted for only a small portion of the variance in the behaviors they have been used to predict (e.g., Argyle & Little, 1972; Bem, 1972; Bowers, 1973; Fiske, 1974; Mischel, 1968, 1973; Peterson, 1965, 1968; Sarason, Smith, & Diener, 1975). Mischel (1968), for example, has reviewed diverse sources of evidence that seem to suggest that measures of consistency in personality (whether they assess the correspondence between test and nontest manifestations of traits, or measures of behavioral consistency across situations) seldom yield correlations higher than .30.

The implications of this last criticism for the dispositional strategy seemed rather devastating. If this criticism were valid, dispositions would, in general, be expected to exhibit only weak predictive validity and only weak consistency across situations. This pessimistic view of Mischel and others was widely publicized and helped contribute to a growing sense of disenchantment with personality research in general and with the trait approach in particular. In essence, it was assumed that if personality traits were generally such poor predictors of behavior, the fault must lie in the specific personality traits or in the trait concept itself, and not in the methods used to measure these traits or test their validity. To believe otherwise was to assume that of the thousands of personality studies conducted over four decades of research, the overwhelming majority were methodologically deficient in one or more respects. It is easy to see why the first of these assumptions would have been preferred over the second; however, the events of recent years suggest that that second assumption is the more correct. It now appears that personality research has been plagued throughout its history by fundamental methodological flaws that are only beginning to receive the attention they deserve.

As researchers and theorists sought reasons for the poor predictive validity of personality traits, it became apparent that traits could not be used to predict the behavior of "all of the people, all of the time" (Bem & Allen, 1974). Instead, the predictive validity of traits was acknowledged to be limited such that accurate predictions could be made only some of the time—that is, for some people in some situations, and then only for some traits and some criterial behaviors. Subsequent theoretical and empirical efforts were therefore directed toward identifying the *moderating variables* that distinguish the instances in which traits do correspond to behaviors from those in which they do not.

In a review of these developments, Snyder and Ickes (in press) have identified four categories of moderating variables that determine the degree of correspondence between personality traits and their criterial behaviors. These categories, as represented in Table 6.1, include: (1) those relating to the *predictor* (i.e., to the particular trait or disposition being studied); (2) those relating to the *criterion* (i.e., to the particular behavior(s) to which the predictor is being applied); (3) those relating to the *person* whose behavior one is attempting to predict; and (4) those relating to the *situation* in which the prediction occurs. Moderating variables in the first category answer the question "Which traits?" by specifying the types of traits and dispositions that will or will not be good predictors of behavior. Moderating variables in the second category answer the question "Which behaviors?" by specifying the types of behaviors that traits and dispositions are or are not likely to predict. Moderating variables in the third and fourth categories answer the questions "Which people?" and "Which situations?" by specifying for which types of people and in which types of situations a given trait or disposition will or will not predict its criterial behavior(s).

Although space precludes a detailed discussion of all of the moderating variables that have been identified to date (see Snyder & Ickes, in press, for a more complete review), some of the more important and/or representative moderating variables are considered, by categories, in the following sections.

Table 6.1. Four Categories of Moderating Variables*

Category	Function	Representative Examples	References
Predictor moderating variables	Specify the types of traits and dispositions that will or will not be good predictors of behavior	Self-reported consistency of the predictor	Bem & Allen (1974)
		Self-reported observability of the predictor	Kenrick & Stringfield (1980)
Criterion moderating variables	Specify the types of behaviors that traits and dispositions will or will not predict	Multiple-act measures of the behavioral criterion	Jaccard (1979)
		Prototypicality of the behavioral criterion	Buss & Craik (1980)
Personal moderating variables	Specify for which types of people traits and dispositions will or will not predict their criterial behaviors	Self-monitoring	Snyder (1979)
		Self-consciousness	Carver & Scheier
Situational moderating variables	Specify in which types of situations traits and dispositions will or will not predict their criterial behaviors	"Weak" versus "strong" situations	Ickes (1982)
		Precipitating versus nonprecipitating situations	Snyder & Ickes (in press)

*Adapted from Snyder & Ickes (in press).

"Which Traits?": Predictor Moderating Variables

The search for predictor moderating variables is based on the assumption that some types of trait or dispositional measures are relatively good predictors of their criterial behavior(s), whereas other trait or dispositional measures are relatively poor predictors of behavior. Two such predictor moderating variables that have been proposed and studied are the self-reported *cross-situational consistency* of the predictor (e.g., Bem & Allen, 1974) and the self-reported *observability* of the predictor (Kenrick & Stringfield, 1980). Regarding the first variable, Bem and Allen (1974) reported that, for individuals who described themselves as cross-situationally consistent in displaying their characteristic levels of friendliness, the correlation between assessed extraversion and actual friendly behavior ($r = .51$) was substantially larger than the same correlation for individuals who reported low cross-situational consistency in their display of friendliness ($r = .31$). They also reported that the actual cross-situational consistency of friendly behavior was greater for individuals in the first group than for those in the second. Bem and Allen concluded that trait measures which take into account the self-reported cross-situational consistency of the trait in question will generally predict their criterial behaviors better than measures that do not (see also Kenrick & Stringfield, 1980; Turner & Gilliland, 1979; and Underwood & Moore, 1981).

A second predictor moderating variable, the self-reported observability of the predictor, was investigated by Kenrick and Stringfield (1980), who asked individuals to rate the extent to which their behavior in each of 16 trait domains was publicly observable. Results indicated that behavioral consistency was reliably greater ($r = .68$) for trait domains that subjects rated high on public observability (e.g., introverted-extroverted) than for trait domains rated low on public observability ($r = .49$, e.g., emotional/stable). Thus, traits whose criterial behaviors are publicly observable may demonstrate better predictive validity than those whose criterial behaviors are not easily verified by outside observers.

Why should self-reported consistency and self-reported observability function as predictor moderating variables? According to Snyder and Ickes (in press):

> Their success derives, in part or whole, from the fact that each procedure solicits evidence of requirements that, of necessity, must be fulfilled before behavior can and will be predictable from measures of traits and dispositions. Behavior must be stable from situation to situation before measures of traits and dispositions collected in one situation will predict behavioral measures of those traits and dispositions collected in other situations. And, public actions must be meaningful reflections of private traits and dispositions before measures of traits and dispositions will predict behavioral manifestations of those traits and dispositions.

"Which Behaviors?": Criterion Moderating Variables

The search for criterion moderating variables is based on the assumption that some criterial behaviors can be predicted relatively well by trait or dispositional measures, whereas other behaviors can be predicted only poorly or not at all by such measures. Two of the more important criterion moderating variables that have been proposed and studied are *multiple-act vs. single-act measures* of the behavioral criterion (e.g., Jaccard, 1979) and the *prototypicality* of the behavioral criterion (e.g., Buss & Craik, 1980).

Perhaps the most intense reaction to Mischel's (1968, 1973) pessimistic reviews of personality research has come from writers who have argued that the generally low personality-behavior correlations of .30 or less are largely artifacts of unreliable measurement. According to this argument, because most of the studies on which Mischel's conclusions were based employed single-act measures of the criterial behavior (i.e., measures for which error of measurement tends to be relatively high and the probability of sampling trait-determined behavior relatively low), the indices of predictive validity obtained in these studies were necessarily of low magnitude. However, as several investigators (e.g., Block, 1971; Epstein, 1979, 1980; Hartshorne & May, 1928–30; Jaccard, 1974, 1979) have demonstrated, when the behavioral measure takes the form of a multiple-act measure (i.e., repeated measures that are aggregated to yield a single summary score), measures of trait-behavior correspondence can yield very high values, frequently in the range of .60 and above. Thus, criteria that assess general patterns of trait-relevant behavior (i.e., aggregated summaries of behavior sampled across time, situation, etc.) can be predicted relatively well from trait or dispositional measures, even though criteria that assess specific, single-act behaviors may be predicted poorly or not at all.

To further improve the predictability of the behavioral criterion, Buss and Craik (1980) have recommended that researchers be sensitive to another criterion moderating variable—the prototypicality of the behavior with respect to the trait being studied. These authors reported that the self-reported behaviors most prototypic (i.e., best examples, central members) of the trait domain of dominance (e.g., monopolizing conversation, taking command of the situation) were highly predictable from measures of the trait of dominance. In contrast, the self-reported behaviors least prototypic of dominance (e.g., asking someone out on a date, using flattery in order to get one's way) were only weakly predictable from the dominance trait measure. In subsequent research, Buss and Craik (1981) have replicated their findings for dominance and extended their approach to the successful prediction of self-reported acts of aloofness and gregariousness.

Why do multiple-act measures of the behavioral criterion and the prototypicality of the criterion both function as effective criterion moderating variables? According to Snyder and Ickes (in press):

> At the very least, it may be the case that multiple-act criteria succeed because they provide more reliable samples of the relevant behavioral domain than do single-act criteria. And, also at the very least, it may be the case that prototypic measures of the behavioral criterion succeed because they provide more valid measures of the behavioral domain than do non-prototypic measures. From this perspective, any and all procedures that augment the reliability and validity of the assessment of behavioral criteria should also enhance the extent to which those behavioral criteria can be predicted from measures of relevant traits, dispositions, attitudes, and other characteristics of the individual.

"Which People?": Personal Moderating Variables

The search for personal moderating variables is based on the assumption that there are some types of individuals whose behavior is predictable from measures of their traits, dispositions, attitudes, etc., whereas there are other types of individuals whose behavior is not predictable from such measures but is guided by situational influences instead. Two of the better-investigated personal moderating variables are self-monitoring (Snyder, 1974, 1979) and *self-consciousness* (Fenigstein, Scheier, & Buss, 1975; for reviews, see Buss, 1980, and Carver & Scheier, 1981). A list of other personal moderating variables that have been identified and studied can be found in Snyder and Ickes (in press).

According to Snyder's (1974, 1979) conception of self-monitoring, some individuals (high self-monitoring individuals) monitor and regulate their behavior on the basis of situational information, whereas others (low self-monitoring individuals) monitor and regulate their behavior on the basis of information provided by their own internalized traits, dispositions, attitudes, self-conceptions, and so on. Consistent with this conception, research has indicated that high self-monitoring individuals: (a) exhibit considerable situation-to-situation specificity in their behavior (e.g., Lippa, 1976, 1978; Rarick, Soldow, & Geiser, 1976; Shaffer, Smith, & Tomarelli, 1982; Snyder & Monson, 1975), and (b) display minimal consistency between their behavior and relevant underlying personal attributes (e.g., Snyder & Swann, 1976; Snyder & Tanke, 1976). By contrast, low self-monitoring individuals have been shown to: (a) exhibit considerable cross-situational stability (e.g., Lippa, 1976, 1978a, 1978b; Lippa & Mash, 1979; Snyder & Monson, 1975) and temporal stability (e.g., Lutsky, Woodworth, & Clayton, 1980) in their behavior, and (b) display substantial correspondence between their behavior and the dispositions presumed to underlie it (e.g., Ajzen, Timko, & White, 1981; Becherer & Richard, 1978; Ickes, Layden, & Barnes, 1978; Lippa, 1978a, 1978b; Snyder & Tanke, 1976; Zanna, Olson, & Fazio, 1980; Zuckerman & Reis, 1978).

The notion that the behavior of some individuals is guided primarily by their traits, attitudes, and other dispositions whereas the behavior of other individuals is guided primarily by situational and social cues is also inherent in Fenigstein, Scheier, and Buss's (1975) conception of individual differences in self-consciousness. According to this conception, individuals who score high on a factor called private self-consciousness are chronically and habitually aware of their attitudes, dispositions, and motives, etc., and the heightened awareness of these dispositions results in their serving as salient cues to guide and channel the individuals' behavior. In contrast, individuals who score low on the private self-consciousness factor are assumed to be relatively unaware of their traits and dispositions, and are therefore much more susceptible to situational, as opposed to dispositional, influences. Evidence supporting these distinctions has been found in studies conducted by Scheier (1976), Scheier, Buss, and Buss (1978), Scheier and Carver (1977), and Turner (1978). For example, Scheier, Buss, and Buss (1978) found that self-rated aggressiveness correlated strongly with actual aggressive behavior for subjects high in private self-consciousness ($r = .66$), but not for subjects low in private self-consciousness ($r = .09$).

What are the criteria that seem to characterize successful personal moderating variables? According to Snyder & Ickes (in press):

> To the extent that we can generalize from the cases of self-monitoring and private self-consciousness, . . . it would appear that a psychological construct will perform successfully as a personal moderating variable to the extent that it validly and reliably taps those processes by which information about the self and information about . . . situations are attended to and utilized in guiding . . . behavior.

In other words, any personal moderating variable will succeed to the extent that it distinguishes individuals on the basis of their preferential attentiveness and responsiveness to dispositional versus situational information as guides to action in particular behavioral domains.

"Which Situations?": Situational Moderating Variables

The search for situational moderating variables is based on the assumption that there are some types of situations in which traits and dispositions will serve as relatively good predictors of their criterial behavior(s), whereas there are other types of situations in which traits and dispositions will serve as relatively poor predictors of their criterial behavior(s).

"Strong" versus "Weak" Situations. According to Snyder and Ickes (in press), the most important situational moderating variable can be conceptualized as the "strength" versus "weakness" of situations as they are experienced by the individual. In general, psychologically "strong" situations tend to be those that provide salient cues to guide behavior and have a fairly high degree of structure and definition. These situations may be regarded as highly "scripted" in the sense intended by Abelson (e.g., Abelson, 1976; Schank & Abelson, 1977). In contrast, psychologically "weak" situations tend to be those that do not offer salient cues to guide behavior, are relatively unstructured and ambiguous, and are only weekly "scripted" if at all.

The methodological implications of the "strong/weak" distinction for research in personality have been explored by Ickes (Ickes, 1982, 1983; Snyder & Ickes, in press), who has made the following observations. First, and perhaps most obvious, measures of traits and dispositions should typically predict behavior better in "weak" situations than in "strong" ones (cf. Mischel, 1977). Ironically, however, the most cursory examination of the published literature in personality suggests that the overwhelming majority of personality studies are conducted in highly structured, psychologically "strong" laboratory situations in which salient and relatively unambiguous cues are provided to guide behavior. Conversely, only a small minority of personality studies are conducted in psychologically "weak," unstructured situations in which individuals are forced to rely primarily on their own internal traits and dispositions to guide their behavior.

Second, Ickes has suggested that the inappropriate reliance of personality researchers on the psychologically "strong" test situation, epitomized by the experiment, has resulted not only from psychology's tradition of training graduate students in this approach but also from the historical lack of alternative paradigms for the study of personality. Because the experiment historically evolved as a procedure for "isolating and measuring the effects" of situational variables, its application in psychology has typically been one in which "the independent variable (a situational manipulation) is designed and programmed to occur in a fixed and constant fashion, independently of the behavior of the subject" (Monson & Snyder, 1977, p. 97). This type of "strong situation" procedure makes sense when the researcher is attempting to study the impact of situational factors on behavior, since it ideally maximizes the variance in behavior due to the particular situational factor(s) under investigation while minimizing the "error" variance due, among other things, to individual differences in personality. It is easy to see, therefore, how researchers who use experimental designs exclusively might forget that individual difference variance need not always be regarded as mere "error" or "noise," since in terms of their research that is all it is.

What is less easy to see is why most personality researchers (who presumably should know better) should have succumbed to the temptation of relying so heavily on the experimental paradigm in their personality research. Obviously, for personality researchers and others who are interested in influence on behavior of dispositional factors, the variance due to individual differences is *effect* variance, not "error" variance. Therefore, unlike the experimentalists, these researchers should prefer to use paradigms in which such variance is not minimized but is maximized instead. The irony is that many personality researchers, by using carefully structured experimental situations, may thereby eliminate much of the same individual difference variance they are in fact purporting to study!

Another reason why traditional research paradigms in personality may not provide optimal situations for demonstrating trait-behavior correspondence has been suggested by Monson and his colleagues (Monson, McDaniel, Menteer, & Williams, 1983). This reason, which appears blindingly obvious in retrospect, is the simple statistical fact that the magnitude of any correlation is restricted to the extent that the range of either or both of the correlated variables is restricted. In typical studies of personality conducted in the field, trait-behavior correlations are obtained in naturalistic situations to which subjects have often self-selected because of the congruence between the "structure" of these situations and the subjects' personalities. To the degree that these naturalistic situations are structured to promote such self-selection, the ranges of both the dispositional predictor variable and the behavioral criterion variable will be restricted, and any resulting correlation will necessarily be relatively low. Similarly, in typical studies of personality conducted in structured laboratory settings, the structure of the task will generally impose normative constraints on behavior that restrict the range of appropriate behavior on the criterion variable and also limit the magnitude of the trait-behavior correlations. Thus, in *both* of the traditional settings for personality research, the statistical artifact of restricted range operates to virtually guarantee the low trait-behavior correlations that have so concerned various researchers and theorists in the field.

Research which addresses these problems associated with the use of psychologically "strong," highly structured test situations has been conducted by Ickes and his colleagues and by Monson and his colleagues. Ickes (1982, 1983) has developed a research paradigm for the study of personality influences on social behavior occurring in a psychologically "weak" (i.e., relatively unstructured and ambiguous) interaction situation. In studies employing this paradigm, two individuals with no past history of interaction whose traits or dispositions have previously been assessed are left alone together in a "waiting room" where they are free to interact or not, as they choose. Because the individuals have not been instructed to interact, and because other external cues to guide their behavior are lacking, they essentially are forced to depend on internalized dispositions to guide their spontaneous interaction behavior.

Theoretically, the correspondence between traits and behavior should be optimal in this type of paradigm, not only because the "weak" situation minimizes the impact of situational cues while maximizing the impact of dispositional ones but also because the researcher can ensure that the ranges of both the predictor and criterion variables are not restricted through subject self-selection or through the operation of powerful situational constraints on behavior. Consistent with this reasoning, studies employing the paradigm have repeatedly demonstrated strong influences on social behavior of trait and dispositional variables such as self-monitoring (Barnes & Ickes, 1979; Ickes & Barnes, 1977), gender and sex-role orientation (Ickes & Barnes, 1978; Ickes, Schermer, & Steeno, 1979; LaFrance & Ickes, 1981; Lamke & Bell, 1982), locus of control (Rajecki, Ickes, & Tanford, 1981), and birth order (Ickes & Turner, 1983). The dispositional influences found in these studies generally yield larger mean differences and F-ratios than those obtained in studies using more structured interaction paradigms (cf. Duncan & Fiske, 1977), and such differences are typically evident across a wide range of behavioral and self-report measures. Moreover, their generalizability to "real-world" social interaction is likely to be enhanced by the spontaneous, unconstrained nature of the behavior that is observed. For detailed reviews and discussions of the paradigm, see Ickes (1982, 1983).

In addition to the findings of Ickes and his colleagues, the results of an independent line of research conducted by Monson and his colleagues (Monson, Hesley, & Chernick, 1982) provide even more direct evidence that the relationship between trait and behavioral measures depends on the strength of situational pressures. In a questionnaire investigation, Monson et al. found that individual differences on the introversion-extraversion dimension correlated more highly with predicted behaviors when situational pressures were weak ($r = .42$) than when they were moderate ($r = .32$) or strong ($r = .13$). In a follow-up study examining actual behaviors, introversion-extraversion scores were found to predict behavior more effectively in a getting-acquainted conversation when situational pressures were weak ($r = .63$), than when there were either strong situational pressures encouraging introversion ($r = .36$) or strong situational pressures encouraging extraversion ($r = .25$). Finally, in an empirical test of their restriction-of-range argument, Monson et al. (1983) demonstrated that when the covariation of trait and behavior is assessed *across* self-selected and non-self-selected situations, the obtained cross-situational correlations is considerably higher than the correlation obtained *within* either type of situation considered by itself.

Taken collectively, the studies by Ickes and his colleagues and those by Monson and his colleagues offer converging evidence that individual differences may have their strongest impact on behavior in relatively unstructured, psychologically "weak" situations. Why, then, have personality researchers persisted for decades in using "strong situation" experimental paradigms that may actually eliminate the very individual differences in behavior which the researchers are attempting to study? Clearly, the orthodoxy of training graduate students in the experimental approach and the historical lack of alternative operational models account for some of this persistence. It is probably also true, however, that at least some "strong situation" paradigms really do work; otherwise, their use would have been subject to extinction long ago. It is therefore important to attempt to distinguish between "strong" situations in which dispositional measures *can* be used to accurately predict behavior and "strong" situations in which dispositional measures *cannot* be used for this purpose.

Precipitating versus Nonprecipitating Situations. Of the "strong situation" paradigms used in personality research, the most effective appear to be those that establish test situations in which behavioral manifestations of the relevant dispositional differences are maximized. These have been termed "precipitating situations" by Snyder and Ickes (in press) because they precipitate or polarize differences in the behavioral manifestations of the particular trait or disposition being studied. In general, the criteria that appear to define a precipitating situation are: (1) it is relevant to the particular disposition being studied, (2) it makes the disposition salient as a guide to behavior, and (3) it permits (as situationally appropriate) specific, alternative modes of responding that individuals should differentially select as a function of their location on the dispositional dimension. As the third criterion suggests, the precipitating situation is, in essence, a kind of behavioral forced-choice that ideally can be resolved only by appeal to the particular disposition to which it is relevant.

Many of the "strong situation" paradigms commonly used in personality research may share some, but not all, of the criteria that define the precipitating situation. To the degree that all of these criteria are met (for an example, see Bem & Lenney's, 1976, study of sex-typing and the avoidance of cross-sex behavior), these paradigms will probably provide relatively good evidence for dispositional influences on behavior. However, to the degree that none of these criteria are met, the resulting test situations should be nonprecipitating and should provide relatively poor evidence for dispositional influences on behavior. For a more extensive discussion of precipitating situations and the criteria used to define them, see Snyder and Ickes (in press).

PRESCRIPTIONS FOR CLINICAL RESEARCH IN PERSONALITY

Because all of the activities included in the application phase of personality research are affected by the correspondence problem, the various "solutions" to this problem suggested by the moderating variable approach can be used as the bases of some general methodological prescriptions for clinical research in personality.

First, consider the importance of predictor moderating variables in selecting, revising, or constructing a measure of the trait or disposition of interest. After you have satisfied yourself regarding the usual psychometric criteria for evaluating the measure's utility (internal consistency, test-retest reliability, convergent and divergent validity, etc.), do not fail to consider additional aspects of the predictor that will affect its ability to predict criterial behaviors. For example, does the measure seek to assess a trait whose behavior manifestations are readily observable? And does it assess the degree to which subjects report their behavioral manifestations of the trait to be consistent across situations? If the answer to such questions is "no," you should typically be able to improve the trait measure's predictive validity by selecting, revising, or constructing a measure that incorporates such features.

Second, consider the importance of criterion moderating variables in selecting or constructing your operational measure(s) of criterial behavior(s). Design and theoretical considerations permitting, you should attempt to measure criterial behaviors that are maximally prototypic of the trait in question. Similarly, circumstances permitting, you should attempt to employ multiple-act measures of the behavioral criterion in order to minimize error of measurement and maximize the probability of sampling trait-determined behaviors.

Third, consider the importance of personal moderating variables with regard to the subject populations from which your research samples are drawn. For some applications of clinical research in personality, it will be of major theoretical importance to distinguish individuals whose behavior reflects their dispositions from those whose behavior does not reflect their dispositions. Thus, Hull and Young (in press), for example, found that high-private-self-conscious men from an alcoholic treatment program were more likely to drink in response to the feelings created by negative self-relevant events than were low-private-self-conscious men from the same treatment program. In this case, separating the subjects on the basis of the personal moderating variable of private self-consciousness permitted the researchers to identify those who were particularly likely to demonstrate a correspondence between the disposition (negative self-relevant feelings) and the clinical behavior (alcoholic relapse) of interest. In an analogous study using a different personal moderating variable called self-motivation, Dishman, Ickes, and Morgan (1980) found that cardiac rehabilitation patients whose self-motivation was high were more likely to keep their commitment to stay in an aerobic exercise program than those whose self-motivation was low.

Fourth, consider the importance of situational moderating variables when choosing or creating an appropriate situational context for your personality research. If the study can be conducted in a relatively unstructured, psychologically "weak" situation, it is likely that dispositional influences will account for more of the variance in subjects' behavior than they would in a relatively structured, psychologically "strong" situation. However, in those instances in which psychologically "strong" situations must be employed, these situations should satisfy, insofar as possible, the criteria for "precipitating" situations. If you can ensure that the "strong" test situations you establish: (1) are relevant to the disposition being studied, (2) make this disposition salient as a guide to behavior, and (3) permit (as situationally appropriate) specific, alternative modes of responding that subjects should select differentially according to their location on the dispositional dimension, you should be able to optimize your chances of "precipitating" disposition-based differences in behavior in spite of the "strong" situational context.

Although it will be useful to consider moderating variables in all four categories when designing any personality study, the relative importance of each of these categories will vary with the type of research being conducted. For example, in research concerned with personality assessment, it is particularly important to consider the role of predictor moderating variables when designing the operational measure (paper-and-pencil scale, structured interview, etc.) of the trait or disposition of interest. Later, in research designed to establish the construct validity of the measure through its ability to predict criterial behaviors, it is particularly important to take criterion moderating variables into account to ensure highly reliable measures of behaviors that are prototypic of the trait domain being studied. On the other hand, when this assessment and initial validation stage is complete and the research has moved into the "bootstrapping" stage, the researcher will often deliberately choose to study low-prototypic criterion behaviors in order to explore some of the more subtle or unexpected behavioral correlates of the trait or disposition. And, since an important goal of the bootstrapping phase is to determine the boundary conditions for the clinical or social psychological phenomenon of interest, the researcher's attention during this phase is likely to focus on the role of personal and situational moderating variables that tend to define those instances in which trait-behavior correspondence is observed.

Space precludes developing more specific prescriptions for the use of the moderating variable approach in personality research; however, the general strategy for using the approach should be clear at this point. To illustrate more concretely some important aspects of this strategy, a brief research example is provided below.

A RESEARCH EXAMPLE

A study conducted by Ickes and Barnes (1978) may be used to illustrate some features of the moderating variable approach to the study of personality. This study is one of a continuing series of studies designed to explore the role of personality variables in defining compatible versus incompatible relationships. Like the other studies in this series, it employed the "weak situation" paradigm which the present author developed to study the influence of personality factors on behavior occurring in initial, unstructured dyadic interactions (Ickes, 1982, 1983).

The immediate purpose of the study was to determine how the sex-role orientations of male and female participants would affect their interactions in mixed-sex dyads. Its broader purpose was to develop testable hypotheses about the compatibility/incompatibility of dyads composed of men and women with traditional (i.e., masculine, feminine) or nontraditional (i.e., androgynous) sex-role orientations. The results were expected to have implications for clinical psychology (specifically, for marital counseling) if socially "compatible" versus "incompatible" dyad types could be identified.

The subjects in the study were 40 male and 40 female undergraduates whose sex-role orientations had been assessed earlier in the semester by means of the Bem Sex-Role Inventory (Bem, 1974). Within the constraints imposed by their gender and sex-role orientation, the subjects were randomly (and without their prior knowledge) assigned to one of four different types of mixed-sex dyads. These dyad types were based on the systematic pairing of: (1) a "masculine" man and a "feminine" woman, (2) a masculine man and an androgynous woman, (3) an androgynous man and a feminine woman, and (4) an androgynous man and an androgynous woman.

After being contacted by telephone and scheduled to participate at the same time, the subjects in each dyad reported to separate waiting areas—a procedure designed to ensure that they would not meet or interact before the session began. The experimenter met them, established that they did not know each other, and escorted them into a "waiting room." There, they were invited to be seated on a large couch. The experimenter then left them alone together, ostensibly to retrieve some questionnaires to be used in the study, and timed a 5-minute interval in which the subjects' behavior was covertly audio- and videotaped. Upon returning to the room, the experimenter explained the need for deception and obtained the subjects' written permission releasing the tapes for use as data. The subjects were then asked to complete posttest questionnaires concerning their perceptions of self and other during the 5-minute interaction period. Following the collection of these self-report data, the subjects were thanked for their participation and released.

Several behavioral measures were subsequently coded from the videotapes by raters who were kept blind to the subjects' sex-role orientations. Analyses of the resulting behavioral and self-report data revealed that the most "traditional" dyad type—the one composed of a masculine male and a feminine female—had interactions that were significantly less involving and rewarding than those occurring in dyads in which one or both participants were androgynous. Subjects in the masculine male/feminine female dyads not only spoke, looked, gestured, and smiled to each other less than did subjects in dyads in the remaining dyad types, but expressed less liking for each other as well (see Table 6.2). The potential clinical significance of these findings is further evidenced by the results of two recent survey studies (one in Australia, the other in the U.S.) involving samples of married respondents (Antill, 1983; Shaver, Pullis, & Olds, 1981). In both of these studies, traditional marriages between masculine males and feminine females were associated with relatively low ratings of marital satisfaction.

The Ickes and Barnes (1978) study contains at least two features that reflect the moderating variable approach to the study of personality. First, the data were collected in a psychologically weak, unstructured situation in which the influence of personality on behavior was not likely to be suppressed or overridden by the influences of strong situational factors (situational moderating variable). Second, the primary behavioral measures of talking, looking, gesturing, etc., took the form of aggregated, multiple-act summaries of the total frequency and duration of these behaviors over the entire 5-minute observation period (criterion moderating variable). Because the study was explicitly designed to explore the possible correspondence of sex-role orientations and low-prototypic social involvement behaviors, the prototypicality moderator (criterion moderating variable) was deliberately not represented in this "bootstrapping" research. Also not represented were personal or predictor moderating variables, and design features reflecting these variables might well have increased the strength and specificity of the obtained results.

As this example suggests, the moderating variable approach should be applied flexibly, not inflexibly, in personality research. It is not essential that

Table 6.2. Differences in Liking and Behavior Between the Male ST-Female ST Dyad Type and the Other Dyad Types over a 5-Minute Interaction Period

	Dyad Type				
Dependent Measure	Male ST-Female ST	Male ST-Female A	Male A-Female ST	Male A-Female A	$F(1, 36)$
Liking	19.2	43.0	42.6	40.8	15.98***
Verbalizations					
Total frequency	21.0	29.7	34.6	28.3	3.03†
Total duration (sec)	46.7	90.2	87.3	67.0	4.80*
Directed gazes					
Total frequency	12.9	19.7	21.7	20.8	2.99†
Total duration	34.9	75.2	74.7	61.1	4.69*
Expressive gestures					
Total frequency	1.6	7.2	4.7	4.0	4.41*
Total duration	1.3	11.4	6.1	4.0	3.58†
Positive affect					
Total frequency	4.0	8.2	9.8	8.4	6.59**
Total duration	11.4	21.5	29.1	23.0	4.10*
Negative affect					
Total frequency	1.2	.7	.9	1.1	<1
Total duration	1.9	.6	1.9	1.2	<1
Pos-neg affect					
Total frequency	2.8	7.5	8.9	7.3	7.26**
Total duration	9.5	20.9	27.2	21.8	4.41*

Note. When dyads, rather than subjects, are the units of analysis, the reported means are based on the averaged scores of each pair of subjects, not on their combined scores. ST = stereotypically sex typed; A = androgynous.

†$p < .10$.
*$p \leq .05$.
**$p < .02$.
***$p < .001$.

all of the moderating variables in the four categories be represented in every personality study. However, it is recommended that the researcher carefully consider each of them in designing his or her research and then implement those which appear to be appropriate with respect to the purposes of the study. When applied in a judicious, informed way, the moderating variable approach can greatly enhance the methodological sophistication of personality research and define more precisely the conditions in which particular dispositions correspond to particular behaviors. Given the importance of these goals, the use of the moderating variable approach is likely to increase in both clinical and non-clinical personality research.

SUMMARY

The *assessment* phase of personality research is typically followed by an *application* phase involving such activities as construct validation, deductive hypothesis-testing, inductive data-gathering, or practical attempts to predict behavior. All of these activities, in one way or another, force the researcher to deal with the problem of the degree of *correspondence* between personality traits and their criterial behaviors. Accordingly, all of these activities tend to share a common set of methodological problems that are addressed by a *moderating variable approach* to the study of personality. This approach seeks to distinguish instances in which traits do correspond to their criterial behaviors from instances in which they do not.

Snyder and Ickes (in press) have identified four major categories of moderating variables that determine the degree of correspondence between personality traits and their criterial behaviors. *Predictor* moderating variables answer the question "Which traits?" by specifying the types of traits and dispositions that will or will not be good predictors of behavior. *Criterion* moderating variables answer the question "Which behaviors?" by specifying the types of behaviors that traits and dispositions are or are not likely to predict. *Personal* moderating variables answer the question "Which people?" by specifying for which types of people a given trait or disposition will predict its criterial behavior(s). And *situational* moderating variables answer the question "Which situations?" by distinguishing situations in which a given trait or disposition will predict its criterial behavior(s) from those in which it will not.

Although it is useful to consider moderating variables in all four categories when conducting personality research, the relative importance of each category will vary with the type of research being conducted. Thus, predictor moderating variables may be especially relevant in personality assessment, criterion moderators may be particularly important in construct validation, and personal and situational moderating variables may play a major role in determining the boundary conditions or generalizability of a specific trait-behavior correspondence. Because a flexible application of the moderating variable approach can greatly enhance the methodological and conceptual sophistication of personality research, the use of this approach is expected to increase.

REFERENCES

Abelson, R.P. (1976). Script processing in attitude formation and decision making. In J. Carroll & J. Payne (Eds.), *Cognition and social behavior*. Hillsdale, NJ: Erlbaum.

Ajzen, I., Timko, C., & White, J.B. (1981). *Self-monitoring and the attitude-behavior relation*. Unpublished manuscript, University of Massachusetts at Amherst.

Alker, H.A. (1972). Is personality situationally specific or intrapsychically consistent? *Journal of Personality, 40,* 1–16.

Antill, J. (1983). Sex-role complementarity versus similarity in married couples. *Journal of Personality and Social Psychology, 45,* 145–155.

Argyle, M., & Little, B.R. (1972). Do personality traits apply to social behavior? *Journal for the Theory of Social Behavior, 2,* 1–35.

Barnes, R.D., & Ickes, W. (1979). *Styles of self-monitoring: Assimilative versus accommodative.* Unpublished manuscript.

Becherer, R.C., & Richard, L.M. (1978). Self-monitoring as a moderating variable in consumer behavior. *Journal of Consumer Research, 5,* 159-162.

Bem, D.J. (1972). Constructing cross-situational consistencies in behavior: Some thoughts on Alker's critique of Mischel. *Journal of Personality, 40,* 17-26.

Bem, D.J., & Allen, A. (1974). On predicting some of the people some of the time: The search for cross-situational consistencies in behavior. *Psychological Review, 81,* 506-520.

Bem, S.L. (1974). The measurement of psychological androgyny. *Journal of Consulting and Clinical Psychology, 42,* 155-162.

Bem, S.L., & Lenney, E. (1976). Sex typing and the avoidance of cross-sex behavior. *Journal of Personality and Social Psychology, 33,* 48-54.

Block, J.H. (1968). Some reasons for the apparent inconsistency of personality. *Psychological Bulletin, 70,* 210-212.

Block, J.H. (1971). *Lives through time.* Berkeley, CA: Bancroft Books.

Bowers, K.S. (1973). Situationism in psychology: An analysis and critique. *Psychological Review, 80,* 307-336.

Buss, A.H. (1980). *Self-consciousness.* San Francisco: Freeman.

Buss, D.M., & Craik, K.H. (1980). The frequency concept of disposition: Dominance and prototypically dominant acts. *Journal of Personality, 48,* 379-392.

Buss, D.M., & Craik, K.H. (1981). The act frequency analysis of personal dispositions: Aloofness, gregariousness, dominance and submissiveness, *Journal of Personality.*

Carver, C.S., & Scheier, M.F. (1981). *Attention and self-regulation: A control-theory approach to human behavior.* New York: Springer-Verlag.

Dishman, R.K., Ickes, W., & Morgan, W.P. (1980). Self-motivation and adherence to habitual physical activity. *Journal of Applied Social Psychology, 10,* 115-132.

Duncan, S., Jr., & Fiske, D.W. (1977). *Face-to-face interaction: Research, methods, and theory.* Hillsdale, NJ: Erlbaum.

Epstein, S. (1979). The stability of behavior: I. On predicting most of the people much of the time. *Journal of Personality and Social Psychology, 37,* 1097-1126.

Epstein, S. (1980). The stability of behavior: II. Implications for psychological research. *American Psychologist, 35,* 790-806.

Fenigstein, A., Scheier, M.F., & Buss, A.H. (1975). Public and private self-consciousness: Assessment and theory. *Journal of Consulting and Clinical Psychology, 43,* 522-527.

Fiske, D.W. (1974). The limits for the conventional science of personality. *Journal of Personality, 42,* 1-11.

Hartshorne, H., & May, M.A. (1928-1930). *Studies in the nature of character* (Vol. 1). *Studies in deceit.* New York: Macmillan.

Hull, J.G., & Young, R.D. (in press). The self-awareness reducing effects of alcohol consumption: Evidence and implications. In J. Suls & A.G. Greenwald, (Eds.), *Social psychological perspectives on the self* (Vol. 2). Hillsdale, NJ: Erlbaum.

Ickes, W. (1981). Sex-role influences in dyadic interaction: A theoretical model. In C. Mayo & N. Henley (Eds.), *Gender and Nonverbal Behavior.* New York: Springer-Verlag.

Ickes, W. (1982). A basic paradigm for the study of personality, roles, and social behavior. In W. Ickes & E.S. Knowles (Eds.), *Personality, roles, and social behavior.* New York: Springer-Verlag.

Ickes, W. (1983). A basic paradigm for the study of unstructured dyadic interaction. In H. Reis (Ed.), *New directions for methodology of behavioral science: Naturalistic approaches to studying social interaction.* San Francisco: Jossey-Bass.

Ickes, W., & Barnes, R.D. (1977). The role of sex and self-monitoring in unstructured dyadic interactions. *Journal of Personality and Social Psychology, 35,* 315–330.

Ickes, W., & Barnes, R.D. (1978). Boys and girls together—and alienated: On enacting stereotyped sex roles in mixed-sex dyads. *Journal of Personality and Social Psychology, 36,* 669–683.

Ickes, W., Layden, M.A., & Barnes, R.D. (1978). Objective self-awareness and individuation: An empirical link. *Journal of Personality, 46,* 146–161.

Ickes, W., Schermer, B., & Steeno, J. (1979). Sex and sex-role influences in same-sex dyads. *Social Psychology Quarterly, 42,* 373–385.

Ickes, W., & Turner, M. (1983). On the social advantages of having an older, opposite-sex sibling: Birth order influences in mixed-sex dyads. *Journal of Personality and Social Psychology, 45,* 210–222.

Jaccard, J.J. (1974). Predicting social behavior from personality traits. *Journal of Research in Personality, 17,* 145–148.

Jaccard, J.J. (1979). Personality and behavior prediction: An analysis of behavioral criterion measures. In L. Kahle & D. Fiske (Eds.), *Methods for studying person-situation interactions.* San Francisco: Jossey-Bass.

Kenrick, D.T., & Stringfield, D.O. (1980). Personality traits and the eye of the beholder: Crossing some traditional philosophical boundaries in the search for consistency in all of the people. *Psychological Review, 87,* 88–104.

LaFrance, M., & Ickes, W. (1981). Posture mirroring and interactional involvement: Sex and sex-typing effects. *Journal of Nonverbal Behavior, 5,* 139–154.

Lamke, L., & Bell, N. (1982). *The influence of sex role orientation on initial interactions within same-sex.* Unpublished manuscript.

Lippa, R. (1976). Expressive control and the leakage of dispositional introversion—extraversion during role-played teaching. *Journal of Personality, 44,* 541–559.

Lippa, R. (1978a). Expressive control, expressive consistency, and the correspondence between expressive behavior and personality. *Journal of Personality, 46,* 438–461.

Lippa, R. (1978b). *Self-presentation and the expressive display of personality.* Paper presented at the annual convention of the American Psychological Association, Toronto, Canada.

Lippa, R., & Mash, M. (1979). *The effects of self-monitoring and self-reported consistency on the consistency of personality statements made by strangers and intimates.* Unpublished manuscript, California State University at Fullerton.

Lutsky, N., Woodworth, W., & Clayton, S. (1980). *Actions-attitudes-actions: A multivariate, longitudinal study of attitude-behavior consistency.* Paper presented at the annual meeting of the Midwestern Psychological Association, St. Louis, MO.

Magnusson, D., & Endler, N.S. (Eds.). (1977). *Personality at the crossroads: Cur-*

rent issues in interactional psychology. Hillsdale, NJ: Erlbaum.

Mischel, W. (1968). *Personality and assessment*. New York: Wiley.

Mischel, W. (1973). Toward a cognitive social learning reconceptualization of personality. *Psychological Review, 80,* 252–283.

Mischel, W. (1977). The interaction of person and situation. In D. Magnusson & N.S. Endler (Eds.), *Personality at the crossroads: Current issues in interactional psychology*. Hillsdale, NJ: Erlbaum.

Monson, T.C., Hesley, J.W., & Chernick, L. (1982). Specifying when personality traits can and cannot predict behavior: An alternative to abandoning the attempt to predict single-act criteria. *Journal of Personality and Social Psychology, 43,* 385–399.

Monson, T.C., McDaniel, R., Menteer, L., & Williams, C. (1983). The self-selection of persons to situations: Its implication for the correlation between dispositions and behavior within a situation. Manuscript submitted for publication.

Monson, T.C., & Snyder, M. (1977). Actors, observers, and the attribution process: Toward a reconceptualization. *Journal of Experimental Social Psychology, 13,* 89–111.

Peterson, D.R. (1965). Scope and generality of verbally defined personality factors. *Psychological Review, 72,* 48–89.

Peterson, D.R. (1968). *The clinical study of social behavior*. New York: Appleton-Century-Crofts.

Rajecki, D.W., Ickes, W., & Tanford, S. (1981). Locus of control and reactions to a stranger. *Personality and Social Psychology Bulletin, 7,* 282–289.

Rarick, D.L., Soldow, G.F., & Geiser, R.S. (1976). Self-monitoring as a mediator of conformity. *Central States Speech Journal, 27,* 267–271.

Sarason, I.G., Smith, R.E., & Diener, E. (1975). Personality research: Components of variance attributable to the person and the situation. *Journal of Personality and Social Psychology, 32,* 199–204.

Schank, R., & Abelson, R.P. (1977). *Scripts, plans, goals and understanding: An inquiry into human knowledge structures*. Hillsdale, NJ: Erlbaum.

Scheier, M.F. (1976). Self-awareness, self-consciousness, and angry aggression. *Journal of Personality, 44,* 627–644.

Scheier, M.F., Buss, A.H., & Buss, D.M. (1978). Self-consciousness, self-report of aggressiveness and aggression. *Journal of Research in Personality, 12,* 133–140.

Scheier, M.F., & Carver, C.S. (1977). Self-focused attention and the experience of emotion: Attraction, repulsion, elation, and depression. *Journal of Personality and Social Psychology, 35,* 625–636.

Shaffer, D.R., Smith, J.E., & Tomarelli, M. (1982). Self-monitoring as a determinant of self-disclosure reciprocity during the acquaintance process. *Journal of Personality and Social Psychology, 43,* 163–175.

Shaver, P., Pullis, C., & Olds, D. (1981). Report on the LHJ "Intimacy Today" Survey. Unpublished manuscript.

Snyder, M. (1974). The self-monitoring of expressive behavior. *Journal of Personality and Social Psychology, 30,* 526–537.

Snyder, M. (1979). Self-monitoring processes. In L. Berkowitz (Ed.), *Advances in experimental social psychology* (Vol. 12). New York: Academic Press.

Snyder, M., & Ickes, W. (in press). Personality and social behavior. In G. Lindzey

& E. Aronson (Eds.), *Handbook of social psychology* (3rd ed.). Reading, MA: Addison-Wesley.

Snyder, M., & Monson, T.C. (1975). Persons, situations, and the control of social behavior. *Journal of Personality and Social Psychology, 32,* 637–644.

Snyder, M., & Swann, W.B., Jr. (1976). When actions reflect attitudes: The politics of impression management. *Journal of Personality and Social Psychology, 34,* 1034–1042.

Snyder, M., & Tanke, E.D. (1976). Behavior and attitude: Some people are more consistent than others. *Journal of Personality, 44,* 510–517.

Turner, R.G. (1978). Effects of differential request procedures and self-consciousness in trait attributions. *Journal of Research in Personality, 12,* 117–132.

Turner, R.G., & Gilliland, L. (1979). The comparative relevance and predictive validity of subject generated trait descriptions. *Journal of Personality, 47,* 230–244.

Underwood, B., & Moore, B.S. (1981). Sources of behavioral consistency. *Journal of Personality and Social Psychology, 40,* 780–785.

Zanna, M.P., Olson, J.M., & Fazio, R.H. (1980). Attitude-behavior consistency: An individual difference perspective. *Journal of Personality and Social Psychology, 38,* 432–440.

Zuckerman, M., & Reis, H.T. (1978). A comparison of three models of predicting altruistic behavior. *Journal of Personality and Social Psychology, 36,* 498–510.

7

Strategies for Psychopathology Research

Michael F. Pogue-Geile
Martin Harrow

INTRODUCTION

The field of psychopathology is concerned with the scientific understanding of abnormal behavior and experiences. Such basic understanding can be valuable in many ways. In addition to the important advantages of understanding behavior disorders, at times major advances in explaining normal human functioning have emerged from studies of abnormal behavior. An excellent example of this is the progress in understanding normal brain-behavior relationships that has come about by studying brain-damaged patients. In addition, such basic understanding has important implications for the improved prevention and treatment of psychopathology.

The present chapter will describe the goals of psychopathology research and will present a schema for evaluating and employing some of the major research strategies. Although examples from the psychological literature will be emphasized, these methods are equally applicable to investigating either the psychological or the biological aspects of psychopathology. In addition, examples from research on schizophrenia will predominate because it is perhaps one of the most intensively researched diagnoses, and because it is our area of special interest.

A Brief History

Since this chapter is concerned with methodology, the following brief history will emphasize general conceptions of psychopathology that influence current investigations. The conception of psychopathology as being caused by disordered bodily functions or by psychological trauma represented an important advance over previous supernatural explanations. In Greece during the 4th century B.C., Hippocrates was among the first to suggest this idea

The writing of this chapter was supported in part by grant MH-26341 from the National Institute of Mental Health and by research grants from the John D. and Catherine T. MacArthur Foundation and the Carnegie Corporation.

and to eschew supernatural explanations. This insight placed psychopathology within the realm of phenomena that are amenable to scientific investigation.

A second influential heuristic in studying psychopathology was also provided by Hippocrates, who was among the first to propose a classification system for psychopathology. He grouped together under a single diagnosis those persons who shared similar symptoms. This general tradition of classification and diagnosis, although not his specific scheme, has had a tremendous influence on research in psychopathology. Indeed, most such research today is framed in these terms and investigates general diagnostic issues.

Following the Middle Ages, psychopathology was slowly re-established as a natural phenomenon, as opposed to a supernatural one, during the Renaissance and the succeeding years. Although during this time there were numerous specific theories of psychopathology, perhaps most important in shaping general ways of thinking were several developments in the fields of general medicine and biology.

During the 19th century in general medicine, the bacteriological causes of numerous diseases (e.g., leprosy, tuberculosis, and cholera) were described, and treatments were devised based on this knowledge. The strategy leading to these discoveries emphasized the careful description of symptom syndromes and their courses. Only by such careful clinical classification were the bacterial agents able to be isolated in the majority of the diagnosed patients. These experiences also reinforced the notion that specific pathogens were necessary and sufficient to cause particular diseases. The remarkable successes of these strategies in general medicine continue to have a tremendous and often controversial impact on current approaches to psychopathology.

Other major influences on the study of psychopathology during the second half of the 19th century were Darwin's theory of evolution, and the "rediscovery" of Mendel's work on genetics. These discoveries provided investigators in psychopathology with an additional etiological agent, namely, individual differences due to genetic transmission. These genetic discoveries complemented those of general medicine, which at that time emphasized specific environmental pathogens.

These developments outside of psychiatry were primarily biological. As a result, the study of psychopathology was influenced and itself emphasized the biological aspect of psychopathology as opposed to the psychological. Within the field of psychopathology, the characterization of the syndrome of general paresis and its association with the syphilis spirochete by Krafft-Ebing (1840–1903) and others was an additional influential argument for the view that psychopathological disorders should be best thought of as diseases of the nervous system. Thus, the predominate Zeitgeist of 19th century psychopathology research emphasized the organic, generally genetic, bases of psychopathology rather than its psychological aspects.

The last two major developments that we will mention both occurred at the turn of the century. During this time Emil Kraepelin (1855–1926), working within the organic tradition, described his classification of the major functional psychoses into dementia praecox and manic-depressive psychosis. With some minor alterations, Kraepelin's diagnoses of dementia praecox (later renamed schizophrenia by E. Bleuler) and manic-depressive psychosis have provided the framework for most research in severe psychopathology since his time.

The other major development at the turn of the century was the work of Sigmund Freud. Although trained in the same organic tradition as Kraepelin, Freud's contribution was in emphasizing the role of psychological factors in psychopathology. In particular, Freud suggested that some psychopathology may have a primarily psychological etiology. This notion continues to be an important contribution. The relative weight given to biological and psychological factors in psychopathology remains an active theoretical issue.

This necessarily brief history has only touched on some of the major conceptual developments and assumptions that are most relevant to current issues in psychopathology research. More detailed histories are available (e.g., Kraepelin, 1962; Maher & Maher, 1979; Zilboorg, 1941).

GENERAL GOALS OF PSYCHOPATHOLOGY RESEARCH

Research methods provide a means for attempting to answer questions. Therefore, the general goals of psychopathology research will be described before discussing the methods that arise from them.

Development of a Valid Diagnostic System

Classification of individuals into groups according to their similarities and differences is an important part of the study of psychopathology for at least two reasons. First, classification serves a communication function and thus allows for the accumulation and application of knowledge, both among investigators and among patients. A second and even more important reason is that a useful and valid classification system can provide more information about a new member of a particular class than just those characteristics that define the class. For example, to the extent that it is valid, a diagnosis of schizophrenia should tell us more than that a person has met the inclusion and exclusion criteria for the diagnosis. Ideally it should imply information about pathology, etiology, course, optimal treatment and other characteristics.

Given that classification is generally useful, one major goal of psychopathology research is to develop a valid diagnostic system based on etiology or pathology. However, in the absence of knowledge about pathologies and etiologies, psychopathology is currently classified only on observable signs and self-reported symptoms. A distinction can be drawn between such syndrome diagnoses, which are based only on observable signs and symptoms, and pathological diagnoses, which are based on the presence of a specific pathology or etiology. In the latter type, observable signs and symptoms may aid in recognizing an individual case, but the diagnosis is defined by the presence of a specific pathology. Syndrome diagnoses in contrast are both recognized and defined by signs and symptoms because pathology and etiology is unknown. Such preliminary diagnostic systems based on "surface" manifestations serve as tools to investigate underlying etiologies and pathologies. The more closely such surface classifications reflect unknown underlying pathology, the easier it is to detect pathological characteristics that are common to most members of the diagnostic class. However, if the symptomatic classification includes a number of hidden subgroups that are etiologically and pathologically heterogeneous, then the search for common characteristics in the diagnostic category becomes very difficult. For example, it may well be the case that our present diagnostic classification of schizophrenia, which is based solely on symptoms and signs, includes a number of subgroups that are pathologically and/or etiologically heterogeneous. If 10% of "schizophrenias" are the result of a defect in enzyme x, then most studies using small samples that compare schizophrenics and controls will lead to the conclusion that enzyme x is irrelevant to schizophrenia (Buchsbaum & Reider, 1979).

One goal therefore is to design a diagnostic system based on observable signs (without knowing pathology) that maximally reflects underlying pathology and etiology. The fact that classification is both a goal and a method is an important characteristic of research in psychopathology.

Description of Pathology

A second general goal of psychopathology research is the description of pathology. The term *pathology* refers to the abnormalities in psychological and biological processes that produce a person's observable symptoms. Pathology therefore refers to characteristics of a person and may reflect a final common pathway arising from numerous etiologies. For example, the defining pathology of diabetes mellitus is insulin deficiency, which may itself arise for various reasons. There are generally multiple levels of these pathological characteristics that form complex causal networks. The goal is to identify those characteristics that are most important and most amenable to treatment.

Description of Etiologies

A third goal involves understanding the etiologies of psychopathology. Etiological influences may be either environmental agents or genetically transmitted characteristics that lead to the development of pathology.

The investigation of environmental influences may be complicated by at least two phenomena. First, many environmental influences may be *correlated* with, but not causally related to, pathological characteristics of a person. For example, should poor social support be considered an etiological environmental influence, or a result of the person's pathology, or both? Because of the difficulty of distinguishing these two types of influence without experimental manipulation, the general term, "antecedents of disorder," which denotes both influences, is often most appropriate. Second, environmental events also often *interact* with characteristics that serve to protect persons or to make them vulnerable. Thus, it is often the case that not every person exposed to some noxious environmental agent develops difficulties. To fully understand such an environmental influence, we need to know the characteristics of those persons who developed difficulties vs. those who did not. The description of genetic influences is similarly complicated by the likelihood of interactions between genetic and environmental influences.

Description of the Courses of a Disorder

This goal attempts both to describe the course of a disorder and to specify person characteristics and/or environmental events that are associated with different courses. It is important to distinguish between such influences that may affect the course of a disorder once it has developed and etiological influences that lead to the development of the disorder in the first place, because they may be quite different. Information concerning the course of a disorder is useful both practically and as a potential validation criterion for diagnostic systems.

GENERAL CHARACTERISTICS OF PSYCHOPATHOLOGY RESEARCH

Most research in psychopathology is essentially correlational, not experimental since, for ethical reasons, psychopathology itself and potential etiological factors generally cannot be randomly assigned and their effects measured. Without such experimental manipulation, it is frequently difficult to rule out rival hypotheses and to make statements concerning causality. Often we must be content with only describing associations among characteristics. The designs to be discussed below reflect this correlational nature of psychopathology research and represent attempts to surmount its limitations.

Although many experimental strategies are not appropriate with humans, subhuman animal experimental studies can be useful adjuncts. However, since much of psychopathology involves subjective experiences (e.g., hallucinations), language abnormalities, and social interactions, the comparison of animal with human findings must be made cautiously. Nevertheless, several potential animal models of psychopathology have been proposed and should eventually prove important.

Although potential etiological factors generally cannot be randomly assigned for ethical reasons, potential treatments can be. Aside from the practical therapeutic effects of controlled treatment studies, such investigations can also shed light on pathology. This approach has provided potentially valuable hypotheses concerning the biological aspects of schizophrenia (e.g., Snyder, Banerjee, Yamamura, & Greenberg, 1974). Thus knowing what helps a disorder tells something about the pathology itself.

Another important characteristic of psychopathology research is the method that is frequently used to identify groups that are homogeneous in etiology or pathology. The strategy most often used involves the correlation among variables, one of which is usually diagnosis. A high correlation depends upon the appropriateness of both the diagnostic variable and the variable of interest. Although such designs are often thought of as investigating the role of the "dependent" variable, they can also be used to shed light on the validity of the diagnosis itself. In this sense there is no "independent" variable, all are "dependent" variables. For example, the finding that schizophrenics generally have more severe courses than affective disorders (Harrow, Grinker, Silverstein, & Holzman, 1978) not only suggests that long-term functioning is relevant to schizophrenia, it also suggests that the diagnosis itself seems to identify some more or less homogeneous group. Although any variable may reflect on the validity of diagnostic distinctions, the following variables are often given particular weight: long-term course, family history of the disorder, and response to treatment (Robins & Guze, 1970).

Up to this point only comparisons between diagnoses have been discussed. Similar methods may be used to investigate potential heterogeneity *within* diagnostic categories. If certain characteristics are correlated *within* a diagnostic group, it may be that all of these variables reflect the effects of some common pathological factor. Although all of the designs discussed below are described in terms of diagnostic comparisons, they are equally applicable to investigating subgroups within a diagnostic category.

A recent study by Sedvall and Wode-Helgodt (1980) is an example of this covariation approach to investigating heterogeneity within diagnostic categories. These investigators correlated the amount of various neurotransmitter substances in the cerebrospinal fluid (CSF) of schizophrenics with whether or not the patients had any first-degree relatives who were schizophrenic. Their finding that schizophrenics with a positive family history had much higher levels of some metabolites than those with a negative family history may suggest the presence of etiological heterogeneity within schizophrenia.

Given the likelihood that current diagnostic categories may be heterogeneous, such studies of subtypes within diagnoses are especially important.

METHODOLOGICAL CONSIDERATIONS IN THE DIAGNOSTIC PROCESS

The process of assigning diagnoses is crucial, as most designs rely on diagnoses in selecting subjects and in forming groups. Although the eventual goal of diagnosis, like any other measurement scheme, is validity (i.e., to reflect a common pathology), reliability is a necessary aid in achieving this end.

There have been two advances in recent years that have improved the reliability of the diagnostic process. First, the structured interview has standardized, across both patients and interviewers, the data base from which diagnostic decisions are made. Although most such instruments rely on clinical judgment to decide when a particular sign or symptom is present, they provide explicit definitions and rating criteria for each item. In addition, they furnish a standard format that ensures that every patient is assessed on the same characteristics. The Present State Exam (PSE) (Wing, Cooper, & Sartorious, 1974) and the Schedule for Affective Disorders and Schizophrenia (SADS) (Spitzer & Endicott, 1979) are two of the most frequently used structured interviews.

The second advance in improving the reliability of the diagnostic process was the incorporation of explicit inclusion and exclusion criteria into diagnostic systems. Inclusion criteria are those characteristics that must be present in order to qualify for a certain diagnosis, whereas exclusion criteria are those characteristics that must be absent. In the case of the Research Diagnostic Criteria (RDC) for schizophrenia, delusions of control and nonaffective verbal hallucinations are two of several inclusion criteria and the absence of a depressive syndrome is one of the exclusion criteria. Such specific criteria allow for more uniform application of the diagnostic system by different investigators.

Prior to the Feighner Criteria, used at Washington University (Feighner, Robins, Guze, Woodruff, Winokur, & Munoz, 1972), diagnostic manuals provided only general descriptions of disorders as guides to diagnosis (e.g., *Diagnostic and Statistical Manual* [2nd. ed.], [DSM II], American Psychiatric Association, 1968). Now several diagnostic systems are available that have explicit criteria and rely on symptoms and behavioral signs that themselves can be reliably rated. Some of the major "objective" diagnostic systems are: the Feighner Criteria (Feighner, Robins, et al., 1972), the Research Diagnostic Criteria, (RDC) (Spitzer, Endicott, & Robins, 1978), the official *Diagnostic and Statistical Manual*, 3rd edition (DSM III) (American Psychiatric Association, 1980), and the New Haven Schizophrenia Index (Astrachan, Harrow,

Adler, Brauer, Schwartz, Schwartz, & Tucker, 1972). The use of such diagnostic systems along with structured interviews has become standard procedure in most research studies of psychopathology. In addition, frequently several of these different diagnostic systems are applied to the same set of patients to investigate their relative validities. The diagnostic system that leads to the greatest between-group differences and within-group similarity may more closely reflect common underlying types of pathology.

RESEARCH DESIGNS

The following presents a conceptual framework for evaluating and utilizing some of the major research designs in psychopathology.

Case-Control Sampling

This first and most common type of subject sampling strategy has been termed the case-control procedure because a group of "cases" (e.g., persons with the diagnosis of interest, such as schizophrenia) is compared to an appropriate control group (such as hospitalized depressives) on some characteristic. This method also has been described as the ex post facto design. If the characteristic, for example, social withdrawal, is more common among cases than controls, then it may be associated in some manner with the disorder.

The most important aspect of this design is that it is correlational not experimental. The condition of interest (e.g., schizophrenia) is not randomly assigned, but is sampled from pre-existing groups. Therefore, without random assignment, case and control groups may differ on many characteristics other than psychopathology that may complicate interpretation of results. For this reason, the following cautions concerning the selection of subjects are necessary.

First, the sampling of cases should be as representative of the population of cases as is possible. The advantages of a representative sample of cases include: (1) improved generalization of findings, (2) increased comparability with other studies, and (3) improved estimation of demographic characteristics of cases. Since truly representative samples are difficult to obtain, it is important to document and to consider potential selection biases when interpreting results.

The first potential selection factor that may affect the representativeness of the sample concerns the selection of treated cases (i.e., inpatient or outpatient) vs. untreated cases (i.e., diagnosable persons in the community with no treatment history). This distinction is only beginning to be appreciated in psychopathology research (Weissman, Myers, & Thompson, 1981) and it is unclear how generalizable results on treated cases are to untreated cases. Among treated cases, a second selection factor is the institution through which they are ascertained. Patients admitted to a state hospital undoubtedly differ from those admitted to a private or Veterans Administration hospital in ways that may affect the study results. A third selection factor is the number of prior treatment contacts that subjects have had. Subjects who have long treatment histories may not be representative of treated cases in general. Not included in such chronic samples are milder cases who have never sought treatment after their original contact. Therefore, studies should generally include as many first admission patients as possible. A fourth selection factor is whether the subject consents to and completes the assessment procedure. Often with complex assessment procedures, the most severe patients are screened out because they cannot complete the task (Chapman & Chapman, 1977).

The decision as to which groups will serve as controls depends on what one is attempting to "control." A sample of normal non-patients provides a general baseline for comparison. In addition, a control group from the same treatment facility that is composed of a specific diagnostic category chosen on theoretical grounds is also useful. Such a patient control group helps control for the factors associated with being hospitalized and can test the specificity of the characteristic being studied (Ritzler & Rinehart, 1981). A specific diagnostic control group is often better than a heterogeneous group of patients because the composition of the group can be more easily replicated, and it can provide substantive information concerning the specificity of a characteristic.

The selection of the individual control subjects is one of the most controversial aspects of this design. Control subjects can be selected to be as representative of their own group as is possible; however, this may result in controls that differ from cases on potentially important variables such as social class or intelligence. Alternatively, controls can be deliberately matched on such characteristics with cases (via selection or statistical adjustment).

The representative control group strategy is frequently considered to lead to problems in inferring the reasons for group differences. For instance, if a sample of schizophrenics is found to be of a lower social class than a control group of depressives, it is unclear whether the schizophrenics' poorer performance on some cognitive task of interest is due to their disorder or to their lower social class. The matching or statistical adjustment strategy (e.g., analysis of covariance) is an attempt to clarify this ambiguity. In the matching case only the lowest social class depressives would be compared with the schizophrenics, thus "controlling" for social class.

However, the matching or statistical adjustment method also presents inferential problems. Perhaps most important, the matching strategy assumes that social class, for instance, is a "nuisance" variable and because it is irrelevant to the disorder it should be controlled (Meehl, 1970, 1971). However, if the schizophrenics and depressives were initially selected to be representative of their respective diagnostic classes, then any demographic differences between the two must reflect some real-world association with the disorders. Therefore, rather than considering lowered social class as being irrelevant to schizophrenia, low social class might in fact be a contributing cause or perhaps some result of the schizophrenic process. In which case, it makes no sense to "control" for some important aspect of the disorder. Thus, matching strategies are based on some implicit causal model of what variables are irrelevant and there are usually plausible alternative causal models that would be obscured by matching.

In addition, matching on one variable often systematically unmatches on another variable. For instance, matching on social class may lead to samples being unmatched on age or some other characteristic. Because of this, even large samples can generally be matched on only a small number of variables at the same time and the end result may be groups of highly atypical subjects. In addition, matching may also lead to regression toward the mean on the variable of primary interest. Given this controversy (see Chapman & Chapman, 1973b; Meehl, 1970), perhaps the best resolution is to analyze the data both with and without matching (or statistical adjustment) and to report any differences in results.

Case-Control Sampling: Cross-Sectional Assessment. This first design employs the case-control sampling strategy to select subjects and then assesses them cross-sectionally, once, at the time of their ascertainment. The goal of this design is generally to identify either pathologies or antecedents of a disorder. This is undoubtedly the most common design in psychopathology research, and can provide some useful information, but in many ways it is not a strong design.

An example of this common design is an important study by McGhie, Chapman, and Lawson (1965) reporting that schizophrenic inpatients performed more poorly than control groups of nonschizophrenic psychotic patients, and normals on a test designed to measure distractibility. The test involved recalling a string of aurally presented digits in the presence of auditory distraction. Although well-designed and carefully interpreted, this study (or any similar one) illustrates the inferential limitations of a cross-sectional design.

The primary difficulty in interpretation is the issue of causal priority. One is presumably interested in distractibility, for example, because of the possibility either that it produces schizophrenic symptoms or that it, along with other symptoms, reflects some central abnormality of schizophrenics' psychological processes. However, since this is a correlational design, it is difficult to know whether distractibility reflects some more central characteristic of schizophrenia or is merely a peripheral effect of the disorder.

In addition to this ambiguity in the direction of causality, there is the possibility that distractibility is associated with schizophrenia through the influence of some nonspecific third variable. Some of these difficulties have been discussed in the section on case-control sampling and matching on demographic variables. Other sorts of nonspecific third variables include general upset, anxiety, and psychotic disorganization. Thus, it is possible that an acute episode of schizophrenia leads to anxiety (which is not specific to schizophrenia), that in turn leads to distractibility. Although such alternative hypotheses are difficult to rule out with a cross-sectional design, longitudinal data (see below) can often be helpful. This ambiguity is equally applicable to biological variables, which also may be sensitive to general activity level, stress, and upset.

Medication status is an additional third variable that is very important in some psychopathology research. For example, comparisons of schizophrenics taking antipsychotic medication with depressives who are not taking such medication are often complex to interpret. Although it is generally difficult to control in actual practice, at least in some situations medication can be manipulated and its potential effects should be evaluated.

The Chapmans (1973a; 1978) have proposed a method that attempts to clarify somewhat the inferential ambiguity involved in this general design. They argue that if some particular difficulty is central to a disorder, then patients should show more of this abnormality than other similar problems. This differential deficit design encourages theoretical parsimony. Although the psychometric aspects are still controversial (e.g., Strauss, 1978), this may prove to be a promising approach that should lead to more specific theorizing.

When it is used to investigate the antecedents of a disorder (e.g., early childhood characteristics, or recent life events) a second major difficulty of the cross-sectional design is the uncertainty of retrospective reporting. Recall is poorest for vaguely defined characteristics and for events farthest in the past. Retrospective reporting has also been shown to be importantly biased by current circumstances in the direction of attempting to "explain" current psychopathology (Yarrow, Campbell, & Burton, 1970).

Case-Control Sampling: Retrospective Assessment. This design, termed the follow-back strategy by Garmezy and Streitman (1974a), attempts to identify the antecedents of psychopathology (i.e., early characteristics and/or environmental influences). The strategy involves case-control sampling and assessment *prior* to subject selection. This prior assessment usually is based on "society's records," such as school reports and birth records.

Watt and associates' (Watt, Fryer, Lewine, & Prentky, 1979) study of the early characteristics of schizophrenics is an excellent example of this approach. Starting with a state-wide list of psychiatric hospital admissions, Watt cross-referenced this list with the roster of a local school district. He was thus able to locate the school records of 30 schizophrenics and a series of control subjects and to blindly rate them on various behavioral characteristics. Briefly, one result was that preschizophrenic boys were found frequently to be aggressive, whereas the girls were more often characterized as being over-inhibited.

This strategy is a clear improvement over the retrospective reporting of the cross-sectional design. Such follow-back data are not based on recall of long past events, are not biased by the knowledge of adult outcome, and are prior to any potential iatrogenic effects of hospitalization.

Although potentially powerful, this design has certain limitations, perhaps the most important of which involves the quality of the records. Obviously, society's records do not cover all the characteristics that might be of later potential interest to a psychopathologist, as the records are generally kept for non-research reasons. Even if the domain of later interest is described in the earlier records, one may question the reliability of the descriptions.

In order to increase the range of data available, one variation on this strategy has been to include only cases for whom child clinic records are available. However, this selection bias presents a distorted view because only cases who had difficulties as children are included.

Another difficulty with the follow-back design is that it can falsely create the illusion of true prediction. Knowing the adult outcome makes the subjects' histories appear directed and inevitable. More formally, this design provides only the conditional probability of having a certain childhood characteristic; *given* being a diagnosed case as an adult. In contrast, most research and treatment questions involve the opposite conditional probability; namely, what is the chance of having adult difficulties *given* some childhood experience or characteristic? In addition, by starting from a single endpoint with a specific adult disorder and tracing backwards, this design may obscure the broad range of potential outcomes that may follow a particular childhood experience. For example, although in Watt's study many preschizophrenic boys were aggressive as adolescents, undoubtedly only a small percentage of aggressive adolescent boys will later become schizophrenic. In fact, adolescent aggression may represent a more potent risk factor for later criminality (Loeber & Dishion, 1983) than for schizophrenia, and many aggressive adolescents will go on to lead normal lives. The follow-back design does not provide either the range of outcomes following adolescent aggressiveness, for instance, or the probability of the various outcomes.

Case-Control Sampling: Retrospective Follow up. This design is primarily concerned with describing and predicting a disorder's course, and not its antecedent characteristics. It involves ascertainment of cases and controls at some time *prior* to the beginning of the study. Generally, hospital records from some earlier time period are searched to identify cases and their controls. Subjects are then located and assessed either in person or through other records.

This design can provide a view of the long-term course of a diagnostic group without requiring many years to pass in order to complete the study.

Tsuang and colleagues' study of schizophrenia, the Iowa 500, is a sophisticated example of this approach (Tsuang, Woolson, & Fleming, 1979). Modern objective diagnostic criteria were applied to the hospital charts of patients admitted between 1934 and 1944. Psychiatric patients, who were retrospectively diagnosed from the original hospital charts (blind to outcome) as either schizophrenic, manic, or depressed, and a sample of normal surgical patients were then relocated in 1976, approximately 30 to 40 years after they were first hospitalized. One of the many findings of this study was that schizophrenics tended to function more poorly on occupational, social, and symptom variables at followup than the depressed patients. Such an association between diagnosis and later course is one strategy to provide evidence for the validity of the original diagnostic distinction.

This design depends to a great extent on the quality of the hospital records that were used to initially diagnose subjects. Hospital records often vary in quality and earlier records may not include information that is needed by current diagnostic criteria. The results will only be representative to the extent that the retrospective diagnoses reflect current diagnostic practices. The use of archival records also restricts the variety of variables that may be used to predict later courses. For example, if reliable ratings of thought disorder were not originally included in the charts, the prognostic value of thought disorder could not be investigated.

Another potential problem in this longitudinal type of study concerns subject attrition. Attrition refers to the number of initial cases who were not able to be located and contacted for followup assessment. Often relocating patients is difficult because no plans were made to recontact the patients when they were initially hospitalized. In studies that cover a long time period, attrition can also be increased by patient deaths, which force one to rely only on available records and interviews with family members (if available) as follow-up assessments.

Aside from reducing sample size, attrition becomes most problematic when it is selective with respect to the variables under study. For example, if most patients who were lost to attrition were not able to be located because they were functioning poorly and had no permanent address, then the results based only on the successfully followed-up patients could be falsely optimistic. One way to attempt to estimate the influence of attrition is to compare successfully followed up patients with those who were lost to follow-up on characteristics from the initial evaluation. Although informative, this analysis cannot completely ensure the comparability of followed up and lost subjects.

Despite the potential limitations of poor record quality and high attrition, this strategy can be an efficient and relatively quick way of evaluating the general long-term courses of various diagnostic groups.

Case-Control Sampling: Prospective Follow up. This design, like the previous one, is primarily concerned with describing the course of a diagnostic group and factors that might be associated with different courses. In addition, the longitudinal aspect of this design can be very useful in investigating pathology. In this strategy, cases and controls are ascertained at the start of the study and are first assessed at that time. Assessments are then repeated over time at generally fixed intervals (e.g., every 2 years) as the sample grows older. This design is termed prospective because subjects are recruited and assessed from the beginning of the study with the intention of later being followed up.

An important example of this design is Harrow and colleagues' Chicago Followup Study of schizophrenia and other diagnostic groups (Harrow, Grinker, Silverstein, & Holzman, 1978; Harrow & Silverstein, 1977; Pogue-Geile & Harrow, in press). In this large project, hospital admissions between 18 and 30 years old were assessed as inpatients with structured interviews and diagnosed blind to other information, using multiple diagnostic criteria (e.g., DSM II, RDC, DSM III). Retrospective assessments of prehospitalization functioning and prospective measures of current specific symptoms, such as positive and negative thought disorder, were also made during the initial inpatient phase. These patients were then located and retested, using a similar comprehensive battery, at 2-year intervals following their discharge from index hospitalization. This project has investigated the longitudinal course of thought disorder, psychosis, functioning and negative symptoms in schizophrenia. (Harrow & Quinlan, in press; Harrow, Silverstein, & Marengo, 1983; Silverstein & Harrow, 1981).

One primary advantage of the prospective follow-up study over the retrospective type is that the initial assessments can be designed to include any measures that will be of later interest. In addition, the reliability of the assessments can be established by using trained raters for all assessments. For similar reasons one can have more confidence in prospectively assigned diagnoses than in ones assigned retrospectively.

A prospective design is also well studied to investigating pathology because it can assess the longitudinal stability of characteristics. Assessing the same patients when they are acutely disturbed and then again when they are less symptomatic is a powerful method for determining whether some potential pathological characteristic merely reflects a general state of disorganization or some more persistent trait.

Like all other longitudinal designs (i.e., those involving more than one assessment), the prospective follow-up design is vulnerable to the potentially biasing effects of sample attrition. In addition, it is particularly important to control the number of prior treatment contacts of patients in this design. If some patients enter the study with already established patterns of chronicity, it is likely that they will continue in this manner. In which case, attempts to predict later functioning from initial characteristics may merely find that characteristics associated with established chronicity predict continued chronicity. For this reason, it is particularly important to have as many first admission patients as is possible and to obtain records of prior treatment.

This prospective follow-up design, coupled with a comprehensive and farsighted assessment battery, is a particularly rich strategy for investigating a variety of research questions. Although it has many advantages over a retrospective follow-up design, it is of course much more expensive and time consuming.

Cohort Sample Designs

In contrast to the strategies discussed thus far, the following designs do not begin with ascertaining a case. Rather, they select a cohort of subjects defined according to some criteria other than diagnosis. Such cohort designs are generally used for one of two purposes.

Cohort Sampling: Theoretical Selection Criteria. In this first case, the prime interest is in evaluating the potential consequences of some particular experience or characteristic. For example, in order to investigate the later effects of a childhood experience, such as early parental loss, a cohort of children whose parents had died before age 10 and suitable control children would be selected and then evaluated over the years. Problems and strengths that were more common among the early loss group than among appropriate control children would be likely candidates to have early parental death as an etiological influence or risk factor.

The cohort design has been used surprisingly infrequently to investigate potential risk factors (i.e., characteristics or experiences) in psychopathology (cf. Buchsbaum, Coursey, & Murphy, 1976). One recent example is the large prospective study being conducted by Chapman and Chapman (Chapman, Chapman, Raulin, & Edell, 1978; Chapman, Edell, & Chapman, 1980). Based on theorizing by Meehl (1962), concerning hypothesized characteristics of "schizotypes" (i.e., persons with the potential, given relevant stresses, to become schizophrenic), the Chapmans have devised potential measures of these characteristics and have selected cohorts and controls from college students based on them. They are currently planning to follow this cohort to evaluate the later rates of schizophrenia and other disorders in the "schizotypes" and controls.

One advantage of this design is that it allows one to assess all the possible outcomes of a particular experience or characteristic, rather than just select outcomes as was the case with the follow-back design. In addition, cohort sampling provides important information, which the follow-back design generally does not furnish, on the probability of later having difficulties *given* some earlier experience or characteristic. Although still correlational and not experimental, this design is a potentially powerful one for investigating antecedents or risk factors and seems to have been under-used in psychopathology research. It is perhaps most useful when investigating some experience that is generally considered important, or when investigating some already partially supported theoretical prediction. Other case-control designs, such as the follow-back, may be less expensive methods for initially evaluating preliminary hypotheses.

Cohort Sampling: Empirical Selection Criteria. Cohort sampling may also be used in order to prospectively describe the antecedents of a disorder. In this case, cohorts may be selected according to criteria purely for practical reasons. For example, it is generally impractical to follow up a series of thousands of consecutive births for 40 years in order to prospectively investigate the antecedents of an uncommon disorder, such as schizophrenia, whose onset of obvious clinical symptoms may be relatively late in life. With such uncommon, late-onset disorders, any initial selection criteria that might increase the number of eventual cases will make the study more efficient. In such situations the primary interest of the study remains in prospectively describing the antecedents of a particular disorder, not in evaluating the potential effects of the selection criteria, which are in fact already known.

Such "high risk" designs became quite popular in the 1960s and 1970s as a means of potentially describing the antecedents of schizophrenia (Garmezy, 1974b). Most of these studies selected the children of schizophrenic parents as subjects, as was first suggested by Pearson and Kley (1957). Other studies have shown that there is an approximate 10–15% risk for developing schizophrenia in the offspring of a mating where one of the parents is schizophrenic (Gottesman & Shields, 1982). This represents a 10- to 15-fold increase over the morbid risk of approximately 1% for schizophrenia in the general population. Consanguinity was used as a selection criterion for most of these studies because no other factor has been shown to increase as much the later risk for schizophrenia.

The first such high risk study of schizophrenia was initiated by Mednick and Schulsinger (1968) in Denmark. They selected a cohort of 207 offspring of schizophrenic mothers. Control children with non-patient parents were matched on age, sex, and other characteristics with the high-risk subjects. The subjects were then comprehensively assessed at intervals of several years. In a recent report of their 10-year assessment, when the subjects' average age was 25 years old, 14 subjects in the high risk group and one of the controls had been diagnosed as being "certain" schizophrenics. Briefly, this preliminary report suggested that those high risk subjects who became schizophrenic (at a young age) tended to have had birth complications, and to be described by their teachers as easily angered and upset (Mednick, Schulsinger, & Schulsinger, 1975).

The advantages of the high-risk design are those of any prospective study. Most important, characteristics that the investigator is interested in may be studied that might not be available in public records, as would be the case with the follow-back design. In addition, since subjects are studied before the onset of florid symptomatology and hospitalization, measures are less likely to be affected by these nonspecific factors (Mednick & McNeil, 1968).

One potential limitation of the high-risk design is its generalizability (Lewine, Watt, & Grubb, 1981). For example, it is not at all certain whether the antecedents of schizophrenics who have a schizophrenic parent are representative of the approximately 90% of schizophrenics who do not have an affected parent. Not only is such a bias possible, but its importance is difficult to evaluate.

A second limitation of this design is that results on the antecedents of schizophrenia must wait until the high-risk group has passed through the majority of the period of risk. For diagnostic groups, like schizophrenia, that have a variable age at clinical onset between adolescence and 60 years old, definitive results on the antecedent characteristics of eventual schizophrenics have to wait a long time.

Until these final results are available, comparisons of the *entire* high-risk group with low-risk controls are often made. Such analyses most properly only reflect the consequences of the selection criterion (i.e., having a schizophrenic parent) and are *not* necessarily related to potential antecedents of the disorder (McNeil & Kaij, 1979). As only a minority (about 10%) of high-risk subjects will eventually develop schizophrenia, an absence of a significant difference between the *entire* high-risk group and controls does not rule out this characteristic as being associated with those few subjects who may eventually become schizophrenic at a later date. Similarly, a significant difference between the total samples of high- and low-risk groups does not imply that the characteristic will be more frequent in that specific subset of high-risk subjects who eventually become schizophrenic.

Such limitations are highlighted in high-risk studies because of the ambitiousness of their goals. Despite these cautions, such designs should provide new information for the field.

Cohort Sampling: Representative Sample. A powerful method for describing the antecedents of a diagnostic group is the prospective study of a cohort representative of the general population. This design avoids the problems in generalizability of the high-risk study and can evaluate the importance of any potential risk factor (if it is measured) as it naturally occurs in the population. However, the expense and logistic difficulties that would be involved in following thousands of subjects restrict the relevance of this design to diagnostic groups that are fairly common and that tend to have clinical onsets relatively early in life. Adult psychiatric disorders that fit these criteria include alcoholism and criminality in males and depression in females. A recent study reported by Vaillant (1983), which approaches this design, involved the long-term follow up of a geographically representative sample of urban, lower socioeconomic status men whose antecedents and courses of alcoholism were described. Although too comprehensive to be summarized here, the importance of findings from such designs seems to justify the effort and expense involved in these studies.

Consanguinity Designs

The last general types of design involve case-control sampling, but in addition to assessing the cases (termed probands) and their controls, a cohort of the probands' relatives is also ascertained and assessed. The general aim of such studies is to understand the transmission of disorders. In particular, most of these designs attempt to assess the importance of genetic influences, although they can often yield unique information on environmental influences as well.

Family Designs. A family study starts with ascertaining cases (or probands) and appropriate controls. The various types of relatives (e.g., fathers, mothers, brothers, etc.) of these probands and controls are then assessed blind to the status of the proband. The best method is to actually locate and interview the relatives in person (the family interview method). In contrast, the family history method gathers information about relatives from one or more informants and not all relatives are actually seen. The family history method has generally been found to underestimate the prevalence of mild disorders in the relatives (Thompson, Orvaschel, Prusoff, & Kidd, 1982). The family study does not explicitly attempt to separate genetic from environmental relationships and therefore the results obtained may often be due to either influence or their combination.

Assessment may focus on several different aspects of probands and relatives. The most common, genetically-oriented, approach emphasizes diagnosing family members. The obtained number of certain types of relatives who have the same diagnosis as the proband may then be compared to the number predicted by various models of genetic transmission. Multigenerational data (i.e., grandparents, etc.) are particularly helpful in these studies. A goal of such studies is to identify the mode of genetic transmission (i.e., dominant or recessive, etc.). They often arbitrarily assume little environmental influence and argue that if obtained results closely fit specific genetic expectations then the genetic explanation is most likely (e.g., Tsuang, Bucher, & Fleming, 1982).

In addition to potential evidence on modes of genetic transmission, this traditional diagnosis-oriented approach also provides information on the genetic/environmental relationships among diagnoses. For example, the finding that the relatives of schizophrenic probands are at increased risk for schizophrenia but not depression compared to the general population and vice versa

(Tsuang, Winokur, & Crowe, 1980) would suggest that these may indeed be different disorders that each tend to "breed true." Similarly, diagnoses other than schizophrenia that are more frequent in the relatives of schizophrenic probands than in the general population might be genetically/environmentally associated with schizophrenia.

Family studies, like most other methods, also lend themselves to investigating heterogeneity within a diagnostic group. Thus, characteristics of probands that distinguish those with and those without a family history of the disorder may suggest that familial and non-familial forms are different. A summary of other methods of investigating heterogeneity using family studies is presented in Rieder and Gershon (1978).

Another approach to family studies comes from an environmentalist orientation. These types of studies generally assess immediate family members of probands and controls on characteristics (often family communication and interaction styles) that are hypothesized to be disorder-inducing (Jacob, 1975). The results of such studies using the family design cannot be attributed solely to environmental transmission any more than they can be attributed solely to genetic influences, because of the complete correlation of genetic and environmental relationships in the family study design. In addition, the direction of causality is difficult to infer in such studies. For example, it may be just as likely that living with a schizophrenic offspring leads to disordered family communication as vice versa.

Twin Designs. Most frequently, twin designs have been used to estimate whether or not genetic influences are important in a disorder's etiology. To this end, the twin study seeks to "keep constant" the degree of environmental relationship while "varying" the degree of genetic relationship. The design of the twin study involves ascertaining a series of cases of a particular diagnosis who are also twins. There are two types of twins. Monozygotic (MZ), or identical, twins arise from a single fertilized egg and thus share 100% of their genes, whereas dizygotic (DZ), or fraternal, twins come from two fertilized eggs and therefore share, on average, 50% of their genes. DZ twins are genetically no more similar than any other pair of siblings. Generally only same-sex DZ twins are studied in order to control for the similarity of sex within a twin pair since all MZ co-twins are the same sex. Zygosity can be determined quite precisely by serological analyses.

After a series of MZ and DZ probands is ascertained, their co-twins are assessed and diagnosed (ideally blind to the proband's diagnosis). Concordance rates (i.e., percentage of co-twins with the same diagnosis as the proband) are then compared for MZ and DZ twins. The estimation of genetic influence depends upon the assumption that MZ co-twins' environments are no more similar to each other than are DZ co-twins' environments in terms of factors that might be relevant to the development of the disorder. Although difficult to conclusively prove, studies that have investigated this assumption generally support it (Plomin, Willerman, & Loehlin, 1976; Scarr, 1968). Given this assumption, the only difference between MZ and DZ twin pairs is their genetic similarity. Therefore, if higher concordance rates are found in MZ twins than in DZ twins this difference may be due to the MZ twins' increased genetic similarity, and thus suggests the importance of genetic influences for the disorder.

A sophisticated example of this classical twin design is Gottesman and Shields' (1972) twin study of schizophrenia. From a series of 45,000 consecutive admissions to the Maudsley Hospital in London, 55 probands were ascertained who were both consensually diagnosed as schizophrenic and were twins. Zygosity determination yielded 22 MZ and 33 DZ twin pairs. The probands' co-twins were extensively assessed and were diagnosed blindly. According to one diagnostic index, 50% of MZ twin pairs were concordant (pairwise) for schizophrenia compared to 9% of DZ twin pairs. The significantly higher MZ concordance was interpreted as indicating the influence of genetic factors in schizophrenia. The fact that MZ concordance was not 100% suggests that environmental influences must also be important.

In addition to evaluating the importance of genetic factors, twin designs can also investigate the potential role of environmental influences. Because they are genetically identical, any differences between MZ co-twins should be the result of environmental differences. Therefore MZ twin pairs who are discordant for a disorder can be assessed for potential differences in experiences that may have contributed to or protected from the development of the disorder. Although it has a long history, this strategy was recently employed by Pollin and colleagues (Belmaker, Pollin, Wyatt, & Cohen, 1974) to investigate potential environmental differences within MZ twin pairs who were discordant for schizophrenia. They reported that the co-twins who later became schizophrenic tended to have slightly lower birth weights and to be more submissive than the co-twins who did not become schizophrenic.

Evaluation of the characteristics of the nonaffected members of discordant MZ twin pairs may also provide information concerning indicators of the genetic predisposition to the disorder. For example, if some abnormality were found both in schizophrenics and in their unaffected MZ co-twins, it *might* indicate a genetic vulnerability to schizophrenia (e.g., Holzman, Kringlen, Levy, & Haberman, 1980).

In addition, the twin design, like the family study, can provide information concerning the genetic relationships between diagnostic groups. Thus, diagnoses that are common in the nonschizophrenic members of MZ twin pairs discordant for schizophrenia may be genetically associated with schizophrenia, whereas the diagnoses that are infrequent in these subjects would appear to be genetically distinct from schizophrenia.

Twin studies also lend themselves to potentially identifying heterogeneity within a diagnostic group. One such strategy would seek out characteristics that differ between concordant and discordant pairs (Rosenthal, 1959). Such a characteristic could potentially identify more genetic forms of the disorder as opposed to more environmental forms. Shields and Gottesman (1972) used a variation of this procedure to investigate the validity of various diagnostic systems. They diagnosed their twins according to several systems and then compared the differences in MZ and DZ concordances. The diagnostic system that maximized the MZ/DZ difference was interpreted as identifying the most "genetic" schizophrenia.

Although twin studies are difficult to conduct due to the rarity of the joint event of both being a twin (about 1 of 83 births) and of having a particular psychiatric diagnosis, it should be clear from this brief summary that such studies can uniquely shed light on a variety of important issues.

Adoption Designs. In the general family study, the degree of genetic relationship and the degree of shared environment are completely confounded. Immediate family members not only share one-half of their genes, but they also generally live in the same household and interact closely with one another. Adoption designs attempt to disentangle genetic and environmental relationships.

The first type of adoption study has been termed the adoptees design. This strategy begins by identifying adoptees with generally one biological parent who is affected with the disorder of interest. Most often those with affected biological mothers are selected because of the potential ambiguity in establishing paternity. In addition, a control group of adoptees with nonaffected biological parents are also studied. In order to disentangle genetic and environmental influences as much as possible, it is important that only adoptees who were separated from their biological parents soon after birth and who were adopted into the homes of non-relatives be included in the study. The adult adoptees of the two groups are then assessed, blind to the status of their biological parentage, and are diagnosed.

The essential assumption in interpreting the results of this design is that there is no systematic difference between the two groups of adoptees in their adoptive environments that might be relevant to the development of the disorder. Selective placement of the offspring of psychiatric patients into the least fit of adoptive families might possibly produce such a difference. However, most potential adoptive parents are carefully screened and are probably above average in mental health. If their adoptive environments do not systematically differ, the most likely explanation for any differences in rates of diagnoses between the two groups of adoptees (i.e., those with and without affected biological parents) is the transmission of genetic influences from their biological parents.

An excellent example of this design is the first adoption study of schizophrenia, which was conducted by Heston (1966). Using hospital records, Heston located 58 schizophrenic women who had given birth while hospitalized during the years 1915 to 1945 and had immediately given up their children for placement in a foundling home. Matched control subjects whose biological parents had no history of psychiatric disorder, were selected from the records of the same foundling homes. Heston was then able to interview and blindly diagnose these foster-reared offspring in 1964 when their average age was 36 years old. Briefly, a morbid risk of about 16% for schizophrenia was found in the "experimental" adoptees in contrast with 0% in the control adoptees. In addition to schizophrenia, a number of other diagnoses were found to be more common in the experimental group, which suggested their possible genetic relationship with schizophrenia or the effect of unknown paternal psychopathology.

A complimentary type of adoption study, the adoptees' family design, starts with adult adoptees with a particular diagnosis and an appropriate group of control adoptees who have no psychiatric history. The adoptive and biological relatives of these two groups of adoptees are then traced and assessed. If genetic influences are important for the disorder, then more biological relatives of the affected adoptees should be diagnosed than the biological relatives of the control adoptees.

This design was first introduced by Kety and colleagues in their Danish-American adoption studies of schizophrenia (Kety, Rosenthal, Wender, Schulsinger, & Jacobsen, 1978). In a complex series of studies using nationwide adoption and psychiatric registers, which are available in Denmark, Kety and his colleagues identified all the adoptees in Copenhagen and in a later study all those in Denmark who were diagnosed as schizophrenic and also a matched sample of control adoptees.

The adoptees' biological and adoptive relatives were then located and eventually interviewed (the Copenhagen sample) or diagnoses were assigned based on hospital records (total Denmark sample). Although complex, the results of these studies found the prevalence of schizophrenia-spectrum disorders to be higher in the biological relatives of the schizophrenic adoptees than in the biological relatives of control adoptees. The rates of diagnoses did not differ between the two groups of adoptive relatives. Such a pattern of results suggests the presence of a genetic influence in schizophrenia-spectrum disorders.

In addition to the investigation of genetic influences noted above, adoption designs also offer unique opportunities to investigate potential environmental influences (e.g., Wender, Rosenthal, Kety, Schulsinger, & Welner, 1973, 1974). One recent method, using subjects from Kety's study, compared those environmental characteristics of schizophrenic adoptees with schizophrenic biological relatives (high genetic risk) versus those of schizophrenic adoptees without schizophrenic biological relatives (low genetic risk) (Kinney & Jacobsen, 1978). The results of this study tentatively suggested that potential early brain trauma was more common among schizophrenic adoptees at low genetic risk than among those at higher genetic risk. Such studies represent a rich source of information concerning potential environmental influences as well as a means of investigating potential gene by environment interactions. (Plomin, DeFries, & Loehlin, 1977).

Although logistically difficult to conduct, it should be clear from this brief discussion that adoption studies represent powerful methods for addressing a variety of important questions concerning the etiology of psychopathology.

RESEARCH STRATEGIES: A SPECIFIC APPLICATION

Until now we have emphasized the generality of various designs and have briefly discussed particular studies only for illustrative purposes. However, since designs are meant to be realized in practice, we will conclude with a methodological discussion of a specific research study.

This recent study by Pogue-Geile and Harrow (in press) investigated the role of a particular type of symptom in schizophrenia. Recent theorizing had suggested that the overt symptomatology of schizophrenia might be usefully divided into two types. "Positive" symptoms would represent behavioral or cognitive excesses, such as hallucinations, delusions, and florid thought disorder. In contrast, "negative" symptoms would include a deficit or the absence of some normal function, such as psychomotor retardation, flat affect or poverty of speech. Some theorists had suggested that schizophrenics with negative symptoms might have a disorder that is distinct from those schizophrenics with primarily positive symptoms.

One of the main goals of the study was therefore to investigate potential heterogeneity within the schizophrenic diagnostic category. Using case-control sampling, subjects were selected from consecutive admissions between the ages of 18- and 30-years-old to a private psychiatric hospital. Within several weeks of admission the patients were assessed with the SADS structured interview (Spitzer & Endicott, 1979) and were diagnosed blind to other test data using the objective Research Diagnostic Criteria (RDC) (Spitzer, Endicott, & Robins, 1978). Because theory suggested that negative symptoms should be more prominent following acute disturbance, these subjects were studied over time in a prospective design and followed up approximately one and one-half years after their index hospitalization discharge. Approximately 75% of the subjects in this study were able to be successfully followed up. Thirty-nine schizophrenic and 33 depressed patients with completed follow ups composed the study sample.

A control group of depressed patients was chosen to control for general factors associated with being a psychiatric patient and in order to investigate the specificity of negative symptoms to schizophrenia as opposed to depression. Depressed patients were not initially matched with schizophrenics on demographic characteristics for those reasons discussed by Meehl (1970). Instead, between-group comparisons were analyzed separately, both for the total unselected groups and for the groups matched on education, sex, or number of prior hospitalizations. The sample was studied early in the course of their disorder in order to minimize any potential effects of established chronicity. Forty-three percent of the sample were experiencing their first hospital admission. Correlational analyses within the schizophrenic group were based both on the total group and on the first-admission patients alone, in order to investigate any potential effects of established chronicity. It was impossible for practical and ethical reasons to control medication. Therefore, we made between-group comparisons of all major variables while matching on medication and investigated the association of negative symptoms with medication status.

Our ratings of positive and negative symptoms were based on standardized, objective, and psychometrically homogeneous rating scales. Inter-judge reliability was assessed for all measures and was satisfactory.

In order to investigate the role of negative symptoms as a potential marker of pathological or etiological heterogeneity within schizophrenia, their associations with other important aspects of the disorder were investigated. The rationale here was that if a particular characteristic co-occurs with many other important characteristics *within* a diagnostic group, then they may all reflect the effects of some common underlying pathological factor that is not present in all members of the diagnostic group. Negative symptom ratings at follow up were correlated with (1) demographic variables, (2) ratings of prehospitalization functioning, (3) concurrent ratings of role functioning at follow up, and (4) concurrent ratings of positive symptoms at follow up. Ratings of overall functioning were multidimensional, covering social, occupational, symptom, and rehospitalization domains.

Briefly, negative symptoms were found to be significantly more common in schizophrenics than in depressed patients at follow up. Negative symptoms at follow up were associated within the schizophrenics with school failure and poor prehospitalization social functioning. Concurrently at followup, negative symptoms were similarly associated with poor social and vocational functioning. At follow up within the schizophrenic group, positive and negative symptoms were found to be statistically independent of each other. The overall results were interpreted to suggest that negative symptoms seem to mark a subgroup of schizophrenics with poor functioning and with the potential for further deterioration. The absence of a negative correlation between negative and positive symptoms within the schizophrenic group was interpreted as evidence against hypotheses that positive and negative symptoms are at opposite ends of a single continuum. Studies of the longitudinal stability of negative symptoms and of their long-term predictive power would be relevant to investigating further whether negative symptoms represent some distinct pathological process.

SUMMARY

In summary, this chapter has sought to highlight the essentially correlational nature of most psychopathology research and some of the inferential limitations of such methods. Along with these cautions, however, we have sought to illustrate the range of methodological possibilities that are available. Obviously, this does not represent an exhaustive listing and in the absence of experimental methods, investigators are limited only by their own ingenuity in taking advantage of nature's experiments and proposing new strategies.

Although we have presented a number of different methodological considerations in this chapter, we want to re-emphasize that research is conducted to advance knowledge, and that methodology in this area is not an end in itself, but represents a means toward the end of increasing our understanding of psychopathology. Knowledge may be advanced by many different approaches and techniques, including ones that still await development by innovative investigators. Carefully designed research methodology thus represents ways to increase the likelihood of valid scientific results and to discourage false leads.

We can also note, somewhat optimistically for young investigators, that in the field of psychopathology there are many opportunities to further knowledge, since there are still many unknowns. In addition, the potential contributions from research in this area can be considerable: both in terms of easing human suffering and in terms of understanding human behavior. Steady progress on these important and difficult problems has been made in the past 25 years. This steady advance thus far suggests that the field of psychopathology is an opportune area for further research in the future and that such progress is likely to continue for some time to come.

REFERENCES

American Psychiatric Association. (1968). *DSM-II, Diagnostic and statistical manual of mental disorders* (2nd ed.). Washington, DC: Author.

American Psychiatric Association. (1980). *Diagnostic and statistical manual of mental disorders* (3rd ed.). Washington, DC: Author.

Astrachan, B.M., Harrow, M., Adler, D., Brauer, L., Schwartz, A., Schwartz, C., & Tucker, G. (1972). A checklist for the diagnosis of schizophrenia. *British Journal of Psychiatry, 121,* 529–539.

Belmaker, R., Pollin, W., Wyatt, R.J., & Cohen, S. (1974). A followup of monozygotic twins discordant for schizophrenia. *Archives of General Psychiatry, 30,* 219–222.

Buchsbaum, M.S., Coursey, R.D., & Murphy, D.L. (1976). The biochemical high-risk paradigm: Behavioral and familial correlates of low platelet monoamine oxidase activity. *Science, 194,* 339-341.

Buchsbaum, M.S., & Reider, R.O. (1979). Biologic heterogeneity and psychiatric research. *Archives of General Psychiatry, 36,* 1163–1169.

Chapman, L.J., & Chapman, J.P. (1973a). Problems in the measurement of cognitive deficit. *Psychological Bulletin, 79,* 380–385.

Chapman, L.J., & Chapman, J.P. (1973b). *Disordered thought in schizophrenia.* Englewood Cliffs, NJ: Prentice Hall, Inc.

Chapman, L.J., & Chapman, J.P. (1977). Selection of subjects in studies of schizophrenic cognition. *Journal of Abnormal Psychology, 86,* 10–15.

Chapman, L.J., & Chapman, J.P. (1978). The measurement of differential deficit. *Journal of Psychiatric Research,* 303–311.

Chapman, L.J., Chapman, J.P., Raulin, M.L., & Edell, W.S. (1978). Schizotypy and thought disorder as a high risk approach to schizophrenia. In G. Serban (Ed.), *Cognitive defects in the development of mental illness.* New York: Brunner/ Mazel.

Chapman, L.J., Edell, W.S., & Chapman, J.P. (1980). Physical anhedonia, perceptual aberrations, and psychosis proneness. *Schizophrenia Bulletin, 6,* 639–653.

Feighner, J.P., Robins, E., Guze, S.B., Woodruff, R.A., Winokur, G., & Munoz, R. (1972). Diagnostic criteria for use in psychiatry research. *Archives of General Psychiatry, 26,* 57–63.

Garmezy, N., & Streitman, S. (1974a). Children at risk: The search for the antecedents of schizophrenia. Part I. Conceptual models and research methods. *Schizophrenia Bulletin, 8,* 14–90.

Garmezy, N. (1974b). Children at risk: The search for the antecedents of schizophrenia. Part II: Ongoing research programs, issues, and intervention. *Schizophrenia Bulletin, 9,* 55–125.

Gottesman, I.I., & Shields, J. (1972). *Schizophrenia and genetics: A twin study vantage point.* New York: Academic Press.

Gottesman, I.I., & Shields, J. (1982). *Schizophrenia: The epigenetic puzzle.* New York: Cambridge University Press.

Harrow, M., Grinker, R.R., Silverstein, M.L., & Holzman, P. (1978). Is modern-day schizophrenic outcome still negative? *American Journal of Psychiatry, 135,* 1156–1162.

Harrow, M., & Quinlan, D. (in press). *Disordered thinking and schizophrenic psychopathology.* New York: Gardener Press.

Harrow, M., & Silverstein, M.L. (1977). Psychotic symptoms in schizophrenia after the acute phase. *Schizophrenia Bulletin, 3,* 608–616.

Harrow, M., Silverstein, M., & Marengo, J. (1983). Disordered thinking: Does it identify nuclear schizophrenia? *Archives of General Psychiatry, 40,* 765–771.

Heston, L. (1966). Psychiatric disorders in foster home reared children of schizophrenic mothers. *British Journal of Psychiatry, 112,* 819–825.

Holzman, P.S., Kringlen, E., Levy, D.L., & Haberman, S.J. (1980). Deviant eye tracking in twins discordant for psychosis. *Archives of General Psychiatry, 37,* 627–631.

Jacob, T. (1975). Family interaction in disturbed and normal families: A methodological and substantive review. *Psychological Bulletin, 82,* 33–65.

Kety, S.S., Rosenthal, D., Wender, P.H., Schulsinger, F., & Jacobsen, B. (1978). The biologic and adoptive families of adopted individuals who became schizophrenic: Prevalence of mental illness and other characteristics. In L.C. Wynne, R.L. Cromwell, & S. Matthysse (Eds.), *The nature of schizophrenia.* New York: John Wiley & Sons.

Kinney, D.K., & Jacobsen, B. (1978). Environmental factors in schizophrenia: New adoption study evidence. In L.C. Wynne, R.L. Cromwell, & S. Matthysse (Eds.), *The nature of schizophrenia.* New York: John Wiley & Sons.

Kraepelin, E. (1962). *One hundred years of psychiatry.* London: Peter Owen.

Lewine, R.R.J., Watt, N.F., & Grubb, T.W. (1981). High-risk-for-schizophrenia research: Sampling bias and its implications. *Schizophrenia Bulletin, 7,* 273–280.

Loeber, R., & Dishion, T. (1983). Early predictors of male delinquency: A review. *Psychological Bulletin, 94,* 68–99.

Maher, B.A., & Maher, W.B. (1979). Psychopathology. In E. Hearst (Ed.), *The first century of experimental psychology.* Hillsdale, NJ: Lawrence Erlbaum Associates.

McGhie, A., Chapman, J., & Lawson, J.S. (1965). The effect of distraction on schizophrenic performance: (I) Perception and immediate memory. *British Journal of Psychiatry, 111,* 383–390.

McNeil, T.F., & Kaij, L. (1979). Etiological relevance of comparisons of high-risk and low-risk groups. *Acta Psychiatrica Scandinavica, 59,* 545–560.

Mednick, S.A., & McNeil, T.F. (1968). Current methodology in research on the etiology of schizophrenia. *Psychological Bulletin, 70,* 681–693.

Mednick, S.A., & Schulsinger, F. (1968). Some premorbid characteristics related to breakdown in children with schizophrenic mothers. In D. Rosenthal & S.S. Kety (Eds.), *The transmission of schizophrenia.* New York: Pergamon Press.

Mednick, S.A., Schulsinger, H., & Schulsinger, F. (1975). Schizophrenia in children of schizophrenic mothers. In A. Davids (Ed.), *Child personality and psychopathology: Current topics* (Vol. 2). New York: John Wiley & Sons.

Meehl, P.E., (1962). Schizotaxia, schizotypy, schizophrenia. *American Psychologist, 17,* 827–838.

Meehl, P.E. (1970). Nuisance variables and the ex post facto design. In M. Radner, & S. Winokur (Eds.), *Minnesota studies in the philosophy of science* (Vol. 4). Minneapolis: University of Minnesota Press.

Meehl, P.E. (1971). High school yearbooks: A reply to Schwartz. *Journal of Abnormal Psychology, 77,* 143–148.

Pearson, J.S., & Kley, I.B. (1957). On the application of genetic expectancies as age specific base rates in the study of human behavior disorders. *Psychological Bulletin, 54,* 406–420.

Plomin, R., DeFries, J.C., & Loehlin, J. (1977). Genotype-environment interaction and correlation in the analysis of human behavior. *Psychological Bulletin, 84,* 309–322.

Plomin, R., Willerman, L., & Loehlin, J. (1976). Resemblance in appearance and the equal environments assumption in twin studies of personality traits. *Behavior Genetics, 6,* 43–52.

Pogue-Geile, M.F., & Harrow, M. (in press). Negative and positive symptoms in schizophrenia and depression: A followup study. *Schizophrenia Bulletin.*

Rieder, R.D., & Gershon, E.S. (1978). Genetic strategies in biological psychiatry. *Archives of General Psychiatry, 35,* 866–873.

Ritzler, B.A., & Rinehart, K. (1981). Psychotic controls in schizophrenia research. *Schizophrenia Bulletin, 7,* 729–735.

Robins, E., & Guze, S.B. (1970). Establishment of diagnostic validity in psychiatric illness: Its application to schizophrenia. *American Journal of Psychiatry, 126,* 983–987.

Rosenthal, D. (1959). Some factors associated with concordance and disconcordance with respect to schizophrenia in monozygotic twins. *Journal of Nervous and Mental Diseases, 129,* 1–10.

Scarr, S. (1968). Environmental bias in twin studies. *Eugenics Quarterly, 15,* 34–40.

Sedvall, G.C., & Wode-Helgodt, B. (1980). Aberrant monoamine metabolite levels in CSF and family history of schizophrenia. *Archives of General Psychiatry, 37,* 1113–1116.

Shields, J., & Gottesman, I.I. (1972). Cross-national diagnosis of schizophrenia in twins. *Archives of General Psychiatry, 27,* 725–730.

Silverstein, M.L., & Harrow, M. (1981). Schneiderian first-rank symptoms in schizophrenia. *Archives of General Psychiatry, 38,* 288–293.

Snyder, S., Banerjee, S.P., Yamamura, H.I., & Greenberg, D. (1974). Drugs, neurotransmitters, and schizophrenia. *Science, 184,* 1243–1253.

Spitzer, R.L., & Endicott, J. (1979). *Schedule for affective disorders and schizophrenia.* New York: Biometrics Research, New York State Psychiatric Institute.

Spitzer, R.L., Endicott, J., & Robins, E. (1978). *Research Diagnostic Criteria (RDC) for a selected group of functional disorders.* New York: Biometrics Research, New York State Psychiatric Institute.

Strauss, M.E. (1978). The differential and experimental paradigms in the study of cognition in schizophrenia. *Journal of Psychiatric Research, 14,* 316–320.

Thompson, W.D., Orvaschel, H., Prusoff, B.A., & Kidd, K.K. (1982). An evaluation of the family history method for ascertaining psychiatric disorders. *Archives of General Psychiatry, 39,* 53–58.

Tsuang, M.T., Bucher, K.D., & Fleming, J.A. (1982). Testing the monogenic theory of schizophrenia. *British Journal of Psychiatry, 140,* 595–599.

Tsuang, M.T., Winokur, G., & Crowe, R.R. (1980). Morbidity risks of schizophrenia and affective disorders among first degree relatives of patients with schizophrenia, mania, depression, and surgical conditions. *British Journal of Psychiatry, 137,* 497–504.

Tsuang, M.T., Woolson, R.F., & Fleming, J.A. (1979). Long-term outcome of major psychoses. *Archives of General Psychiatry, 36,* 1295–1301.

Vaillant, G. (1983). *The natural history of alcoholism.* Cambridge, MA: Harvard University Press.

Watt, N.F., Fryer, J.H., Lewine, R.R.J., & Prentky, R.A. (1979). Toward longitudinal conceptions of psychiatric disorder. In B.A. Maher, (Ed.), *Progress in experimental personality research* (Vol. 9). New York: Academic Press.

Weissman, M.M., Myers, J.K., & Thompson, W.D. (1981). Depression and its treatment in a U.S. urban community: 1975–1976. *Archives of General Psychiatry, 38,* 417–421.

Wender, P.H., Rosenthal, D., Kety, S.S., Schulsinger, F., & Welner, J. (1973). Social class and psychopathology in adoptees: A natural experimental method for separating the roles of genetic and experiential factors. *Archives of General Psychiatry, 28,* 318–325.

Wender, P.H., Rosenthal, D., Kety, S.S., Schulsinger, F., & Welner, J. (1974). Cross-fostering: A research strategy for clarifying the role of genetic and experiential factors in the etiology of schizophrenia. *Archives of General Psychiatry, 30,* 121–128.

Wing, J.K., Cooper, J.E., & Sartorious, N. (1974). *Measurement and classification of psychiatric symptoms.* New York: Cambridge University Press.

Yarrow, M.R., Campbell, J.D., & Burton, R.V. (1970). Recollections of childhood: A study of the retrospective method. *Monographs of the Society for Research in Child Development, 35,* No. 138.

Zilboorg, G. (1941). *A history of medical psychology.* New York: W.W. Norton & Co., Inc.

8
Psychotherapy

Juris I. Berzins

INTRODUCTION

This chapter examines a number of issues associated with research into the outcomes of psychotherapy. Following a brief overview of the history of psychotherapy research, detailed attention is devoted to a well-known study comparing psychotherapy with behavior therapy (Sloane, Staples, Cristol, Yorkston, & Whipple, 1975). Critical evaluation of that study serves as a vehicle for appraising broader issues in evaluating individual studies as well as in attempting to integrate the results of a number of outcome studies. In this connection, the recent meta-analytic methodology for integrating the results of psychotherapy outcome studies (e.g., Glass, 1976; Smith & Glass, 1977; Smith, Glass, & Miller, 1980) is discussed, with the aim of discerning promising lines of theoretical and empirical progress.

PSYCHOTHERAPY: REVIEWED, COMPARED, STUDIED

A Brief History of Psychotherapy Research

Although quite a few of the early practitioners of psychotherapy may have kept personal records of the outcomes of their treatment of various patients, the scrutiny of psychotherapy with the aid of the scientific method is probably less than six decades old. When I entered graduate school in the late 1950s, what transpired in the consulting rooms of psychodynamic therapists was a matter shrouded in mystery. Even though the pioneering efforts of Carl Rogers in "actually recording sessions" for subsequent coding and analysis were hailed by many as a daring challenge to therapists' reluctance to expose their conduct to examination by researchers, many psychoanalytically-oriented therapists maintained that the very act of recording might have deleterious transference-countertransference implications, much as a therapist's having a pet dog present during sessions might complicate the transference (Wolberg, 1954, p. 188).

It was also not clear in the mid-1950s that conducting research into the effectiveness of psychotherapy was apt to be a rewarding professional experience. After all, Eysenck (1952) had aroused great controversy with his provocative charge that, according to his selective review of the literature, there was no good evidence that psychotherapy with neurotic patients was more effective than no treatment at all. However, Eysenck's challenge did stimulate a great many rebuttals and constructive research efforts, and the espirit of psychotherapy researchers was aided greatly by a series of three formal conferences on psychotherapy research. Conducted over roughly a decade under the sponsorship of the American Psychological Association with the support of the National Institute of Mental Health, they brought together eminent researchers and clinicians to share findings, experiences, and research strategies (Rubinstein & Parloff, 1959; Shlien, 1968; Strupp & Luborsky, 1962). To be sure, some research efforts seemed to skirt the issue of outcome by restricting their focus to "process" variables; that is, aspects of the behavior of the therapist and the patient during sessions. (For a compendium of systems of process measurement, see Kiesler, 1973.) In retrospect, some of the early process studies seem rather amazing. For example, some researchers affixed electrodes to various parts of the therapists' and patients' anatomies in hopes that recorded fluctuations in various channels might afford an insight into "what really goes on" in psychotherapy.

Some process variables, such as the Rogerian "therapist-offered conditions" (e.g., Truax & Carkhuff, 1967), gained ascendancy in the 1960s by suggesting that, regardless of "average" outcomes in comparisons of treated and control groups, therapists who offered high levels of accurate empathy, positive regard, and personal genuineness obtained good results with their patients, whereas low levels of these conditions were thought to lead to deterioration (e.g., Bergin, 1966). Subsequent research with these variables, however, has suggested that these claims require considerable attenuation. There seems to be little evidence that the therapist-offered conditions are sufficient for psychotherapeutic improvement, even if they may be necessary in client-centered and similar therapies (e.g., Mitchell, Bozarth, & Krauft, 1977).

Pursuant upon the publication of Wolpe's *Psychotherapy by Reciprocal Inhibition* (1958), the greatest impetus to outcome research was probably occasioned by the rise of behavior modification and behavior therapy during the 1960s. Just as Eysenck himself, while remaining the foremost critic of "traditional" (psychodynamic and eclectic) psychotherapy (Eysenck, 1961, 1965), championed therapy based on "learning theories" as an effective means for alleviating neurotic problems, many like-minded researchers conducted studies of the effects of behavioral interventions (especially systematic desensitization) upon neurotic-like problems, (particularly phobias). With the concurrent emergence of interventions such as token economies based on Skinnerian principles of operant conditioning, behavior therapy gained many adherents eager to prove its superiority to traditional psychotherapy (for an excellent review of the history of behavior modification, see Kazdin, 1978). Gordon Paul's (1966) dissertation research, comparing the effectiveness of "insight therapy" with systematic desensitization in the amelioration of public speaking anxiety, has been regarded by many as the classic study of behavior therapy, conferring distinction not only on its author but also seemingly forming the basis for the belief that the race between "traditional" and behavioral therapies had clearly been won by the latter.

Whatever the ultimate judgment regarding this race might be, there is little question that studies like Paul's inspired subsequent outcome researchers to show much greater methodological rigor and theoretical specificity than had been characteristic of most outcome studies conducted during the preceding several decades. Moreover, behavior therapy brought with it other methodological advances such as the intensive study of the single case through ABAB designs, multiple baseline designs, and so on (cf. Kazdin, 1982). The rallying cry for the emerging perspective on outcome research was Paul's (1967, p. 111) question: "*What* treatment, by *whom*, is most effective for *this* individual with *that* specific problem, and under *which* set of circumstances?" This question was also consistent with Kiesler's Grid Model for psychotherapy research, according to which the possibility of detecting interactions as well as main effects should be enhanced by factorial designs which included several homogeneous groups of patients, homogeneous groups of therapists or types of therapy, multiple occasions of measurement, and multiple measures of change (Kiesler, 1966, 1971).

A general consequence of this quest for specificity was that the evaluative standards for outcome research increasingly emphasized internal validity (Campbell & Stanley, 1966; Cook & Campbell, 1979) at the possible expense of external validity. Thus, the failure of a researcher to control for possible alternative interpretations of the putatively causal relationship between some specific therapeutic intervention and some particular dependent measure (e.g., by failing to control for alleged "nonspecific" effects by including attention-placebo control groups in the design) could form the basis for impeaching the results of the study as inconclusive, whereas the extent to which the findings of a well-controlled laboratory analogue study could be generalized to everyday clinical practices or settings was simply considered an empirical matter to be resolved by further research. Thus, well-controlled studies of behavior modification with college student volunteers who admitted to being fearful of snakes were considered valid contributions to our knowledge of behavior change, even if few practicing therapists had ever encountered a single patient seeking relief from snake phobia.

Adherents of psychodynamic or other non-behavioral approachers, however, tended to criticize such studies either on theoretical grounds (e.g., behavior therapy addresses only "superficial" problems) or on the grounds of external validity. In that fashion, research results which did not meet these evaluators' standards for "real" therapy conducted by real therapists with real patients, and so on, could be excluded from reviews regarding the research evidence on the outcomes of psychotherapy.

Space limitations preclude a discussion in which varying emphases on internal and external validity have interpenetrated the bewilderingly discrepant conclusions drawn by scholarly reviewers of the literature on the outcomes of psychotherapy (e.g., Bergin, 1971; Eysenck, 1952, 1961; Luborsky, Singer, & Luborsky, 1975; Meltzoff & Kornreich, 1970; Rachman, 1971; Smith et al., 1980). It is obvious, however, that an outcome study which simultaneously displays an acceptable degree of internal validity (the indispensable criterion for both behavioral and "traditional" evaluators) *and* external validity (the standard cherished by psychodynamic and other clinicians) should highlight the controversies associated with these evaluative polarities.

Psychotherapy versus Behavior Therapy: The Sloane et al. (1975) Study

This study had four main aims: (1) to compare the effectiveness of behavior therapy, analytically-oriented therapy ("psychotherapy"), and minimal contact (waiting list) treatment; (2) to examine the similarities and differences between behavior therapy and psychotherapy; (3) to investigate the effect on outcome of therapist experience levels and certain other therapist attributes; and (4) to see which kinds of problems or patients might be differentially amenable to one or the other type of psychotherapy.

The design of the study required outpatients at the Temple University Psychiatric Outpatient Clinic to be randomly assigned to each of the three conditions of the study. Three experienced therapists in each of the active treatment conditions saw at least 10 patients each, for a duration of 4 months. Selection of patients for the study was accomplished by three psychiatrists ("assessors") who evaluated the patient's suitability for the study, determined the patient's main problems ("target symptoms"), rated the severity of these problems, and rated the patient's adjustment in other areas of life as well. The assessors reevaluated each patient after 4 months of treatment and again approximately 1 year after the initial contact. A research assistant prepared patients for their assessments, maintained telephone contact with waiting-list patients (the latter had been told that crisis help was available if needed) to reassure them that treatment would be forthcoming, and, at the time of each assessment, also interviewed a close friend or relative of the patient ("informant") to obtain additional perspectives on the patient's status.

The two main measures of treatment outcome consisted of: (1) changes in the severity of three target symptoms (determined individually for each patient in the initial assessment session), and (2) changes in general adjustment (as rated by the assessor, the patient, the therapist, and the informant). Because the assessors could be regarded as the most impartial evaluators of the patient's status, their ratings were accorded greater weight than the ratings of the other sources.

Patients were accepted into the study if: (1) they were appropriate candidates for outpatient psychotherapy (excluded were relatively normal or situationally disturbed persons, on the one hand, and psychotic, drug-abusing, suicidal, or brain-damaged persons, on the other); (2) they were willing to participate in 4 months of "talking therapy" (rather than in some other treatment or drugs); (3) the assessor felt psychotherapy to be the treatment of choice (as versus the need for medication); and (4) they were between 18 and 45 years of age. Some 29 patients were excluded by these criteria; 94 were retained. (Data for four of the latter were not used subsequently.)

The patients retained for the study were predominantly in their early 20s, female (60%), and white. They averaged 14 years of education and had an estimated (probably underestimated) verbal IQ of 99. Fifty-four percent of the sample were students. On the Minnesota Multiphasic Personality Inventory (MMPI), the average patient showed elevations above $T=70$ on scales 2 (Depression), 4 (Psychopathic Deviate), 7 (Psychasthenia) and 8 (Schizophrenia). With the exception of scale 5 (Masculinity-Femininity), the other clinical scales averaged above $T=60$. On the Eysenck Personality Inventory, patients' mean neuroticism score placed them at the 86th percentile, and the mean extraversion score at the 39th percentile, of American college norms. Data from the California Psychological Inventory depicted the sample as low in self-control, sociability, and socialization. About two-thirds of the sample were diagnosed as carrying neurotic (primarily anxiety reaction) diagnoses; the remaining third were judged to exhibit personality disorders.

Categorization of the rated target symptoms showed that, in decreasing order, they concerned anxiety (20%), inability to perform in some area of behavior (17%), unwanted habits (12%), and bodily complaints (11%); six other categories each included from 4 to 9% of the remaining symptoms. The average severity of these symptoms were rated by assessors as being between "moderately severe" and "severe" in all three groups of patients at the outset of therapy.

Sloane et al. wanted the three groups of patients to be matched on three dimensions: (1) number per group (30); (2) level of neuroticism (high and low groups were formed by a median split of neuroticism scores on the Eysenck Personality Inventory); and (3) sex (60% of the patients were female). Because of the investigators' interest in the effects of therapist experience, the six white male therapists were considered to represent different levels of experience. High, intermediate, and low levels of experience were represented in the behavior therapy group by 20, 13, and 6 years, and in the psychotherapy group by 35, 20, and 8 years.

The design of the study thus basically involved nine subgroups of patients

(3 treatment conditions × 3 levels of therapist experience): Two male and three female patients with high neuroticism scores, and the same numbers with low, were assigned randomly to each subgroup.

In the conduct of treatment, therapists were free to employ whatever techniques they deemed appropriate for particular patients. To assess differences in the way behavior therapists and psychotherapists interacted with their patients, however, Sloane et al. secured tape recordings of the fifth therapy interview. The tapes were subsequently rated on a number of process dimensions, most notably those of the Rogerian "therapist-offered" conditions.

Results. After 4 months of therapy, Sloane et al. assessed the changes in two main areas: changes in the severity of the three target symptoms and changes in the levels of adjustment in other areas of functioning. As noted earlier, the assessors' perspective was accorded the principal weight.

The severity of target symptoms (1 = absent; 2 = trivial; 3 = mild; 4 = moderate; 5 = severe) had decreased significantly in both the behavior therapy and psychotherapy groups, relative to changes in the minimal treatment group. The two treated groups did not differ from one another. In terms of the labels associated with the 5-point scale, both active treatments had reduced the severity of symptoms from moderately severe to trivial-to-mild, whereas the severity of symptoms in the minimal treatment group remained within the mild-to-moderate range.

With regard to general adjustment, changes were examined on the basis of two factor-analytically derived item domains based on the structured interview conducted by assessors. These two item domains, termed work inadequacy and social isolation, showed less clearcut results. Although patients in all three groups showed decreases in problems in both areas over the 4-month period, an overall analysis of variance showed no reliable intergroup differences. Neither were the factors of patient neuroticism or sex implicated in significant main or interaction effects. (The latter had been nonsignificant in the target symptom analysis as well.)

To assess whether therapists' experience levels might have played differential roles in the two treated groups, a 2 (treatments) × 3 (experience) × 2 (patients' neuroticism) analysis of variance was performed across target symptom, work inadequacy, and social isolation change scores. In all three analyses, no main or interaction effects proved significant, indicating that the levels of therapist experience obviously had no demonstrable bearing on the outcomes obtained. The authors acknowledge, however, that even their "least experienced" therapist had treated approximately 300 patients during the preceding 6 years.

To facilitate comparison of their results to those of other studies in the literature, Sloane et al. also tabulated the percentages of patients who could be considered to have improved or worsened to varying degrees. An original

13-point rating scale was collapsed into a 5-point scale: 4 = completely recovered; 3 = improved; 2 = no change; 1 = worse; 0 = very much worse. In terms of target symptom severity, 80% of the patients in each of the active treatment groups were rated by assessors at 3 or 4 (improved or recovered) compared with only 48% of the patients in the minimal treatment group. With respect to assessors' ratings of overall adjustment, the percentages of patients rated at 3 or 4 in the behavioral, psychotherapy, and minimal treatment groups were 93, 77, and 77, respectively. (Incidentally, only two patients were rated as having become worse during the 4 months and only one patient was rated as having become worse symptomatically—a very low incidence of "deterioration effects.")

What about the perception of the patients themselves? Analysis of their self-ratings of target symptom severity on a comparable 5-point scale showed that self-ratings of 3 or 4 characterized 74%, 81% and 44% of the patients in the behavioral, psychotherapy, and minimal treatment groups, respectively. On self-ratings of overall adjustment, the respective percentages for the behavioral, psychotherapy, and minimal treatment patients were 93, 80, and 55. (Note that, in the minimal treatment group, assessors saw more patients as improving in overall adjustment than reported by patients themselves, viz. 77% vs. 55%.)

In analyses of variance comparing the four sources of ratings available in this study—assessor, therapist, patient, informant—it was found that the behavior therapists tended to perceive greater improvement in work adjustment than did assessors or informants, and greater improvement in sexual adjustment than did all three other sources. There were no significant intergroup differences in ratings of social adjustment. Sloane et al. also report intercorrelating the ratings across sources, using for this purpose a composite score based on rated improvements in work, social, and sexual adjustment. Because, for example, some informants might not have known details of the patient's adjustment in the sexual area, completeness of data varies across sources (no degrees of freedom reported). Nevertheless, the intercorrelations are shown in Table 8.1

Since the assessors' ratings were considered the most credible in this study, it is somewhat reassuring that they correlated significantly with those of patients and informants. Therapists' ratings, which in many studies have been regarded as acceptable measures of outcome, appear to be the most idiosyncratic in this study. The impression should be tempered, however, by recognition of several methodological issues: each therapist, after all, rated only the 10 patients he treated; each assessor rated a presumably greater (unstated) number of patients; each patient and informant rated only one target person. The correspondences in rank order are thus obviously complicated by intersource differences in means, variances, levels for "anchoring," and reasons for missing data.

Table 8.1. Intersource Correlations for Composite Improvement Scores

	Source of Rating		
Source of Rating	T	P	I
Assessor (A)	.13	.65*	.40**
Therapist (T)		.21	−.04
Patient (P)			.25
Informant (I)			

Note. Table entries are taken from the text of Sloane, Staples, Cristol, Yorkston, & Whipple (1975), p. 112.
*$p < .01$.
**$p < .001$.

Sloane et al. were able to obtain follow-up data on all but two of the original participants who once again met with their assessors and were evaluated by them. Although several factors complicated clear-cut group comparisons (e.g., patients had undergone differing amounts of subsequent therapy), the overall impression of the 1-year data is that the changes evident at 4 months had continued in a favorable direction or had been maintained. (A 2-year follow-up effort located 61 of the original 90 patients; by this time, the minimal treatment group had obtained as much therapy as the treated groups and, like the latter, had maintained its gains.)

The remainder of the original report by Sloane et al. focused on differences between the two types of active treatment on various process measures. One of the surprising findings was that behavior therapists exceeded psychotherapists in rated accurate empathy, self-congruence, and depth of interpersonal contact (no differences in unconditional positive regard); therapists' scores on these dimensions, however, did not predict the degree of patient improvement in this sample. With regard to the relationship between various patient characteristics and improvement, one of the interesting findings was that, whereas psychotherapists performed more effectively with patients who showed low rather than high levels of initial distress on the MMPI, the behavior therapists showed no differential outcomes with patients varying in initial distress. In fact, there was a suggestion that behavior therapy might be especially helpful with patients who showed relatively *elevated* MMPI scales suggestive of acting-out tendencies such as scale 3 (Hysteria) and scale 9 (Mania).

Sloane et al. concluded:

> It is remarkable that all three groups of patients significantly improved in four months. The control group was by no means "untreated," but it improved considerably without any formal therapy. Nevertheless, both groups of formally

treated patients improved significantly more than the control patients on their target symptoms. This is rather clear evidence that therapy in general "works." (pp. 223–224)

Critique of the Sloane et al. Study

Whereas no single study may ever be perfect, the study by Sloane et al. certainly passes minimal standards of adequacy by a wide margin. The study embodies obvious strengths in the areas of internal validity (e.g., treatment groups were compared with an equivalent control group; random assignment of patients to groups was successful; no attrition occurred over the 4-month period) and external validity (e.g., therapists were experienced practitioners; patients were genuine applicants for outpatient therapy and were selected to be representative of the types of patients who most commonly obtain treatments of the sort offered; therapies were conducted without artificial constraints, and so on). The investigators also commendably sought information regarding patient improvement from multiple sources (but accorded the major weight to the presumably most objective source, viz. the assessor), tailored outcome measures (target symptoms) at least in part to the salient concerns of each patient as an individual, conducted extensive process analyses to assure themselves that the behavior therapists and psychotherapists indeed behaved in sessions as their "school" allegiances would lead one to expect, and showed high levels of ethical concern, e.g., by keeping in contact with waiting-list patients and offering them crisis help if needed. In short, this is a very good study of the outcomes of psychological treatment. One can certainly understand the sentiments of one of the behavior therapists in this study, Joseph Wolpe, who wrote in the preface of the book by Sloane et al.:

> Although I was involved as a "behavior therapist" in the study I did not realize what a splendid piece of research had been in the making until I saw the final manuscript. In the perceptiveness of its planning, the variety and rigor of its comparisons, and the care of its execution, it is unmatched by any other clinical study in the history of psychotherapy. (p. xix)

Similarly, Bergin and Suinn (1975), invoking an obvious comparison with Paul's (1966) study of insight versus desensitization in the treatment of public speaking anxiety, declared the study by Sloane et al. to be "clearly superior in the sense of involving clinical cases representing a number of syndromes and treatment by experts in a natural setting" (p. 511). In their book reporting on their meta-analysis of the results of 475 psychotherapy outcome studies, Smith et al. (1980) referred to the study by Sloane et al. as "the best single outcome evaluation of psychotherapy ever accomplished" (p. 26).

But now, as Smith et al. (1980) did in their book, it may be appropriate to consider an evaluative comment from Albert Bandura:

> A widely publicized study (by Sloane et al.) comparing the relative efficacy of behavioral therapy with psychotherapy, similarly contains the usual share of confounded variables, unmatched mixtures of dysfunctions, and inadequately measured outcomes relying on amorphous clinical ratings rather than on direct assessment of behavioral functioning. As is now predictable for studies of this type, the different forms of treatment appear comparable and better than nothing on some of the global ratings but not on others. With such quasi-outcome measures even the controls, who receive no therapeutic ministrations, achieve impressive improvement. Based on this level of research, weak modes of treatment are given a new lease on life for those who continue to stand steadfastly by them. (Bandura, 1978, p. 87)

Similarly, after designating the study by Sloane et al. as the "best controlled study *of its kind* yet conducted" (p. 52, italics added), Kazdin and Wilson (1978) took a dim view of the fact, for example, that Sloane et al. included a variety of clinical syndromes in their study:

> The inclusion of different types of problems treated by widely differing techniques compounds the difficulties involved in answering *the outcome question*, namely, determining the specific effect of a specific treatment on a specific problem. (pp. 56–57, italics added)

Kazdin and Wilson (1978) likewise regarded as unfortunate the fact that Sloane et al. permitted therapists to select technical interventions according to their own clinical judgments of appropriateness, since such "omnibus packages" do not permit the researcher to identify critical change-producing variables.

Before discussing some of the reasons for these startlingly discrepant evaluative perspectives on the merits of this study, some fairly specific as well as more general comments appear appropriate.

(1) Almost every reviewer of this study has commented on the high improvement rate shown by the minimal treatment group: It seems too good to be true. Although with regard to target symptoms, only 48% of the minimal treatment patients were rated as improved over 4 months, 77% of these patients were rated as improved in overall adjustment (the same percentage as in the psychotherapy group even if lower than the 93% in the behavior therapy group). Were assessors uncommonly lenient in their judgments? A more likely explanation, and one favored by the authors themselves, is that the lengthy interview with impressive psychiatric assessors, the opportunity to sort out their problems, the telephone contacts by a "warm and friendly" research assistant, etc. comprised a quasi-therapeutic package which, in the context of a prestigious university-sponsored research project, exerted stronger demands and encouraged hopes for improvement than implied in a "control" designation for this group. But, since assignment to groups was random and since

both the behavioral and psychotherapy groups exceeded this group with respect to target symptom relief, one would have to conclude that the active treatments were "powerful" indeed to have overcome such "attention-placebo" effects.

(2) Although it is difficult to imagine that patients, especially those on waiting-list status, might not have emitted spontaneous remarks suggesting their group membership at the 4-month reassessment, the assessors were reported to have remained blind to the group membership of patients "with surprising success" (p. 85). Since this null hypothesis is not capable of proof, the authors presumably base this allegation on their failure to detect biases favoring one therapy over another (or, given the improvement of patients in the minimal treatment group, favoring therapy over no therapy). But there is no documentation of the mean ratings involved in such comparisons. In fact, it is not clear how many patients in the study were rated by each assessor.

(3) The operationalization of therapist experience in this study does not seem meaningful. Analyses of variance were applied as though the three therapists in each group could be regarded as representing one of three different "fixed" levels of experience. But all therapists had at least 6 years of experience and the actual years in the two groups were only roughly comparable (e.g., the "high" behavior therapist had the same 20 years of experience as the "intermediate" psychotherapist). Had therapist experience proven to have had main or interactive bearing upon the outcome data, such effects would have probably been more readily explicable as adventitious differences among six particular therapists than the effects of differing amounts of prior clinical experience.

(4) In this connection, since each therapist administered only one of the two types of therapy (rather than both, as in Paul, 1966, for example), formal attempts should have been made to demonstrate that this therapist × treatment confound did not bias the results, e.g., by showing by *F* tests that differences between treatments (even if these were infrequent) overrode differences between specific therapists nested within treatments. There are indications in the analyses for therapist-offered conditions, for example, that the "significant" differences between behavior therapists and psychotherapists might have been due almost exclusively to the lower ratings assigned to only one of the psychotherapists (p. 167). The authors acknowledge this problem in the context of process measures but it applies with equal cogency to outcome measures.

(5) With regard to the measures of outcome employed, the most face-valid and persuasive information regarding the efficacy of the two therapies came from the assessor-rated changes in target symptom severity (for a recent review of individualized outcome measures, see Mintz & Kiesler, 1982). Whereas Kazdin and Wilson (1978) have criticized the assessors' "dependency" on information supplied by the patient, it is difficult to imagine a more valid source of problem definition than the patient who is seeking help for the problems.

Although Sloane et al. could have added some standardized outcome measures to the ones they actually used (e.g., retesting with the MMPI was suggested by Garfield, 1976), they in fact added specially constructed rating scales addressing adjustment in vocational, social and sexual areas. On these and similar rating scales (with generally untested psychometric properties), it is true that all sources of ratings (assessors, therapists, patients, and informants) tended to see the patients as improving but there were not only disagreements as to mean levels of adjustment among sources but also with regard to the rank-ordering of patients on these dimensions of adjustment (cf. Table 8.1 above). Although some of the reasons for these disagreements are purely methodological, the fact remains that therapists' ratings of improvement, for example, which in some reviews of psychotherapy have been considered acceptable measures of outcome (cf. Luborsky, Chandler, Auerbach, Cohen, & Bachrach, 1971), correlated significantly with *no* other source in this study!

To be sure, there have been serious efforts to develop a "core battery" for measuring the outcomes of psychotherapy (e.g., Waskow & Parloff, 1975) but the use of ad hoc measures of outcome has been and continues to be characteristic of the vast majority of outcome studies. I have argued elsewhere that the systematic study of agreements and disagreements among sources of outcome evaluation on measures that show psychometric promise is a matter of high priority if the efficacy of therapeutic interventions is to be evaluated against reasonably consensual standards (Berzins, Bednar, & Severy, 1975). Such research probably would require extensive collaboration among investigators in a variety of clinical settings. But in the meanwhile, I would certainly underscore the observation that "the measurement of outcomes seems to have been abandoned at a primitive stage in its development" (Smith et al., 1980, p. 187; see also Bergin & Lambert, 1978, pp. 171–179).

Turning now to a more general discussion of the reasons for the sharply discrepant evaluative reactions by the critics cited at the beginning of this section, it seems appropriate to examine them under two related headings. One explanation concerns differences regarding conceptual and methodological priorities in outcome research; the other involves ideological commitments and worldviews or "world hypotheses" (Pepper, 1942).

Cook and Campbell (1979) point out that investigators with theoretical interests differ from theorists with applied interests in the priorities they assign to various forms of validity in evaluating research studies. (The distinction between research and evaluation, or elucidatory and evaluative inquiry, as drawn by Smith et al., 1980, is also applicable.) Whereas both groups assign the highest weight to the internal validity of a study, psychotherapy researchers whose main interest lies in delineating specific causal relationships between specific therapeutic interventions and specific changes in problem behaviors, for example, will be much more concerned with the construct validity of causes and effects and with statistical conclusion validity than they will be with external validity. The behavioral critics of Sloane et al., accordingly, have acknowledged the acceptable internal validity of the study (random assignment, no attrition, etc.) but then their focus shifts immediately to such aspects of statistical conclusion validity as the reliability of measures (global clinical ratings), the reliability of treatment effects (e.g., Why were treatments not strictly standardized?) and such aspects of the presumable construct validity of causes and effects as the possible presence of mono-operation biases (Why were no behavioral measures used?) or mono-method biases (Why was observable problem behavior not studied?).

On the other hand, the applied researcher or the practicing clinician, after determining that the internal validity of the study is indeed satisfactory, looks immediately for external validity and only then considers other "niceties." (Cook and Campbell suggest that, for these evaluators, the probable order of concerns, after internal and external validity, would be: the construct validity of effects, statistical conclusion validity, and the construct validity of causes. This ordering is debatable.) In this light, the lack of standardization in administering treatments—allowing therapists to select interventions appropriate to their clinical judgment—would emerge as a strength of the study by Sloane et al., because this is the way most practicing therapists operate. And, even if Paul (1966) was able to avoid a therapist × treatment confound by having his therapists perform *both* insight and behavioral interventions, in the "real world" therapists do not tend to use techniques inconsistent with their beliefs regarding effectiveness or techniques in which they had not been trained. With regard to the omission of behavioral measures by Sloane et al.: How could one realistically expect to observe 90 patients in problem situations unless one intentionally recruited patients whose problems were easily observed and were homogeneous (e.g., snake phobics)? In this manner, one can appreciate that what to one group of evaluators comprises "unmatched mixtures of dysfunctions" (cf. Bandura, 1978, quoted earlier), to the other group is a realistic sample of patients with presenting complaints common to most outpatient settings.

Consequently, one can appreciate that evaluative reactions that seem almost embarrassingly at variance with one another may have a basis in genuine convictions regarding "good" clinical research. Besides, as Kazdin (1980) has observed:

> As a general rule, design features that make an experiment more sensitive to a test of the independent and dependent variables tend to limit the generality of the findings. Conversely, features of an experiment that enhance generality tend to decrease the sensitivity of the experimental test. (p. 53)

A second perspective for explaining how the results of this study could be evaluated so differently concerns the evaluators' ideological and metaphysical commitments. After all, the main conclusion of this study (if accepted as valid) is that *both* behavior therapy and psychotherapy are (relatively equally) effective in alleviating the severity of target symptoms in neurotic patients and *both* are superior in this regard to a minimal treatment condition. One cannot imagine that "traditional" psychodynamic therapists would be disturbed by this conclusion. But to the behaviorally-oriented evaluator who believes that the race between behavioral and "traditional" therapies has been long over, this conclusion could arouse dissonance. Even though behavior therapists could point to this study as contradicting the stereotypes of behavior therapists as cold and manipulative and of behavior therapy as appropriate only to monosymptomatic phobias or "superficial" problems, to rejoice over such victories in the context of a "tie" is difficult. It is not surprising, consequently, that in spite of his favorable evaluation of this study cited earlier, Wolpe (1981) in a later publication reported only differences favoring behavior therapy and omitted mention of "ties" (e.g., he cited percentages of overall improvement ratings rather than improvement in target symptoms).

In a broader sense, it is probably accurate to characterize most of the behavioral evaluations as grounded in the world hypothesis of mechanism (Pepper, 1942). In his classic volume, *World Hypotheses,* Pepper contended that there are only a few relatively (but in principle equally) adequate "world hypotheses," each of which was based on a different root metaphor. The relevance of the four relatively adequate world hypotheses explicated by Pepper—formism, mechanism, contextualism, organicism—to psychological theory and research has emerged in a number of recent publications (e.g., Jenkins', 1974, documenting his shift from a mechanistic to a contextual framework for studying human memory, or Sarbin's, 1977, advocacy of contextualism as the most appropriate theoretical model for psychology). Most of the evaluative clashes regarding the merits of the study by Sloane et al. have involved clashes between mechanism and the other three hypotheses. But, if there are such marked methodological, theoretical, and ideological schisms in evaluating a single study, how can one hope to attain clarity regarding what is known in a series of psychotherapy outcome studies?

Meta-analysis of Psychotherapy Outcome Studies

The serious student of psychotherapy research who has looked for guidance to senior scholars in the field for the most rigorous or thoughtful appraisals of the results of the literally hundreds of studies inevitably has found contradictions of the most glaring sort between the opinions of these scholars. (For a review of the reviews of psychotherapy outcome studies, see Smith et al., 1980, especially Table 2.1 on p. 23.) Those of us who teach graduate students, to be sure, have observed with disquiet that when different graduate students undertake to write evaluative reviews of particular sub-areas of psychotherapy research, their usually excellent papers often reach diametrically opposite conclusions regarding "what is clearly known" in that area of research. In their reviewing methodology the graduate students (like their teachers) have tended to use either narrative integrations or "box score" integrations (Smith et al., 1980). As regards narrative integrations:

> This method of research integration may have emanated from an epistemology of uniformity, an expectation of consistent findings from homogeneous materials such as a physicist might expect to see. The method was ill-equipped to cope with the variability of the social sciences. As time passed and literature grew to enormous proportions, the problems of narrative integration became more acute. The impossibility of reading several hundred experiments, reflecting on their findings, and then writing a narrative description was clearly apparent. (Smith et al., p. 37)

To reduce the literature to a manageable set of studies, narrative reviewers typically rely on a set of "arbitrary" stipulative definitions and judgments of quality. Some reviewers, for example, may exclude all unpublished dissertation research or all analogue studies. Obviously, each reviewer's biases can have full play under these circumstances.

As concerns the "box score" integration, the basic procedure usually is as follows:

> All studies which have data on a dependent variable and a specific independent variable of interest are examined. Three possible outcomes are defined. The relationship between the independent variable is either significantly positive, significantly negative, or there is no significant relationship in either direction. The number of studies falling into each of the three categories is simply tallied. If a plurality of studies falls into any one of these three categories, with fewer falling into the other two, the modal category is declared the winner. This modal category is then assumed to give the best estimate of the direction of the true relationship between the independent and dependent variable. (Light & Smith, 1971, p. 433)

As Smith et al. point out, the most serious problem with the "box score" approach is that it ignores sample size (making, say, five small-scale studies outweigh one large-sample study). This method also ignores the strength of experimental effects, thus in essence making statistical significance the only criterion of "truth."

The methodological advances that led Glass (1976) and his colleagues to propose that the limitations of narrative and "box score" reviews could be overcome by the method termed meta-analysis are still controversial and in process of refinement. The February 1983 issue of the *Journal of Consulting and Clinical Psychology*, for example, contained a special invited section on meta-analysis, no doubt in response to the desire of many researchers to have its merits and limitations discussed (e.g., Garfield, 1981).

Meta-analysis of psychotherapy outcome studies (Glass, 1976; Smith & Glass, 1977; Smith et al., 1980) basically involves: (a) aggregating detailed summaries of psychotherapy outcome studies in which a treated group has been compared with an untreated control group on one or more measures of outcome; (b) determining the effect sizes associated with each dependent measure in the study, with effect size defined as the mean difference between the treated and the control group on an outcome measure, the difference being divided by the standard deviation of the control group on that measure; (c) averaging effect sizes across studies (to yield an overall estimate of the effectiveness of psychotherapy) or averaging them within interesting subsets of studies (e.g., behavior therapy vs. psychodynamic therapy; neurotic vs. psychotic patients, and so on).

In their major work entitled *The Benefits of Psychotherapy*, Smith et al. reported that the average effect size across a total of 475 outcome studies, encompassing some 1,761 effect sizes, was .85, indicating that the difference between the mean of the groups receiving some form of therapy and that of the untreated control groups was .85 standard deviation units. Put in terms of the normal curve, this finding indicates that

> The average person who receives therapy is better off at the end of it than 80 percent of the persons who do not. Stated differently, but equivalently, the average person, who would score at the 50th percentile of the untreated control population, could expect to rise to the 80th percentile with respect to that population after receiving psychotherapy. (pp. 87–88)

Beyond this global testimony to the effectiveness of psychotherapy as reflected in this "sample" of outcome studies, Smith et al. also conducted extensive analyses of the extents to which effect sizes varied with different types of therapy (variously subgrouped into 18, 6, or 3 subclasses), patient diagnostic categories, types of outcome measures and their reactivity, internal validity of the studies, and so on. To consider only the findings associated with the broadest grouping of therapeutic orientations, behavioral therapies initially appeared more effective than "verbal" ones (mean effect sizes of .98 and .84 respectively). However, analyses which took the reactivity of outcome measures into account eliminated the difference, because behavioral studies generally had employed more reactive outcome measures, e.g., by requiring snake phobics to pick up and handle the snake in the presence of the therapist or experimenter (cf. Bernstein & Nietzel, 1973, on this issue). In an additional analysis of only those 56 studies in which behavioral, verbal, and control groups had been compared directly ("same experiment analysis"), the behavioral group again proved superior (mean effect sizes of .96 and .77 respectively), but Smith et al. deemphasized the significance of this finding because the ostensible superiority of behavioral therapies was associated primarily with measures of fear/anxiety and global adjustment rather than with "less tractable" outcome measures such as changes in addictive or sociopathic behaviors. At any rate, as Glass and Kliegl (1983) stated subsequently:

> This difference (.19 sigma units) between verbal and behavioral therapies struck us as being quite small, and our saying so appears to have offended those who seem to believe that the psychotherapy Olympics were long since over and the laurels were theirs (e.g., Rachman & Wilson, 1980), even as it pleased those (Freudians and Rogerians) who once believed the race had been lost. (p. 32)

There are obvious parallels between the findings of Sloane et al. and this "tie" between behavioral and verbal therapies in the meta-analysis by Smith et al. In the final chapter of their book (which also included a meta-analytic study of the effects of drug therapy and psychotherapy), Smith et al. concluded that the evidence overwhelmingly supported the efficacy of psychotherapy but that different types of therapy did not produce different types of benefit:

> We did not expect that the demonstrable benefits of quite different types of psychotherapy would be so little different. It is the most startling and intriguing finding we came across. All psychotherapy researchers should be prompted to ask how it can be so. If it is truly so that major differences in technique count for little in terms of benefits, then what is to be made of the volumes devoted to the careful drawing of distinction among styles of psychotherapy? And what is to be made of the deep divisions and animosities among different psychotherapy schools? (p. 185)

Evaluation of Meta-analysis

Ever since Eysenck (1978) characterized the initial meta-analysis by Smith and Glass (1977) as "an exercise in mega-silliness," meta-analysis has attracted a great deal of critical attention. In their extended (1980) report, Smith et al. outlined the principal objections to their work: meta-analysis mixes apples and oranges; it seems to advocate low standards of judgment; it lumps studies into gross categories and fails to separate treatments that should not be grouped together; and it has admitted shortcomings in its definitions of effects inasmuch as it necessarily relies on selective reporting, insufficient or incorrectly conducted primary data analyses, and inadequate descriptions of the original studies.

The first and third objections (termed the "uniformity" and "incommensurability" problems, respectively, by Glass & Kliegl, 1983) appear to emanate primarily from behaviorally-oriented critics who, as we saw in connection with the study by Sloane et al., understandably prefer not to be "lumped" with approaches to lesser specificity, homogeneity, or uncongenital philosophical commitments. To these objections, Smith et al. respond that the distinctions which psychotherapy theorists deem important may not be sacrosanct if one wishes to obtain an overview of the general efficacy of psychotherapy, just as it is appropriate to combine apples and oranges if one is studying fruit.

The charge that meta-analysis does not adhere to high standards of scientific judgment ("garbage in, garbage out"), however, warrants more serious attention. The studies selected for meta-analysis obviously vary considerably in their quality; overall conclusions would necessarily have to reflect the average quality of studies examined. To those who object to even considering studies which, in their view, represent flawed work, Smith et al. have replied that indices of the quality of studies (e.g., their rated validity) have been included in the meta-analysis along with many other study characteristics such as therapist experience, patient diagnosis, and so on. The empirical (if post hoc) answer to the quality problem, Smith et al. reported, is that effect sizes tended to vary positively rather than negatively with the quality of studies; studies of lower quality, thus, would merely attenuate the magnitude of effects and make the overall conclusions conservative. (Incidentally, dissertation research, included in the meta-analysis by Smith et al. but impugned by some critics, did *not* show greater effect sizes than did published articles.)

It is true, however, that demonstrating that the effectiveness of psychotherapy is not inferred primarily from studies of poor quality does not mean that the quality of studies is unimportant (cf. Mintz, 1983). This demonstration also does not settle the question of whether studies of dubious quality should have been included in the first place. But, because prior narrative and "box score" reviews all too often have abounded in arbitrary, capricious, nonconsensual, or dogmatic judgments regarding the quality of studies, Smith et al, by *not* excluding large numbers of studies on a priori grounds, have been able to submit at least some aspects of internal and external validity of studies to an empirical test, and that is no small accomplishment.

To give just one example of the problems with a priori judgments of quality, Beutler (1979) reviewed 52 comparative outcome studies for their bearing on some interesting hypotheses concerning which specific therapies might be best for which types of problems. To select a methodologically sound group of studies, Beutler relied:

> on the 13 criteria of adequacy outlined by Luborsky et al. (1975). Failure on 5 or more of the criteria eliminated a study from consideration, whereas fewer failures earned increasingly higher grades. Grades potentially ranged from A to D among included studies, although in practice most studies scored toward the low end of the qualitative scale. The most frequent failing included use of non-clinical populations, minimally trained therapists, and no follow-up data. (Beutler, 1979, p. 885)

This procedure of assigning grades to studies as though they were students in one's class certainly appears reasonable. But is rejecting studies that do not reach the D grade more reasonable than rejecting studies which fail to make a C grade? In Beutler's tabulation, it emerged that the retained studies ranged in quality from D minus to only B plus! Should the studies then be "graded on a curve"? The study by Sloane et al., incidentally, was one of only two studies to attain the lofty B plus plateau. Suffice it to add that, were an alternate reviewer "more rigorous" by excluding studies which did not reach a grade of C, then the classic study by Paul (1966) would have been excluded: It earned a grade of C minus.

Turning now to the methodological problems of meta-analysis, such as having to rely on insufficiently reported or even misanalyzed primary studies, the lack of independence among outcome measures taken within one study, the fact that studies using multiple outcome measures may carry more weight than studies using only a few measures, and so on, these problems and others are receiving empirical scrutiny. For example, while some investigators recommend using studies rather than effect sizes cumulated across studies as a means of circumventing the problem of nonindependence of effect sizes drawn from the same analysis (e.g., Miller & Berman, 1983), there is no reason why researchers cannot and should not conduct both sorts of analyses to see how much of a practical difference possible divergences entail. Thus, Landman and Dawes (1982) reanalyzed a subset of the Smith et al. studies and found not only that the original conclusions were sustained but also that the practice of using effect sizes rather than studies as the units of analysis, if anything, attenuated the inferred effectiveness of psychotherapy. Other matters, such as whether the denominator for effect sizes should use a pooled within-group standard deviation rather than that of the control group (e.g., Miller & Berman, 1983), whether integrations across studies should be corrected for sampling error introduced by the inclusion of small samples (e.g., Stoffelmayr, Dillavou, & Hunter, 1983), and whether the quasi-experimental nature of meta-analysis requires the cautious use of certain inferential statistics (e.g., Strube & Hartmann, 1983), are all open to investigation and refinement.

The only major problem with meta-analysis of the currently available outcome literature seems to be the matter of external validity. Examination of Appendix 3 in Smith et al. (pp. 204–205) reveals, for example, that over a third of the effects (35%) were based on changes in patients classified as "simple phobic," the mean age of patients was 23, the mean experience level of therapists was 3 years, systematic desensitization was the most common form of treatment, and so on. Shapiro and Shapiro (1983) have quite accurately suggested that too many studies in the psychotherapy outcome literature have tended to sacrifice external and construct validity for the sake of internal validity. Mintz (1983) has pointed out that perhaps the entire *population* of psychotherapy outcome studies lacks external validity.

But these very observations regarding the problematic external validity of the available literature are also obvious guides to further research. In this regard, the conduct of more ecologically valid psychotherapy studies would certainly comprise an important priority for further research. (In this connection, it is unfortunate that the comprehensive mental health centers which service enormous numbers of patients around the country have virtually no research programs associated with them.) Meta-analysis may also serve to modify future research in hitherto sacrosanct areas of methodology such as the importance of obtaining follow-up measures on all patients in a study: Nicholson and Berman (1983) have shown recently that, when meta-analytic procedures are applied to studies which have included both post-therapy and follow-up measurement, the conclusions based on follow-up measures do not really differ from those based on post-therapy ones. If the gains achieved during psychotherapy are indeed quite durable, it makes sense to reserve the costly procedures of follow-up assessment for clinical problems which are known to be associated with high rates of relapse (e.g., weight control, smoking) rather than to include them simply on prescriptive grounds.

Overall, meta-analysis has provided the research community with a new attitude toward the systematic integration of the results of two or more studies in any area of research. (See Rosenthal, 1983, for a lucid presentation of computational formulas and for the "binomial effect size display" as a guide for communicating the practical consequences of "new" interventions.) While it may be true, as Mintz (1983) points out, that meta-analysis, like the previous modes for summarizing research, does contain elements of subjectivity (e.g., in the selection of variables for coding, the definition of coding categories, the extensiveness of sampling of certain types of studies, etc.), its basic procedures are public, explicit, objective, and replicable. Thus, criticisms of Smith et al. for inappropriately excluding certain studies of behavior therapy (e.g., Wilson & Rachman, 1983) can readily be evaluated for their tenability by the critics themselves—by conducting an "expanded" reanalysis.

Perhaps the best summary of the contributions of meta-analysis to contemporary research is this succinct statement by Fiske (1983):

> One part of science generates research reports. The other part, the integration of these reports, has been made systematic and scientific by the intervention of meta-analysis. (p. 65)

SUMMARY

Although, at the conclusion of their volume Smith et al. speculated that the absence of differing benefits associated with widely differing techniques might cast doubt on the importance of the theoretical distinctions held dear by various schools of psychotherapy, Glass and Kliegl (1983) later amended this suggestion by noting that, whereas meta-analysis necessarily assumes that *practical* commensurability of differing therapeutic interventions, it can say nothing definitive regarding the *theoretical* commensurability of differing approaches:

> No matter what Smith et al. might have found, their conclusions would not have provided anything but the most dubious evidence for or against the validity of any theory of human behavior, whether biological, behaviorist, cognitivist, or what-have-you. The equality of benefits—if that were observed—surely would say nothing about the equality of theories in respect to heuristic power or capacity to grow. Nor, one must add quickly, would the superiority of effects for A versus B imply the theoretical superiority of A. (p. 39)

Even more generally, it should be remembered that, although theories of psychotherapeutic change could well be *disproven* by well-conducted outcome research, no theory in the area of psychotherapy, as in any other area in science, can be proven experimentally to be the *only* or preemptive explanation of a given pattern of facts (e.g., Popper, 1959; Rychlak, 1968). The very same therapeutic intervention may, after all, be explained plausibly by several theoretical accounts; systematic desensitization may effectively alleviate phobias without restricting theoretical explanations to the concepts of counterconditioning, reciprocal inhibition, or changes in felt self-efficacy.

Although the results of meta-analysis should mute the dogmatic claims of certain theoretical positions, it is not clear whether pluralistic or eclectic models should be encouraged in the training of future practitioners. It is apparent, however, that there is room for theorizing regarding *how* psychotherapeutic interventions accomplish their effects. It may be that factors common to most systems of psychotherapy should receive greater theoretical weight than factors which are considered to be their distinguishing features; it may be that the theoretical locus of causality might have to be shifted from therapist to patient or perhaps to the dyad. But meta-analytic demonstrations of the benefits of psychotherapy in no way preclude the need for theoretical innovation in trying to understand how psychotherapy accomplishes its benefits.

Finally, whereas meta-analysis may have shown that therapy is better than no therapy, it has *not* established that different therapies engender equivalent benefits with respect to particular clinical problems or types of patients. While Smith et al. may rightfully claim to be interested primarily in "unconditional" rather than "conditional" value claims (corresponding, respectively, to the main and interaction effects in the analysis of variance), the intrinsic importance of interaction effects, indicative of which therapies might be better for which types of problems, presumably led Smith et al. themselves to cross-classify therapies by types of patients, types of outcome measures, and so on (cf. Abeles, 1981). Even if the small number of studies or their confounded nature in certain areas may have precluded confident conceptual or statistical conclusions, the objective of improving clinical practice by matching therapists and patients, or therapies and problems, on the basis of sound research which incorporates some version of Kiesler's (1966, 1971) Grid model remains a pragmatic goal (cf. Berzins, 1977). Such research, exemplified by such studies as the ongoing research sponsored by the National Institute of Mental Health comparing several promising approaches to the treatment of unipolar depression, is clearly still in its infancy. Despite promising rational analyses like that of Beutler (1979), much empirical work remains to be done before certain meta-analyses might be appropriate. In the meanwhile, the design of more ecologically valid outcome studies, and the study of convergences and divergences among measures of outcome, have already been cited as important priorities in research which examines the effectiveness of psychotherapy.

REFERENCES

Abeles, N. (1981). Psychotherapy works! *Contemporary Psychology, 26,* 821–823.

Bandura, A. (1978). On paradigms and recycled ideologies. *Cognitive Therapy and Research, 2,* 79–103.

Bergin, A.E. (1966). Some implications of psychotherapy research for therapeutic practice. *Journal of Abnormal Psychology, 71,* 235–246.

Bergin, A. E. (1971). The evaluation of therapeutic outcome. In A.E. Bergin & S.L. Garfield (Eds.), *Handbook of psychotherapy and behavior change.* New York: Wiley.

Bergin, A.E., & Lambert, M.J. (1978). The evaluation of therapeutic outcomes. In S.L. Garfield & A.E. Bergin (Eds.), *Handbook of psychotherapy and behavior change* (2nd ed.). New York: Wiley.

Bergin, A.E., & Suinn, R.M. (1975). Individual psychotherapy and behavior therapy. *Annual Review of Psychology, 26,* 509–556.

Bernstein, D.A., & Nietzel, M.T. (1973). Procedural variation in behavioral avoidance tests. *Journal of Consulting and Clinical Psychology, 41,* 165–174.

Berzins, J.I. (1977). Therapist-patient matching. In A.S. Gurman & A.M. Razin (Eds.), *Effective psychotherapy: A handbook of research.* New York: Pergamon.

Berzins, J.I., Bednar, R.L., & Severy, L.J. (1975). The problem of intersource consensus in measuring therapeutic outcomes: New data and multivariate perspectives. *Journal of Abnormal Psychology, 84,* 10–19.

Beutler, L.E. (1979). Toward specific psychological therapies for specified conditions. *Journal of Consulting and Clinical Psychology, 47,* 882–897.

Campbell, D.T., & Stanley, J.C. (1966). *Experimental and quasi-experimental designs for research.* Chicago: Rand McNally.

Cook, D.T., & Campbell, D.T. (1979). *Quasiexperimentation: Design and analysis issues for field settings.* Chicago: Rand McNally.

Eysenck, H.J. (1952). The effects of psychotherapy: An evaluation. *Journal of Consulting Psychology, 16,* 319–324.

Eysenck, H.J. (1961). The effects of psychotherapy. In H.J. Eysenck (Ed.), *Handbook of abnormal psychology.* New York: Basic Books.
Eysenck, H.J. (1965). The effects of psychotherapy. *International Journal of Psychiatry, 1,* 99–144.
Eysenck, H.J. (1978). An exercise in mega-silliness. *American Psychologist, 33,* 517.
Fiske, D.W. (1983). The meta-analytic revolution in outcome research. *Journal of Consulting and Clinical Psychology, 51,* 65–70.
Garfield, S.L. (1976). All roads lead to Rome. *Contemporary Psychology, 21,* 328–329.
Garfield, S.L. (1981). Psychotherapy: A 40-year appraisal. *American Psychologist, 2,* 174–183.
Glass, G.V. (1976). Primary, secondary and meta-analysis of research. *Educational Researcher, 5,* 3–8.
Glass, G.V., & Kliegl, R.M. (1983). An apology for research integration in the study of psychotherapy. *Journal of Consulting and Clinical Psychology, 51,* 28–41.
Jenkins, J.J. (1974). Remember that old theory of memory? Well, forget it! *American Psychologist, 29,* 785–795.
Kazdin, A.E. (1978). *History of behavior modification: Experimental foundations of contemporary research.* Baltimore: University Park Press.
Kazdin, A.E. (1980). *Research design in clinical psychology.* New York: Harper & Row.
Kazdin, A.E. (1982). Single-case experimental designs. In P.C. Kendall & J.N. Butcher (Eds.), *Handbook of research methods in clinical psychology.* New York: Wiley.
Kazdin, A.E., & Wilson, G.T. (1978). *Evaluation of behavior therapy: Issues, evidence, and research strategies.* Cambridge, MA: Ballinger.
Kiesler, D.J. (1966). Some myths of psychotherapy research and the search for a paradigm. *Psychological Bulletin, 65,* 110–136.
Kiesler, D.J. (1971). Experimental designs in psychotherapy research. In A.E. Bergin & S.L. Garfield (Eds.), *Handbook of psychotherapy and behavior change.* New York: Wiley.
Kiesler, D.J. (1973). *The process of psychotherapy: Empirical foundations and systems of analysis.* Chicago: Aldine.
Landman, J.T., & Dawes, R.M. (1982). Psychotherapy outcome: Smith and Glass' conclusions stand up under scrutiny. *American Psychologist, 37,* 504–516.
Light, R.J., Smith, P.V. (1971). Accumulating evidence: Procedures for resolving contradictions among different research studies. *Harvard Educational Review, 41,* 429–471.
Luborsky, L., Chandler, M., Auerbach, A., Cohen, J., & Bachrach, H. (1971). Factors influencing the outcome of psychotherapy: A review of quantitative research. *Psychological Bulletin, 75,* 145–185.
Luborsky, L., Singer, B., & Luborsky, L. (1975). Comparative studies of psychotherapies: Is it true that "Everyone has won and all must have prizes"? *Archives of General Psychiatry, 32,* 995–1008.
Meltzoff, J., & Kornreich, M. (1970). *Research in psychotherapy.* Chicago: Aldine.
Miller, R.C., & Berman, J.S. (1983). The efficacy of cognitive behavior therapies: A quantitative review of the research evidence. *Psychological Bulletin,* 39–53.
Mintz, J. (1983). Integrating research evidence: A commentary on meta-analysis. *Jour-*

nal of Consulting and Clinical Psychology, 51, 71–75.

Mintz, J., & Kiesler, D.J. (1982). Individualized measures of psychotherapy outcome. In P.C. Kendall & J.N. Butcher (Eds.), *Research methods in clinical psychology*. New York: Wiley.

Mitchell, K.M., Bozarth, J.D., & Krauft, C.C. (1977). A reappraisal of the therapeutic effectiveness of accurate empathy, nonpossessive warmth and genuineness. In A.S. Gurman & A.M. Razin (Eds.), *Effective psychotherapy: A handbook of research*. New York: Pergamon.

Nicholson, R.A., & Berman, J.S. (1983). Is follow-up necessary in evaluating psychotherapy? *Psychological Bulletin, 93*, 261–278.

Paul, G.L. (1966). *Insight versus desensitization in psychotherapy: An experiment in anxiety reduction*. Stanford, CA: Stanford University Press.

Paul, G.L. (1967). Strategy of outcome research in psychotherapy. *Journal of Consulting Psychology, 31*, 109–118.

Pepper, S. (1942). *World hypotheses: A study in evidence*. Berkeley, CA: University of California Press.

Popper, K.R. (1959). *The logic of scientific discovery*. New York: Basic Books.

Rachman, S. (1971). *The effects of psychotherapy*. Oxford: Pergamon Press.

Rachman, S.J., & Wilson, G.T. (1980). *The effects of psychological therapy* (2nd ed.) Oxford: Pergamon Press.

Rosenthal, R. (1983). Assessing the statistical and social importance of the effects of psychotherapy. *Journal of Consulting and Clinical Psychology, 51*, 4–13.

Rubinstein, E.A., & Parloff, M.B. (Eds.). (1959). *Research in psychotherapy* (Vol. 1). Washington, DC: American Psychological Association.

Rychlak, J.F. (1968). *A philosophy of science for personality theory*. Boston: Houghton-Mifflin.

Sarbin, T.R. (1977). Contextualism: The world-view for modern psychology. In A.W. Landfield (Ed.), *Nebraska symposium on motivation: 1976*. Lincoln: University of Nebraska Press.

Shapiro, D.A., & Shapiro, D. (1983). Comparative therapy outcome research: Methodological implications of meta-analysis. *Journal of Consulting and Clinical Psychology, 51*, 42–53.

Shlien, J.M. (Ed.). (1968). *Research in psychotherapy* (Vol. 3). Washington, DC: American Psychological Association.

Sloane, R.B., Staples, F.R., Cristol, A.H., Yorkston, N.J., & Whipple, K. (1975). *Psychotherapy versus behavior therapy*. Cambridge, MA: Harvard University Press.

Smith, M.L., & Glass, G.V. (1977). Meta-analysis of psychotherapy outcome studies. *American Psychologist, 32*, 752–760.

Smith, M.L., Glass, G.V., & Miller, T.I. (1980). *The benefits of psychotherapy*. Baltimore: Johns Hopkins.

Stoffelmayr, B.E., Dillavou, D., & Hunter, J.E. (1983). Premorbid functioning and outcome in schizophrenia: A cumulative analysis. *Journal of Consulting and Clinical Psychology, 51*, 338–352.

Strube, M.J., & Hartmann, D. P. (1983). Meta-analysis: Techniques, applications, and functions. *Journal of Consulting and Clinical Psychology, 51*, 14–27.

Strupp, H.H., & Luborsky, L. (Eds.). (1962). *Research in psychology* (Vol. 2). Washington, DC: American Psychological Association.

Truax, C.B., & Carkhuff, R.R. (1967). *Toward effective counseling and psychotherapy.* Chicago: Aldine.

Waskow, I., & Parloff, M. (1975). *Psychotherapy change measures.* Washington, DC: U.S. Government Printing Office.

Wilson, G.T., & Rachman, S.J. (1983). Meta-analysis and the evaluation of psychotherapy outcome: Limitations and liabilities. *Journal of Consulting and Clinical Psychology, 51*, 54–64.

Wolberg, L. (1954). *The technique of psychotherapy.* New York: Grune & Stratton.

Wolpe, J. (1958). *Psychotherapy by reciprocal inhibition.* Stanford, CA: Stanford University Press.

Wolpe, J. (1981). Behavior therapy versus psychoanalysis: Therapeutic and social implications. *American Psychologist, 36,* 159–164.

9
Test Construction

Charles J. Golden,
Robert F. Sawicki, and
Michael D. Franzen

INTRODUCTION

Research in test construction and general assessment has had wide fluctuations in popularity in recent years. This has been due initially to a feeling in the late 1960s and early 1970s that testing was not a useful enterprise and that time could be better spent on the development of treatment strategies. In recent years, however, the pendulum has returned and the importance of testing is again recognized, especially in areas such as neuropsychology. One unfortunate by-product of the decrease of interest in testing was a deemphasis in many clinical training programs on the research methods and critical analysis of testing issues. Multiple classes on assessment and the statistical basis of tests were dropped from many programs or condensed into a smaller series of classes.

As a result, the sophistication of many psychologists in the area of test construction has been reduced considerably. Many myths about tests and test research have developed (particularly in regard to the meaning of reliability and validity) that are generally inaccurate.

The present chapter is an attempt to explore the research approaches to test construction and to examine realistically what is sought when examining an existing test or test battery or when developing a new instrument. The chapter is organized along the steps that one could take in designing and validating a new test approach. Some of the initial data may not be relevant for the validation of an already existing test. Otherwise, the material may be applied to either the development of a test or to the evaluation of an existing test. Since the authors of this chapter are most familiar with neuropsychology, many of the examples will be drawn from that field; however, the discussion is broad enough to be applicable to other areas of psychology in which test construction is an issue.

TEST CONSTRUCTION

There are at least three approaches to scale construction (Wiggins, 1973). The *analytic* approach relies most heavily on theory to determine the selection of items, procedures, and criteria for assessing individuals. Within this approach, items are selected on the basis of whether they appear to tap an aspect of the construct under consideration. For example, if the theory specifies that an important aspect of the construct of interest is the age at which a person was toilet trained, then a question regarding that information would be included in the scale.

Within the *empirical* approach, the first step in scale construction is to define an operational index of the construct to be measured. For example, in devising the Minnesota Multiphasic Personality Inventory (MMPI) the authors of the test used psychiatric diagnosis as the operational index. The second step was to select items that were assumed to be associated with the index. The authors of the MMPI asked clinicians to generate items that reflected the psychiatric diagnoses. Next, the method of contrasting groups was used to determine which items discriminated between diagnostic groups. It is clear that under this approach, items are chosen on the basis of empirically demonstrated relationships with the criterion. Theory plays less of a role here in comparison to the analytic approach.

A third strategy is the *rational* approach or, as Jackson (1970) has labelled it, the sequential system approach. The sequential system model tries to combine the features of the analytic and the empirical approaches in a logical sequence as well as evaluating the psychometric properties of the resultant scales. It operates under the guidance of four principles, which are: (1) the importance of psychological theory; (2) the necessity for suppressing variance due to response style; (3) the balance of scale homogeneity with generalizability; and (4) the evaluation of convergent and discriminant validity. Items are originally generated on the basis of a coherent theory but are retained on the basis of their psychometric properties and empirical relationships. Because of its flexibility and applicability, the sequential system model is the method most often used today in scale construction. Therefore, it is the approach which provides a broad outline for the discussion in this chapter.

Initial Item Selection

The first step of test development is to determine the domain which test responses will represent. A thorough understanding of what the test is expected to measure will guide both initial validation research and clinical interpretation of individual results. Such theoretical comprehension of what a given test is expected to measure also guides the selection of the initial item pool.

Since the initial item pool is expected to maximize data gathering along some trait or skill dimension, it is useful for persons who are designing their first test to construct a Table of Specifications (Hopkins & Antes, 1978) in order to increase their chances of identifying an item pool which will represent their domain of interest. Initially, many more items are selected than are actually necessary, but they will be pared down by the validation process.

The Table of Specifications may be described as a two-dimensional matrix, where one dimension represents the skills or traits of interest while the other dimension represents the behaviors representative of these characteristics. This blueprint can be used to determine both the number of items which will be selected to represent each aspect (behavior) of the domain of interest and the type of items which will be used. Thus, a comprehensive test battery may include diverse and seemingly unrelated items. A limited purpose test may include only very specific and highly similar items.

Items are most often chosen by face validity. In the best of cases, items are derived from a comprehensive theory which dictates the types of items that may be necessary for a given test. In other instances, item selection may be based on "professional nomination," the result of suggestions by experts, or simply by sampling many items used in other tests or clinical practice. In general, since some items will probably be dropped subsequent to validation, it is better at this stage to be overinclusive in the selection of items. It is recommended that the original item pool include from two to four times the number which one wishes to include in the final version of the test. Overall limitations on the number of items in the initial pool will occur as a function of practical issues: Tests which will require individual administration (e.g., IQ tests) will probably start out with a smaller pool than those which permit group administration (e.g., personality inventories).

Clearly, the choice of items can be quite subjective and dependent on the desires of the researcher and the goals of the research. There is no correct approach so we cannot say that a scale or test which is limited is necessarily better than one which is broad. The real question arises after this stage of work when we ask not whether a test item has been "properly chosen" for inclusion into a scale, but instead ask what a scale measures and what are its limitations as well as advantages. For example, the MMPI uses many items that are not face valid in its clinical summary scales; other approaches to the same item pool have put together alternative scales with a requirement of face validity. Neither approach is better, and indeed an ideal compromise may be a situation like that of the MMPI, in which a general pool of items used to produce both a set of clinical scales and a set of subscales.

Item Formats

Items may be either open-ended or restricted in terms of response options. Restricted items are defined here as forced choice (e.g., true/false) or multiple choice items. Such items are popular with group tests. Open-ended items allow variable responses from patients; however, by necessity, they must be individually administered and scored. Open-ended item construction requires careful selection due to the amount of interpretation which will be required of an examiner to accurately score such items. These items are less likely to automatically meet requirements for standardization.

Item content or presentation is not limited by the type of response format chosen. For example, although inkblots are generally used in tests which are open-ended, we could design an inkblot test which was multiple choice. For example, Is the above inkblot: a. bat? b. a person? c. two persons? or d. a dying swan? Whether such a test would measure the same thing as the more open-ended format is, of course, a question of construct validity that must be empirically explored.

Open-ended/projective items are more useful when the clinician wishes to observe and analyze the process which a patient uses to arrive at a response, while forced choice and multiple choice items are more concerned with the resulting pattern of responses than the process. The meaning of such a pattern is defined by empirically derived correlates.

Items may also be classified as objective or projective. Objective items include not only the forced choice and multiple choice items but also items that allow more flexible responses for which correct answers are consensually determined. An example of the latter is the question, "What does the word 'summer' mean?" Projective items, on the other hand, are deliberately vague and ambiguous. There is a wide range of correct responses to which an interpretive system must be applied in order to derive meaningful scoring. Some would exclude such projective material from standardized tests, but there is no reason to do this as long as the set of items meets the general criteria for standardization.

Limitations to Item Formats

In deciding the item format to use within a test, one must be cognizant of the limitations of each format type. Such limits must be weighed against the amount of useful information which a particular format will generate. Though multiple choice items can be scored quickly, provide greater interrater reliability, and sample a larger content area, they are open to interpretive error due to guessing and random response sets. Such tests also take longer to construct since both test items and distractors must be designed. In the initial stages of test construction such items may also be misplaced on a scale since the researcher must intuitively determine the level of difficulty of each item before it is seen by a patient (Hopkins & Antes, 1978). Similar criticisms may be applied to the true/false format. In addition, the true/false format is greatly affected by the wording used within items. Poorly stated items undermine a test's clinical usefulness.

Though the open-ended/projective items may be constructed more quickly, provide fewer stimulus cues for guessing, and allow the clinician to observe the problem solving process, they require that examiners have extensive training in a scoring system so that responses may be validly interpreted. In addition, scoring takes much longer and "styles" of scoring may limit the overall reliability of the open-ended test.

An important problem in the construction of the open-ended question is choosing ahead of time the correct scoring/recording approach so that the item may be investigated during initial research. As a rule, it is best to start out with overly broad and detailed recording and instructions. As the test development progresses, these broader, more detailed analyses may be broken down into simplified categories depending on the findings with a given item. By recording responses in detail, one can change the process of scoring as it becomes evident that a given approach may be inadequate or fail to derive the information of interest. The more flexibilty that one can maintain in early stages, the easier it will be to make changes in item scoring in later stages as the result of validity or reliability studies. Such approaches will enable one to salvage items without having to repeat extensive preliminary work.

When generating items, it is necessary to consider the influence of method and response style on the stimulus value of the item for the subject. Item characteristics are those quantifiable but nonsubstantive aspects which may influence the response of the subject. Wiggins (1973) discusses some of these characteristics.

The first of these is social desirability. Depending upon the wording of an item, endorsement of the item has variable social desirability. For example, the items "I believe that children should be raised with a firm hand" and "Corporal punishment for children is necessary" both seem to tap the same attitude. However, the wording of the items affects the social desirability and hence, the probability that a subject would endorse the item.

Another item characteristic is the keying direction in which the item is written. Keying direction interacts with an acquiescent response style to result in measurement of a construct other than the one under study. In a scale in which all of the items are keyed true, the scores reflect both the construct under study and acquiescence. The best approach is to balance true keyed items with false key items.

Other item characteristics include item ambiguity, item objectionability, item stability, item serial position,and grammatical dimensions such as sentence length and structure, tense, voice, and person. Not all of these item characteristics will impinge on the validity of all tests. However, it is important to be aware of the possibility of their influence, to assess the magnitude of the influence and to attempt to minimize the influence of the level of item writing.

Standardization: Administration

At this point in the test construction process, there are two major requirements for standardization: (a) standard administration, and (b) standard scoring. Forced choice and multiple choice items meet such criteria without difficulty. The patient is read or reads the item and chooses a response alternative or states his answer. If additional material is used (e.g., pictures), these are identical for all patients.

Open-ended items can present more difficulties for standard administration. Standardization is achieved by having the examiner state the "key" demands in a standard manner. Each subject uses the same set of test materials. Problems arise with open-ended items on two occasions: (a) when an examiner attempts to elicit further information, and (b) when the patient produces an entirely novel response. Open ended questions are also more open to questioning by a patient, which may disrupt the administration procedure.

The first difficulty usually arises when an examiner does not completely understand the intent of an item. Such a problem raises the possibility that the item itself may contain unintended ambiguity. Thus, an individual examiner's interpretation of the item's intent may break standard administration and invalidate the item.

This problem can be handled in one of several ways. The most common approach has been to demand strict adherence to rigid administration rules regardless of outside concerns. Examiners are instructed to adopt testing-the-limits procedures after eliciting a scoreable response in order to gain sufficient additional information which is needed to avoid interpretive difficulties.

A second, more complex, approach is to allow more flexible examination procedures within a standard administration format. For example, the administration of an item requiring a motor response (e.g., finger tapping) may begin with the standard verbal demand, and, if the patient does not comprehend the task requirements, the examiner may follow up with an alternative verbal explanation, followed by an actual demonstration until the patient understands what is necessary to make a scoreable response to the item. The major issue for the test developer is clarity on the intent of an item and the extent to which assistance may be given without invalidating the item. By writing such procedures into the administration instructions, one can offer both flexibility and standardization. It should be noted that in clinical use, such alternate procedures will arise on their own if not specified in the test manual.

In writing such procedures, the item author must be aware of the intent of an item. For example, a demonstration would not be allowed when testing a patient's ability to follow spoken instructions, but is quite appropriate when assessing motor speed. Written instructions could be used as an additional procedure for an item measuring verbal comprehension, but not for an item measuring auditory comprehension.

In all cases, item materials must be identical. Small differences in legibility, color, shape, size, or other stimulus dimensions can create wide, artifactual variations in response to items. In cases where identical materials cannot be easily or reliably employed (such as visual items for the partially sighted), research must identify the effect of such differences, identifying the salient aspects of stimuli in order to aid interpretation.

Standardization: Scaling

A number of scaling methods may be used with items, depending on the domain of interest which the test is intended to measure. Scaling methods can roughly be characterized into three types: nominal, ordinal, or interval scales. Ratio scales are not ordinarily applied to psychological data.

Nominal scaling reflects regrouping responses into arbitrarily defined categories, which are only meaningful in the context of the measure within which they were created. Such categories are not assumed to have characteristics of counting numbers. It is usually the frequency of responses within a given category that provides the focus of interest for the clinician. This method of scaling is most often used when scoring represents an analysis of the process used to achieve an answer rather than the tabulation of the answer alone. The scoring system of the Rorschach Inkblot Test (Exner, 1974) is an example of such a scaling system. Responses may be regrouped under such category headings as "Form," "Location," "Shading," and so forth. Some neuropsychological tests may count the number of responses which may be classified as "perseveration," "neglect," or "impulsiveness."

Ordinal scaling reflects a ranking of responses along some underlying dimension (e.g., adequacy of performance). Thus, an item may be scored as "0" (normal), "1" (borderline), and "2" (impaired). Ordinal scaling does not assume that the distance between numbers is equal, only that the ranking is meaningful. Thus, the change in severity from 0 (normal) to 1 (borderline) is not assumed to have similar magnitude as the change in severity from 1 (borderline) to 2 (impaired). Since there is generally a lack of empirical support for quantifiable parallel increases between psychometric data and behavioral changes, most psychological data could be classified as ordinal in nature.

Interval scaling is also ordered, but the distances between data points are assumed to be equal. The distances between points is meaningful; that is, the difference between "1" and "3" is twice as large as the difference between "1" and "2". The zero point is determined arbitrarily and does not necessarily indicate the absence of the quality measured. Psychophysiological measures serve as the best example of such scaling. Though one would be hard pressed to identify assessment instruments which meet such a scaling criteria, most psychological data can be treated as though it were on an interval scale.

Gaito (1970) defends the assumptions which indicate that a set of scores may take on the characteristics of more than one type of scaling. He suggests that scaling descriptions are guidelines and rigid adherence only promotes the wasting of data. In an example he states,

> The same data may be considered to have the properties of two or more scales, depending on the context in which it is considered. For example, if we look at the response of one subject (*S*) to a single item, the properties of the data are

> those of a nominal scale, i.e., right or wrong. However, if we concentrate on the total score for one *S* or the total scores for a group of *S*'s, we have at least an ordinal scale. (p. 65)

Gaito emphasizes that it is not the property of a given scale which has overriding importance but the degree to which items produce data that is normally distributed in a large sample of subjects. This is an important point to the use of parametric tests to describe the reliability and validity of a set of items which have undergone a scaling transformation. It may be that few of the assumptions underlying parametric tests need be met with any great accuracy, although this point is debated by some (e.g., Hays, 1973).

Item Analysis: Administration Difficulties

After the initial items have been designed and written, it is best to administer them to several normal individuals to see how they "work." This can be a valuable step, saving much time later, as one will find that some of the items simply do not perform as expected. In some cases, administration as envisioned is demonstrated to be impossible on a practical level. This may be because subjects cannot comprehend the instructions, the administration is too difficult for an examiner without three arms, or other related possibilities.

Different examiners may be unable to agree on scoring. For example, in the development of the Luria-Nebraska, we initially had an item, "Show me how to frown." While it appeared simple on the surface, we were unable to come up with scoring criteria from which to get reliable data. In addition, items may require more time than expected. Subjects may balk at an item's content or fail to comprehend an item no matter how it is presented.

In all of these instances, items may be revised or eliminated prior to starting a full validation project. Many of these difficulties are much less frequent with group administered tests like personality inventories.

Item Analysis: Item Efficiency

After these initial steps have been completed, the test may be administered to a sample of interest. This step should include a minimum ratio of two to three times as many subjects as test items. If the test is aimed at several different groups, testing with a sample from each group will be necessary. In administering the items, it is important to ensure that the conditions of testing, as well as the items, are standardized. Lighting conditions, ambient noise, distractions, and other environmental conditions should be closely controlled.

Items ought to be administered in the same order to all subjects. Examiners must be thoroughly trained. Subjects selected for initial pilot studies of the new item set should be cooperative and encouraged to provide their most valid, honest, and accurate performance. An attempt must also be made to select an initial subject pool which is representative of the population to whom the test will later be applied.

After this step has been completed, several analyses may be used to further evaluate items. The *Item Difficulty Index* results from a simple analysis that demonstrates the relative efficiency of items in groups which do and do not possess the characteristic of interest. In its simplest form, the *Difficulty Index* represents the percentage of a given group which fails an item. If one were testing a given ability which was assumed to be randomly distributed within a population and one was using a sample randomly drawn from that population, the expected item difficulty for any given item would be .50. As the item difficulty level moves toward 1.0, a given item is too difficult since at 1.0 no one is passing the item. As the item difficulty approaches 0.0, a given item is too easy, since hardly anyone is missing the item. Both items which are too easy and items which are too difficult are useless in a test, since they offer no discriminations among subjects. Understanding what is communicated by item difficulty in a psychological test is a little more complex.

When analyzing items from a psychological instrument, it is useful to compute difficulty indices for both the sample of interest and the comparative or control sample. Before performing the computations, one must understand that passing or failing an item must be redefined as responding in the scoreable direction or responding otherwise. Thus, if one has designed a set of true/false items which are expected to identify depression, the scoreable direction is the way in which a depressed person would endorse an item. Therefore if one has designed a perfect set of items, one expects that difficulties for the depressed group approach 0.0 while difficulties for the comparison (nondepressed) group would tend toward 1.0, suggesting that the items discriminate between the two groups. The total sample (both depressed and not depressed) difficulty indices would approach .50 given the within group disparities and a sample composed of one-half depressed individuals and one-half nondepressed individuals.

For a neuropsychological test where items also involve some ability dimensions, one expects that item difficulty in a heterogeneous sample of brain impaired will be at .50 or greater, while unimpaired controls ought to have difficulty indices of .30 or less. The latter may be expected in a heterogeneous group of unimpaired normals due to the biological variance for performance measures which is assumed in the general population. Thus one may see that item difficulty is computed by dividing the number of persons who responded in the scoreable direction by the total number of persons who responded to the item. The formula (Hopkins & Antes, 1978, p. 187) would be applicable to an item which can be scored correct/incorrect, and by the nature of the test it is the incorrect response which serves to discriminate among subjects:

$$\text{Item Difficulty} = \frac{\text{Number of subjects who failed the item.}}{\text{Number of subjects who responded to item}}.$$

Since the *Item Difficulty Index* is severely affected by the characteristics of the sample, the initial subject pool must be carefully screened for underlying characteristics which may bias the findings. Thus, deriving such an index from an impaired sample which has a great proportion of Alzheimer's patients will produce a set of results which are an artifact of the sample rather than descriptive of item efficiency in a generalizable sense. Similarly, using a sample of normals with below average cognitive abilities will also create incorrect impressions about item difficulty.

In an appropriate sample those items with difficulties below .2 and above .8 must be closely examined before inclusion in the final test. Again in an appropriate, heterogeneous sample, item difficulty ought to approach .5 for maximum discrimination on the variable of interest. In order to include a broad base of items, item difficulties should be gathered from samples which contain greater and lesser amounts of the variable of interest. Thus, one would intentionally test very bright and less bright people as separate groups if one were creating a test of cognitive efficiency in order to select items which would discriminate accurately along the full spectrum of cognitive abilities.

In examining the item difficulties for neuropsychological tests one expects that in a heterogeneous sample of brain impaired, item difficulties will approximate .5. One may use such knowledge to observe item difficulties in more homogeneous samples of brain impaired persons in order to get a sense of the functions which are impaired within such a homogeneous group. Items which showed difficulty indices above the .7 to .8 range would indicate a localized impairment, which hopefully would be consistent with the known impairment of the homogeneous group. Such findings could then be used to support the construct validity (which will be discussed later in the chapter) of sets of items.

The *Discrimination Index* is a method of differentiating persons high on a given variable from those low on such a characteristic. Thus, if one assumes that a high overall score on the motor scale of the Luria-Nebraska indicates greater impairment in the higher cortical functions associated with motor movements, one would select two sets of subjects from the sample: those having the highest one-third of the scores on the Motor scale and those having the lowest one-third of the scores on the Motor scale, and compare item efficiency in these two groups. The formula for the discrimination index (Hopkins & Antes, 1978, p. 189) is:

$$\text{Discrimination Index} = \frac{\begin{matrix}\text{Number} & & \text{Number} \\ \text{in the} & & \text{in the} \\ \text{Upper Group} & - & \text{Lower Group}\end{matrix}}{\text{Number of Subjects in Either Group}}.$$

When a greater number of subjects in the upper group respond in the scoreable direction than the number of subjects in the lower group, the discrimination index is positive. On the other hand when a greater number of subjects in the lower group respond in the scoreable direction, the discrimination index is negative, and one may assume that there is either something wrong with the item or with the sample on whom it is being tested. According to Hopkins and Antes (1978) the discrimination index may take on values from − 1.0 to + 1.0; values above .40 suggest effective items, while values between + .20 and + .39 are considered satisfactory. It must be remembered that items with negative discrimination indices are discriminating in the wrong direction and ought to be reconsidered.

An alternative way to compare high and low scoring groups is to compute a Phi-coefficient. This coefficient is based on a correlation between group membership (high score and low score) and item score (pass, fail). Like all correlation coefficients it may vary between − 1.0 and + 1.0, with higher scores indicating greater discrimination. A high negative score indicates substantial discrimination but in the wrong direction. This may suggest a scoring or criterion problem. Tables for calculating this coefficient may be found in Jurgensen (1947).

The *Validity Index* is a correlation between a score on a given item and some criterion variable. For example, one may dummy code a criterion variable as 1 = unimpaired and 2–impaired, and correlate each item response with such a variable. In this case, items correlating positively would be related to impairment, while items correlated negatively would be related to peformance by the unimpaired group. If the test is intended to describe impairment, negatively correlated items will need to be reconsidered. It is up to the researcher to determine the level at which a validity coefficient is acceptable. Since it is a correlation coefficient, one may square it to determine the approximate shared variance between the criterion variable and any given item.

A final method used by test developers to evaluate item efficiency is to calculate a point biserial correlation between an item and the overall test score in order to discern the degree to which an item represents what the test measures as a whole. Since the item contributes to the general test score, the test score must be recalculated without the given item before the computation is performed. This avoids artificially inflating the item-test relationship.

Items should be positively correlated with the overall test performance. The exact size of the ideal correlation again varies with the intent of the test. In a test measuring a broad skill or personality category, correlations may be in the .4 to .6 range; in a test which purports to measure a single, highly specific skill, correlations should be substantially higher. In the actual selection of items for the final form, intercorrelations among items must also be considered in the manner discussed later in this chapter.

Within multiple choice tests, analyses may also be performed on the distractors from which the subject must select the correct alternative. One may compute a discrimination index for each distractor. In general, alternatives which are not endorsed are useless, and alternatives which are endorsed to a high degree by subjects who do not contain the characteristic of interest also need to be reevaluated. Obviously such indices will again vary with the characteristics of the subject pool and the overall item difficulty.

A much more complex model of item analysis has been suggested by various theorists based on latent trait models (Anastasi, 1982; Baker, 1977; Weiss & Davison, 1981; Wright & Stone, 1979). These models assume nothing more than a mathematical existence for the characteristic being measured. Based on theoretical models which differ in underlying assumptions, these models can be used to establish item characteristic curves which represent a comparison of item difficulty against the expected scores of the hypothesized trait (usually estimated by the total test score). From these curves, several parameters of item difficulty may be established. In particular, the one parameter logistic model (Rasch model) holds promise for future developments (Rasch, 1966). A more detailed discussion of such methods is not within the scope of this chapter.

Scale Development

A major difference between tests relates to the number of subscales which may be generated within a given test. Item scores may be assembled in a variety of ways, each of which has examples in the literature and in clinical and research applications. More recent tests (e.g., Millon Personality Inventory, Luria-Nebraska Neuropsychological Battery), as well as modifications over the years of tests like the MMPI, illustrate a growing recognition that one may recombine items which were initially validated and created by different methods.

The most intuitive method of scale construction is simple face validity. The most basic case of this method is a scale which is assumed to describe a single dimension. (It should be noted that this is rarely true in reality.) Items are chosen because they are assumed to measure this dimension, and such items usually only vary in difficulty levels. In some cases, there is the assumption that items may be ranked according to difficulty within the scale, so that missing a simpler item implies that more difficult items will also be failed. An example of such a test is the Bender-Gestalt Test (Bender, 1938). Each item is assumed to be a measure of basic visuo-integrative skill which is also related to visual-motor integration. While items vary in complexity (difficulty), they are assumed all to measure the same ability. Thus, items appear to be arranged in order of difficulty.

A face valid depression scale could be put together by picking items which represent the apparent symptoms of depression (e.g., "I feel sad."; "My appetite has decreased."). In this method, the scale may be put together based simply on the impressions of the test developer, other experts, or may reflect an underlying theory of what "depression" is assumed to be. In general, scales which have a strong theoretical background are preferred since this allows the application of more sophisticated validation techniques, as well as facilitating interpretation and understanding of the results of the testing.

If one intends to sum items within a scale, all items must be represented on the same scaling system. This may necessitate transforming answers or scores so that they are all similarly scaled, since an item which is only scored "right/wrong" cannot be meaningfully added to another item which represents the number of correct responses within a given time limit. In addition to the type of scaling already discussed, linear transformations of data may also be performed in order to make individual item results more comparable. One may use z-scores or, if one wishes to avoid negative values, t-scores. This may not work as well if small score differences create a wide range of standard scores.

Further, frequencies within nominal categories may be summed to form scales drawn from responses to all items. Thus, on the Rorschach the scale "Pure Form" represents the total number of occurrences of unmodified form responses across all responses. Similarly, in neuropsychology, one could identify a "Perseveration" scale. Although the initial data is nominal, the summing process creates at least ordinal data (Gaito, 1970).

In addition to the face validity approach to scale formation, scales may also be identified on the basis of empirical properties of the items. These scales are usually based on three basic methodologies: (a) a set of items which discriminate maximally between two groups; (b) a set of items which show high correlations with an external representation of the variable of interest; and (c) a set of items which group together empirically as the result of a factor analytic procedure.

The first methodology may be illustrated by the construction of the original Depression scale of the MMPI. This scale was formed by comparing the responses of a group of psychiatrically diagnosed depressed patients with the responses derived from a control group. Items selected for the scale were those which maximally discriminated the two groups. Another example would be a screening test for brain damage, which could be put together from a set of items which are observed to maximally separate the brain impaired from unimpaired persons.

In the second case, items are selected on the basis of their correlation with an outside criteria. Thus, a depression scale may be formed by correlating item performance with psychiatric ratings of depressed persons on a scale from 1 to 7. If one were more biologically inclined, correlations could be calculated between the results of the dexamethasone suppression test and a set of items assumed to measure depression. This would link the diagnosis of depression to a specific biological marker rather than clinical impression alone.

The validity of the scales developed by these first two methods is thought to be dependent on the adequacy of the group or the external criteria selected. This, however, is not always the case. The MMPI is a perfect example of a test which has been criticized for its method of group definitions but has been found to have enormous clinical value as the result of later empirical study. However, in such cases the empirically based method of interpretation may not resemble the original procedures envisioned by the test developers.

In the third method, scales are factor analytically derived based on the intercorrelations among items within an item pool. It is assumed that items which load on the same factor relate to an underlying trait which can be represented by a factor score. By orthogonally rotating the initial solution and employing some criterion factor loading, sets of items will be identified which form a scale. The whole factor matrix represents a group of independent scales.

An additional factor analytic method which may be used to create a scale includes the use of marker variables; that is, variables which are known to be representative of a given trait. With this method, a depression scale may be constructed from a general pool of items by factor analyzing these items along with a set of variables known to be associated with depression. Items which share factors with the marker variables can then be included in the depression scale.

There are several limitations to the factor analytic procedures which must be considered in using such a methodology. First, one must thoroughly understand the theory which guided the initial item selections or constructions, since the resulting factors can only be interpreted accurately within the context of a theoretical base. Second, each factor solution and rotational method carries with it a set of theoretical assumptions which guide its meaningful application. It is up to the test designer to determine which analysis will create the least distortion in the original data while producing interpretable results. Thus, in choosing a rotational method one must understand, for instance, that the computational method in a Varimax rotation conserves variance down columns. This creates a large first factor partially as a consequence of the computational procedure.

Third, an exploratory (initial) factor analytic solution may be unstable across groups. Therefore, it is important to replicate factor analytically derived dimensions across groups in order to discover whether or not one is observing a stable (reliable) structure; that is, that items are not simply going together as an artifact of the current sample.

A fourth limitation to the factor analytic method results from the sample employed. Since dimensions are formed based on how items (variables) covary, the presence of subgroups in the sample which show both great within group similarity on a set of items and great between group differences on the same set of items offer the possibility of identifying dimensions which reflect the a priori group differences. This is a problem if it is unintended by the investigator. It can be a benefit if within-group characteristics are being used as marker variables.

Underlying characteristics which bias responses may also create artifactual factor dimensions. Thus, factors may actually reflect such variables as scoring approach, age, education, socioeconomic status, cultural, or gender differences.

Finally, the results of a factor analysis are influenced by the items available for the analysis. Underrepresentation of certain skills or traits in the item pool will prevent such variables from emerging as meaningful factors, even if such skills are important to the domain of the test. The best way to avoid such difficulties is to start with the Table of Specifications, which was described earlier in this chapter, as a blueprint for item construction.

Scales may, of course, be created by a combination of any of these methods. For example, original items may be chosen by screening based on face validity; then confirmed by correlational analysis. The resultant items may then be factor analyzed in an attempt to validate assumptions about the structure of the test. This would be an example of Jackson's (1970) sequential model which was referred to earlier.

The latter process may also be used to create new scales from the existing pool of items within a test. For example, on the Luria-Nebraska the original items were selected based on face validity and validated by item-scale correlations. Localization scales were derived from comparisons among groups with known characteristics (localized brain injury), and factor scales were identified from the test item pool.

After initial creation of scales, further item analysis can be performed. For example, items within a scale that are redundant (highly intercorrelated) may be eliminated. Other items may be eliminated due to their overall lack of relationship with the total score of the scale. For scales validated against outside criteria, items showing the least relationship with these criteria may be removed from the scale. Factor analytically derived scales may be shortened by determining the fewest number of items which maximize prediction.

The final decisions regarding scale length must result from several considerations: (1) theoretical concerns, which are an attempt to insure that the domain of interest is being adequately sampled; (2) practical concerns, e.g., time for administration; (3) procedural concerns, that is, the elimination of items which create excessive administrative difficulty while yielding limited clinical information; (4) psychometric concerns or the need to maintain adequate levels of reliability and validity. Though we are speaking about making some final decisions about an instrument at this point, it is optimally useful to enter the next phase of study with several versions of a scale (differing usually only in length) to see which is the most useful for the intended purpose of the test.

Reliability

After tentative scales have been established, initial investigations into reliability and validity can be made. During this phase, scales can still be modified, and this data may cause one to return to earlier stages of construction in order to maximize the usefulness of the particular test. We will first deal with the issues related to reliability.

Reliability research has generally taken a back seat to validity research in the psychological literature. Despite the importance of these issues, few, if any, reliability studies can be identified for many tests. Reliability refers to the stability, consistency, predictability and dependability of a test measure (Kerlinger, 1973). A test can be reliable and still useless. A useful test may have low reliability under some circumstances, however. For example, a test which measures a trait which is constantly fluctuating would not be expected to show test-retest reliability, although alternate form reliability should be demonstrable. A neuropsychological test may show low reliability in normals if score variance is severely restricted. Thus, it is important to understand each type of reliability and to consider each type in relationship to the test and the theory underlying the test. If the wrong form of reliability is applied, or a poor population employed, this research can be highly misleading.

Test-Retest Reliability. The most obvious type of reliability deals with the *stability* of test scores over time. In this method, scores from an initial administration are correlated with scores on the same instrument after some interval. To use this method of describing the reliability of a test, one must start with the assumption that the characteristic measured by the test has temporal stability. Thus, the test-retest method would be a poor estimate for an instrument used to assess state anxiety or for an instrument designed to assess degree of acute impairment after a head injury. No test, even of a stable trait, should be expected to demonstrate perfect test-retest reliability, as there are many factors which influence test scores other than what the test purports to measure. These include: (a) fatigue, which may create differential concentration and motivation levels between two administrations; (b) differential environmental conditions, such as temperature, outside noise, ambient distractions, scheduling demands, or unexpected personal events between sessions; (c) administration errors on the part of the examiner. Test-retest reliability will also be affected by the sample. If homogeneous samples showing either very high or very low scores on the initial administration are used for the second administration, the extremity of their initial scores will capitalize on chance fluctuation and will in all likelihood underestimate the stability of the test.

In interpreting a test-retest coefficient the following limitations must be taken into account. The experience of the first administration may affect the subject's performance during the second administration. Such carry-over effects can work to either underestimate or overestimate an instrument's stability (Allen & Yen, 1979). The length of time between tests creates differential effects depending on the characteristic being measured. Allen and Yen (1979) indicate that short intervals may be subject to effects due to memory, practice, or mood, while longer intervals may be affected by the possibility of acquiring new information and changes in mood. In summary, test-retest estimates of reliability are most appropriate for tests involving abilities rather than achievement or for personality traits which are assumed to be variable.

Alternate-Form Reliability. This is similar to test-retest reliability except another form of the test is administered at the second session. Thus, this coefficient represents both temporal stability as well as the degree of redundancy across forms. One must remember that the maximum alternate-form reliability will be limited by the test-retest reliability. In order to minimize the variance due to time, one can shorten the time between administrations. However, one must keep in mind that this will increase the possibility of carry-over effects.

Adequate alternate form reliability suggests that the items on the two forms are both samples from the same population of items which represents a hypothesized trait or skill. Low alternate form reliabilities suggest that the two test forms are not measuring the same thing. If the tests sample from the same item population, but different components of that population, the correlation may also be small. As an example, let us hypothesize alternate form scales which sample from the universe of anti-social behaviors. If one scale is weighted heavily with items involving criminal activities and the other scale is weighted with items involving the manipulation of other people, then the two scales may exhibit smaller correlations.

Alternate-form reliability has many of the same limitations as test-retest reliability. One may expect this computational type to show effects from both carry-over and length of interval between sessions. These latter factors may be most evident in a test which requires a specific cognitive style for problem-solving or demands a cognitive set which is applicable to both forms.

Split-Half Reliability. In split-half reliability, a type of alternate form reliability is produced by dividing a single scale into two halves. This computational method estimates the degree of consistency across items. Though it does not measure temporal stability, it offers the advantage of a single administration. This method assumes that all of the items contribute equally to the measurement of a central construct.

The major problem with this method rests on the issue of how to split the items. In general, the most convenient method is to correlate odd numbered items with even numbered items (odd-even split). Alternatively, one may correlate the first half of the test items with the latter half; however, this method is inadequate with speeded tests, where the subject may not reach the second half, or with tests which arrange their items by degree of difficulty, where the latter part of the test is much more difficult than the first part. Halves may also be created by random selection, without replacement, but this is a cumbersome and usually unnecessary procedure.

Since this method uses only one-half of the items that are seen in the other reliability measures, split-half reliabilities may be lower than other reliability estimates. The Spearman-Brown formula may be used to estimate the correlation if the number of items has not been reduced.The estimated correlation is equal to:

$$\frac{2r}{(1+r)},$$

where r represents the correlation of the two halves.

The more general form of the Spearman-Brown formula can be used to estimate the effects on reliability by increasing or decreasing the number of items for a scale. The general formula is:

$$\frac{nr}{1+(n-1)r},$$

where n is the ratio of the number of items in the full form to the number of items in the shorter form. Thus, if the number of items started at 60 and $r = .05$ and one is interested in the effect on reliability of increasing the number of items to 150, n would equal 150/60 or 2.5 and the estimated increased reliability would be .71. Such calculations allow one to quickly estimate the effects on scale reliability from either adding or removing items before going to the work of actually constructing the items.

Internal Consistency Reliability. Although split-half reliability is a measure of internal consistency, it only looks at one possible division of items instead of all possible splits. Other formulas have been developed to make more conservative estimates of internal consistency reliability. These are the Kuder-Richardson 20 formula (KR20) and coefficient alpha (Kuder & Richardson, 1937; see also Cronbach, 1951; Ebel, 1965; Kaiser & Michael, 1975).

The KR20 formula is generally intended for tests with items which only have two possible alternatives (e.g., true/false), while coefficient alpha is usually applied to tests whose items have multiple possible answers. The results of these techniques represent an average of all possible split-half reliabilities formed by all possible combinations of items. Formulas for these coefficients may be found in the above references.

Coefficient alpha has a number of additional properties which are useful to note for the purposes of test construction. Alpha is a low estimate of the reliability of a test, which is a less than perfect estimate of the true score for the characteristic of interest; and it is the upper estimate of the variance accounted for by the first factor, when the test is factor analyzed (Allen & Yen, 1979). It is this latter characteristic of alpha which allows one to infer the degree of homogeneity among test items. Obviously, as the first factor accounts for a greater amount of variance (larger alpha reliability), the test may be described more unidimensionally. This is also one of the limits of the alpha reliability estimate. It will tend to underestimate the reliability of a heterogeneous test.

It should be emphasized, however, that there is no particular virtue in raising or lowering the results of these calculations. If the domain of interest is multidimensional, a heterogeneous scale may be more useful. Perfectly homogeneous sets of items would not exist since multiple skills or traits influence the score of any item. Often an extremely homogeneous scale will fail to correlate well with external criterion variables. Usually, there is a need to compromise between a desire to make the scale as internally consistent as possible and demands that the test be useful in the real world.

Inter-Scorer Reliability. Another estimate of a test's reliability may be derived by the use of multiple examiners to score the same protocol of responses. It is useful in most tests except for the simplest to analyze the effect on the test created by a variety of scorers. This is especially important for standardized tests as discussed here, since we are assuming that administration and scoring will provide a consistent base across clinicians for interpretive purposes. This becomes a crucial issue for projective tests of personality and open-ended tests, both of which require the examiner to perform subjective analyses of behavior.

Inter-scorer reliability can be determined from either: (a) obtaining protocols and having them scored by two different investigators; (b) having two examiners observe and score the performance of the same patient at the same time; or (c) having two scorers independently evaluate data from the same patient. In the latter case, a better evaluation of the effects of different administration techniques is achieved but a poorer measure of scoring errors occurs because of complications by test-retest effects. The first two methods do not estimate the effects of different administrators at all, since the test is only given a single time.

In summary one may note that all of the above methods of evaluating reliability assume a univariate structure underlying the test; however, many scales are multidimensional. For example, Galassi, Delo, Galassi, and Bastien's (1974) assertion scale can be broken down into expression of positive affect, expression of negative affect, and asking one's needs to be met. If one wishes to observe the internal consistency reliability of such a test, one may apply Bentler's (1975) procedure, which is applicable to these multidimensional situations.

Analyzing Variance. Anastasi (1982) has observed that these different estimates of reliability can be used to parcel out test variance among subjects which is "true" variance (due to the characteristic of interest) from that attributable to error variance (effects unrelated to the characteristic of interest). She identifies the following techniques as measuring specific types of error variance: (1) test-retest—variance due to time interval; (2) alternate form, immediate administration—variance due to content; (3) alternate form, delayed administration—variance due to both time and content; (4) split-half—variance due to content sampling; (5) KR20 and alpha—variance due to content sampling and heterogeneity; and (6) inter-scorer—variance due to examiner and administration style.

Since the difference between the square of a reliability coefficient and 1.0 represents the percentage of variance we can attribute to a specific factor, we can calculate the total amount of explained and error variance from this information, if we assume that the test under consideration is perfectly reliable. For example, if the test-retest reliability is .9, we can calculate that $1.0-(.9)^2$ or $1.0-.81$ or an estimated 19% of the variance is due to time. If in the same test, the KR20 is .8, we can calculate that item content and heterogeneity account for $1.0-(.8)^2$ or 36% of the total variance. Finally, if the inter-scorer reliability is .95, we can estimate that the examiner effect is responsible for 9.75% of the variance. If one sums these percentages, the total amount of variance attributable to error factors is 64.75%, which leaves, theoretically, 35.25% as true variance.

Further, since true variance can be translated into a theoretical reliability for this scale, the correlation would be the square root of .3525 or just less than .6. Since most test designers find a test with a reliability in the .7 to .8 range to be adequate, it may be inferred that the amount of error variance in most tests is at least 30% to 50% and may be more. However, one must note that the previously described method of estimating error contributions to a test may inflate the error estimate since components of that error effect may overlap between estimation methods (i.e., both alternate form and test-retest are affected by time interval).

Limits of Correlational Estimates. Since all measures of reliability are correlational in nature, all are affected by the way variance is distributed across both items and subjects. First, as the sample being tested becomes more homogeneous, the correlation between measures will decrease due to the restricted range of variance available in one or both measures. Second, tests for which speed is a factor (only subsets of items are completed due to the test's time limitations and the subject's abilities) make calculation of inter-item and internal consistency measures impossible. Anastasi (1982) suggests that procedures like correlating item performance during one time period (the first 10 minutes) with performance in another time period (the last 10 minutes) as a way to get around such difficulties. Correlational estimates will also differ within ability levels when score ranges are restricted.

Validity

The most researched and the most "glamorous" area of research in test construction and assessment is validity research. Certainly, such studies are of the utmost importance: Validity research tells us empirically what a test can and cannot do, its limitations as well as its advantages. Such research comprises the bulk of the papers published in this topic area in the major journals, and attracts the most attention from clinicians. Despite this, the understanding of this research is at a low level. Most frequently, there is a tendency by researchers and by readers to overgeneralize from validity research. A study suggesting a predictive relationship between two parameters in Population A is immediately assumed to be equally true in Population B. Tests developed in one country are borrowed without additional research and used in a second country. Conversely, failure of a test in Population B as opposed to A is seen as indicating that the test is no good, rather than recognizing that one is simply elucidating the limits of the test's usefulness.

As we will see below, the process of test validation is a long and tedious process when done correctly, ranging far beyond the work done for the initial establishment of a test. Indeed, it is safe to say that such work is never completed: Changing times as well as investigations of myriad populations and other factors make this an endless process rather than something limited to a test manual. Ideally, such research is undertaken to delimit the usefulness of each test: No test is usable in all circumstances, no matter how enthusiastic the developer is. Equally so, it is rare to find a test that does not have specific (albeit limited) uses. The point of validity research is to define these uses and limitations as precisely and accurately as possible.

Types of validity can be divided into three major areas: content validity, criterion-related validity, and construct validity. Each is important to any test and all should be established to the appropriate degree. Unfortunately, there is always great controversy over what the term "appropriate degree" means. This is a subjective question, and the problem lies in the fact that none of these can be absolutely established with any amount of research. Rather, it is only possible to determine the presence of these types of validity in a test by an overall weighing of the evidence, as the test does not exist in which all research comes up with the same answers and conclusions. These differences can often be traced to such factors as design, underlying population, and execution style of a study. Properly interpreted, such differences yield valuable information about tests. However, when overgeneralizations in conclusions occur, such differences can be misleading and confusing to the user.

Bias. Before going into the forms of validity in greater detail, it is important to consider whether the test in question is affected by bias. Bias refers to the effect on a test created by some variable other than the characteristic of interest. Bias may be either internal or external. Internal bias refers to the differential interaction of the test with specific examinee characteristics other than the characteristic of interest. This interaction is assumed to be nonrandom.

External bias, also called situational bias (Jensen, 1980), refers to the nonrandom interaction between the test and such variables as race, age, or sex of the examiner; emotional atmosphere created by the testing procedures; or test instructions. The effect of either of these forms of bias is to systematically overestimate or underestimate the meaning of test scores drawn from specific samples in comparison to the meaning of such scores when derived from a large sample randomly selected from the population. This issue becomes especially important when one is designing a test which will be used to make diagnostic decisions.

In considering bias, one must place such concerns in the context of several fallacies (Jensen, 1980) which have grown up in the political climate that has surrounded testing bias in recent history. Jensen (1980) describes three inadequate concepts of bias.

The egalitarian fallacy assumes that all human populations are basically identical. Thus, test results on measures of traits or abilities should never be related to group memberships. In accepting such a premise, the investigator is caught in the position of never being able to accept group differences as being meaningful. The culture-bound fallacy is based on subjective opinion; that is, items are identified as biased by a critic's definitions rather than scientifically. The standardization fallacy suggests that a test is only valid on the sample or combination of samples on whom it was standardized. The validity of a test for any population is an empirical question which needs to be resolved in a research context.

Tests may be observed for bias by several simple methods. Most commonly, regression lines based on a criterion variable may be compared across several samples. In such an analysis, the slopes, intercepts, or standard errors of estimate may be compared between groups. Statistically significant differences on any of these parameters suggest systematic bias in a test (Jensen, 1980). An alternative way of observing the performance of a test between groups is to compare the ranks of within-test item difficulty indices across groups. Ranks ought to remain stable across groups. These issues of bias must be kept in mind as test validity is examined.

Content Validity. Content validity is a measure of the extent to which test items adequately sample from the universe of interest. Content validation starts as the initial items are selected for a test. Content validity is easiest to demonstrate when the test has been built from a well defined theoretical orientation and the designer has started from a Table of Specifications in order to adequately sample a representative group of items.

Subsequent analysis of content validity may differ markedly from the original validation. Future investigators may assume a different underlying theory or support a different set of representative items. When items or scales are shown to have limited content validity, it is usually a result of either incomplete understanding of the underlying theory, lack of a theory, or a tendency to overgeneralize in item construction. Thus, for example, one may assume that a person capable of doing short term memory tasks is also capable of doing tasks requiring long term storage: an assumption which is not accurate. Selection of items which only demonstrate long-term storage will not be effective in determining short-term memory impairment. However, if one is not interested in short term memory, this would not be a problem.

One of the major problems with content validity is the subjectivity of the concept. Clearly, whether a test has content validity depends greatly on the theory used to generate that test. In cases where researchers approach the same concept area with a different theory, the tests will be different. Yet each will be equally valid as long as they follow their underlying theory. For example, if a theory says that intelligence is an underlying dimension which cuts across all tasks, a test may be designed with a wide variety of tasks looking for an underlying "g" factor. If, however, one believes that there is no such thing as an intelligence "g" factor, one will put together a test which yields specific scores for limited areas. On the other hand, if one believes that there are a combination of specific and general factors, then the test organization will follow a different structure and content. In each case, widely disparate but equally content valid tests will be designed. The tests may not have equal construct and criterion related ability, but those need to be established separately.

Overall, content validity is most appropriate for tests of ability (cognition) or achievement. It is generally less of a concern for empirically derived tests where there is no theoretical base, and tests of personality where too high content validity may compromise the usefulness of the test.

Face Validity

Content validity is commonly confused with a form of validity called "face validity." Face validity does not deal with what a test actually measures but rather with what a scale appears to measure based on the reading of various items. The researcher will often find that what an item appears to measure on the surface will differ considerably from what the scale measures in actual practice. What an item actually measures in a test will depend not only on the structure of the item but the conditions under which it is administered and scored. Changes in timing, instruction, and scoring procedures can cause relationships with external correlates to vary considerably. Thus, face validity is essentially a limited concept which may not reflect intended content.

Despite this fact, however, face validity does play a role in test construction. While it is not important to the professional, it is through face validity that the subject receives an impression of what the test is measuring. If a test appears too easy, too hard, inappropriate to what the patient wants, or unnecessarily intrusive, it may affect the patient's test-taking attitude (e.g., level of cooperation, honesty, etc.). These factors should also be taken into account in order to insure the widest usefulness for the test.

Criterion Based Validity. Criterion validity is extremely important and used widely throughout the construction of psychological tests. This form of validity deals with the ability of test scores to assess behavior, either as represented by other test scores, observable behaviors, or other accomplishments such as grade point averages.

Criterion validity can be subdivided into two types: concurrent and predictive. The difference between these forms of criterion validity lies primarily in the temporal relationship between the test and the external criterion. Concurrent validity involves prediction to an alternative method of measuring the same characteristic of interest, while predictive validity attempts to show a relationship with future behavior. For example, concurrent validity would assume a relationship between a new test and an existing test if both are assumed to be sensitive to a dementing process. On the other hand, a design involving predictive validity would attempt to identify future dements based on their performance on the new instrument. The accuracy of such a classification over time would serve as the measure of predictive validity. Since designs involving concurrent validity are generally easier to implement due to the absence of the temporal constraint, concurrent procedures are occasionally substituted though the intent is clearly predictive. Thus, we may assess anxious students already referred to a college counseling center to validate a test of anxiety in students. Patterns identified during such a study could then be used to predict which freshman students are likely to develop anxiety disorders during their college experience. Care must be taken in such cases, since the assumed predictive relationship is not confirmed by the current data and awaits the passage of time.

The existence of concurrent relationships between criterion variables and the results of psychological tests is important to demonstrate. For example, one may note that the presence of brain damage can be determined reasonably well by collecting an incisive history, a CT scan, EEG, PET scan, NMR, and regional cerebral blood flow measures, along with other appropriate biochemical tests; however, such a work-up costs thousands of dollars. Thus, the existence of concurrent relationships between the results of a neuropsychological battery and the results of such broadbased physiological measures allow the possibility of saving both time and money. Further, predictive relationships between neuropsychological findings and changes in function after brain injury provide information in addition to the information delivered by the physiologically based tests.

Tests should be validated against as many criteria as there are behaviors which may be reasonably predicted from the data. Generally such research will identify the limits of a test; that is, test scores will be better predictors of some events and worse for others. Such a pattern of findings helps to identify the appropriate test for a given need. Both clinical users and research users must recognize that no test is appropriate in all circumstances or for all purposes, and it is the purpose of assessment research to clarify those limits for each test.

Both predictive and concurrent validities are accepted by deciding the appropriate level of validity coefficient or correlation between a test score and some criterion variable. The appropriate acceptance level depends on the intended use of the test.

Criterion validity can be established through several alternate research designs. The most common is the correlational design, in which the two separate measures are given to each participant. A related design is the use of ANOVA techniques in which the criterion variables are group membership or levels of a particular noncontinuous variable. One problem with such designs results from the effects of mediator variables. This is usually corrected by the use of partial correlations, or in ANOVA designs, by the use of covariates. For example, two tests may correlate with one another because they both correlate with age or education rather than the variable under question. Two tests of brain damage sensitive to age may correlate with one another despite measuring different aspects of brain dysfunction.

This becomes more complicated when the mediator variables correlate with such factors as group membership; that is, when there is a significant correlation between the independent variable and the mediating variable. For example, if the brain injured group averages 60 years in age and the normal group 20 years, it is impossible to tell whether the differences are due to age or to brain injury. In such cases, partial correlation methods or using covariates are ineffective because the correction for age also corrects for the presence of brain damage. In such conditions, the correction for age needs to be generated on a separate control population with a larger distribution of ages and then this correction can be applied to all subjects. If this is not done, the results are largely meaningless and often inadvertently support the null hypothesis.

In the case of concurrent validity, the tests should be given as closely together as possible unless doing so will make the results worse, such as when the tests are so long that fatigue will result or so similar that some learning will take place. The time period between testing is also affected by how stable or unstable the traits being examined are: If we are testing for situational anxiety, the tests need to be almost simultaneous. If we are testing for degree of brain damage in a normal person without any injury, the time is of little matter. If we are testing a person with a fast-growing tumor, however, tests need to be administered within short periods of time.

A related design is the prediction of group membership. In these cases, whether the patient belongs to the "brain damaged" group or the "normal" group is the criterion variable, for example. In these cases, discriminant analysis may be employed. Such an analysis identifies the components or items of a test which maximally discriminate criterion groups. The items which most discriminate between groups are then used in an ancillary classification analysis to assign group membership. The hit rate derived from the ancillary analysis describes the ability of the most effective parts of the test to relate to the criterion. Thus, low hit rates in such a context are especially damaging to test validity. Such designs are quite powerful, and must be carefully employed (as is generally true of all multivariate techniques). In these cases, in general, the greater the number of subjects in comparison to the number of variables, the less the results capitalize on chance variables (assuming of course that the groups do not differ on other important variables which influence the data.) In general, the number of subjects should be at least five times the number of variables, although in preliminary studies one may have as few as three times as many subjects.

Of more importance, however, than the subject/variable ratio is the ability to cross-validate the discriminant formula derived from the above analysis in another population. A common technique is to collect a population large enough to be split into two groups: The discriminant formula is generated on group 1, and then cross-validated on group 2. In using such a design, the issue becomes: What is an acceptable level of shrinkage between samples? Shrinkage in this case refers to the expected decrease in hit rate between studies. An investigator must discriminate what is a chance difference between samples and what suggests a weakness in the test.

Another important issue is the question of base rates. If the population under study is 90% normal and 10% abnormal, a formula calling everyone normal has a 90% accuracy rate. In such a case, the accuracy would have to be statistically greater than 90% in order to be important. This does not hold, however, in cross-validation studies where the base rates in the cross-validation groups vary considerably from the original. If the formula works at 90% accuracy in a group divided 50-50 as well, then the researcher can rely on the usefulness of the formula in general. However, one still needs to examine how useful the formula is in reality: If a formula gives 90% accuracy but the sample already has a 95% rate of normality (or other group membership), the incremental validity of the formula may be nonexistent. By examining the base rate of the population and the accuracy rate of the formula in each population, one can determine the incremental validity (if any) contributed by the test. It is not unusual to find that the test is appropriate for probems in some populations, but not others. This, however, is more a question of clinical usefulness of a test as opposed to research accuracy and design.

One way to avoid the problem in discriminant analysis is to use rules to classify subjects derived from previous work or even clinical experience with other subjects (never the same subjects used in the study). Such data is not subject to the problems caused by capitalization of the discriminant formula on error variance, although base rate problems will still remain. These can be generally overcome in both instances by examining accuracy rates for each group separately rather than overall. Thus, in the 90-10 example above, a rule or formula which classifies everyone as normal would have accuracy rates of 100% and 0%. The discrepancy is easily used to identify the problem. If the accuracy rates are 90 and 90 for each group, however, then the overall rate of 90% is meaningful and useful.

Construct Validity. Construct validity is the newest type of validity which has been recognized (see Cronbach & Meehl, 1955). This approach is much more complex than the other forms of validity, requiring an accumulation of data over a long period of time. Construct validity involves studying test scores in their relationship not only to variables which the test is intended to assess but also to variables which should have no relationship to the domain underlying the instrument. One builds a *nomothetic net* or inferential definition of the characteristics which a test is measuring. Hypotheses may be generated in a wide variety of ways depending on the characteristic of interest.

For example, when cognitive skills are studied, theories can be used to predict developmental changes that are expected in a trait over time. Such changes are then sought in test scores given at different age levels. This research can obviously be extended over the total life span and not just limited to children.

A second approach includes predictions to other tests which are assumed to measure the same underlying trait as well as those measures which describe unrelated traits. We may predict that a specific intellectual skill should have a moderate correlation with a measure of general IQ, little or no correlation with a measure of hypochondriasis, and a strong correlation to another test measuring the same intellectual skill. It should be clear that in examining such interrelationships the efficacy of the research depends on the accuracy of the original hypothesis, which in turn is related to the investigator's comprehension of the trait under study. Researchers and consumers must be careful not to confuse a researcher's misunderstanding of either the intention of an instrument or the underlying theory with the inefficiency of the instrument itself.

In a major paper, Campbell and Fiske (1959) expanded these notions into an analytic model which includes the concepts of *discriminant* and *convergent* validity. To demonstrate discriminant validity, one needs to show that the test is unrelated to tests which measure different constructs. To demonstrate convergent validity, we need to show that the test is related to tests which measure the same construct. Based on this model, they proposed the use of a multitrait-multimethod design. In such a design, the trait under study is measured in a number of alternative ways, which includes the test that is being evaluated. At the same time measures of assumed unrelated traits are also included. The pattern of intercorrelation among the various measures creates a multitrait/multimethod matrix. The validity of a test is supported if it shows moderate to high relationships with instruments assumed to measure a similar characteristic, while demonstrating low to zero correlations with instruments measuring unrelated characteristics.

Although the Campbell and Fiske (1959) article represents an important consideration in the evaluation of a psychological test, their suggested methodology can be improved. Jackson (1969) has raised criticisms of the methodology and has suggested an alternative evaluation model. Most of Jackson's (1969) criticisms center around the fact that Campbell and Fiske's (1959) methodology compares individual criterion correlations and does not examine the overall structure. Pattern correlations between traits may be influenced by the method variance engendered in measuring the traits under consideration.

Jackson (1966, 1975) instead recommends a factor analysis of the monomethod matrix. In such an analysis, the matrix is first orthogonalized and submitted to a principal components analysis, followed by a varimax rotation. The expected number of factors is set equal to the number of traits under consideration. Although Jackson's analysis helps meet certain shortcomings of the earlier methodology, it is also open to criticism. Because Jackson's procedure capitalizes on the discrepancy between the characteristics of interest, it is not useful for conceptually related traits. Because it uses a monomethod matrix, one may not use it to examine the influence of different methods. Therefore these two methods of validational analysis (cf. Campbell & Fiske's and Jackson's) may be seen as being complementary to each other, and it is advisable to use both in the complete analysis of an assessment instrument.

A further development in the evaluation of multitrait-multimethod matrices involves the use of the structural equations approach. Kallenberg and Kluegel (1975) describe three advantages of this method. The structural equations approach provides a mechanism for describing the correlation trait and method factors. It provides a mechanism for describing the relationships of both trait and method factors under consideration. Finally, in order to use the structural equations method, one must first specify one's assumptions regarding the construct under consideration.

Another way to study construct validity is through factor analysis. One may postulate a factorial structure for a specific instrument given one's assumptions about both the trait which is being measured and the theory from which it was derived. A confirmatory factor analysis is then performed to test the hypothesis. Thus, for example, in our own work with the Luria-Nebraska, predictions were made from Luria's theory of brain functioning. Such predictions were operationalized in terms of item interrelationships and the factoring process is used to test such hypotheses (see Golden, Hammeke, Purisch, Berg, Moses, Newlin, Wilkening, & Puente, 1982, for an example).

In the case of tests in which a limited number of scores or a single score is generated, marker variables whose meaning is more completely understood may be included in the analysis. Factorial relationships with such marker variables can then be used to determine the meaning of the new test scores. In such analyses and in all factor analytic procedures, it is useful to perform a series of factor analyses, in order to determine if the factor structure and the factorial relationships are stable across time and across groups.

Normative Data

After the test has reached an acceptable initial form, normative data may be established. In some cases, this may be done as an integral part of the previously mentioned validation investigations or in a separate phase. Such a decision usually depends on the constraints which the test designer faces as well as the initial results of validation efforts. Several approaches may be taken to form normative data.

Norms will differ depending on the scaling scheme used for a scale or for individual items, a topic which has been discussed earlier. As indicated, a given scaling approach is dependent on the type of information desired and the inferences which will be drawn from the data. Similarly, the eventual scoring system employed, whether percentiles, *t*-scores, *z*-scores, or the like, will depend on many of the same factors. Of greater importance for researchers is recognizing the relativity of norms.

Norms for a given test may differ considerably depending on the characteristics of the standardization sample which was used. In addition, the future sample to which the instrument is applied may differ considerably from the group on whom it was normed, even though both may be from the same general population. This presents serious problems for the test designer.

Although attempts are made to gather representative samples whose characteristics will be appropriate to a wide variety of subjects, this is essentially a futile task in that any limited sample cannot hope to adequately represent a broad population like "the American student," for example, or even more restricted groups like "all 10-year-olds." Individuals within such groups are simply too diverse. A large number of factors will affect individual scores: motivation, environment, culture, age, developmental level, language, training, educational quality, personal experience, gender, and attitude, to name a few. Although such factors may average out across a large group, they grossly affect the interpretation of an individual protocol. Thus, even if a sample of 3,000 subjects were to include the same percentage of American Indians as exist in the population as a whole, to argue that the mean scores of such a sample are as representative of an individual American Indian's performance is of questionable validity. The degree to which such an assumption is accurate may only be determined by norming the test within subgroups that exist within the overall population. The investigator should keep in mind that no single set of norms can be used in all circumstances, and that norms must take into account both individual and group factors in order to be meaningful.

Such an understanding results in a greater emphasis on the use of local or specific norms aimed at individual groups. The degree to which these groups must be precisely described is determined to a great extent by the trait or skill which is being measured. For example, if we wish to look at the population of college educated individuals, fewer persons are necessary in the sample and less discrimination in subject selection is needed if the task to be measured is reading the word "cat," a skill for which there will be limited within-group variation in such a population. On the other hand, a complex skill requiring the comprehension of nuclear engineering will be strongly affected by individual coursework and will, in turn, affect the norms which are derived. Care must be taken in situations where different cultures or language backgrounds will limit exposure to the domain which a test is intended to assess. Thus, in selecting samples in order to create norms, one must consider the factors which will affect the characteristic which is being measured.

Local or specific group norms may be established in two ways. First, norms may be defined in reference to a given subgroup. Thus, on an IQ test, one may establish that Group A has a mean score of 92 and a standard deviation of 18 rather than the more general mean of 100 and a standard deviation of 15. For a member of such a group, we would consequently define a score of 65 as within two standard deviations of normal (92 ± 36), while we would not have done so using the more general norm (100 ± 15). Alternately, we could equate an IQ of 92 in our group with an IQ of 100, using appropriate tables to redefine every other score within our group in a similar manner. This latter method has the advantage of allowing similar interpretive statements to be applied to members of the subgroup; however, one loses the relative information conveyed by the difference between the scores of our group and the more general norm group.

For example, on the Luria-Nebraska, though standard scores are used across all scales, interpretations regarding the absence or presence of brain impairment are modified based on the presence or absence of certain demographic factors. A score of 70 on the Reading scale generally suggests poor reading in English but is not interpreted as "impaired" in an individual who has never been formally educated. The same score does indicate impaired performance in a college graduate with a degree in English Literature. Such a system based on a common scoring scheme has the advantage of allowing one to simultaneously correct for multiple extraneous factors without the need to create tables which anticipate every novel subject characteristic.

In such a system, the reference group serves only to anchor the norms and need not be representative of any specific population. Interpretation is not based on any assumption regarding such a norm group, or its representativeness. Rather, interpretations are modified based on research with subjects with characteristics similar to the patient's. The comparison reference group should not have any unusual characteristics which would mitigate against accurate comprehension of resulting protocols. For example, if the reference group were individuals with an average IQ of 12, too many groups will score many standard deviations from the reference norms, creating interpretive difficulties due to the exaggerated differences between individuals.

Another advantage of such a system is the ease with which other investigators may develop local or specific group norms, which may be communicated to other researchers in simple and understandable terms. This also permits one to develop alternate test forms whose scores can be related to the original reference group, which further insures comparability of scoring across forms.

The use of such locally derived subgroup norms in relation to a fixed reference group produces a situation in which one is never finished collecting normative data. Future investigators may develop norms for their own samples of interest, which may be quite divergent from the original reference sample. They may also investigate the effects of variables such as age, education, anxiety, and so on in order to further refine the limits of interpretation.

A related issue is the use of a national anchor group to insure comparability of scores across tests (rather than within a single test form only). Such an anchor group insures comparability by defining scores on an alternative measure in terms of the scores of the original test. Scores on the new test are assumed to be equal to the scores achieved on the earlier test.

SUMMARY

As the reader can see, research in testing offers a number of alternatives depending on the level one wishes to begin the analysis. It is important to emphasize that any test can be reanalyzed at any of the levels presented at any time. Even after a test has become "accepted" by users, there is a continuing need to evaluate whether the test continues to do what it is supposed to do and whether items continue to serve the function for which they were intended. Since no test is perfect, there is always a better way to formulate the test or to develop methods more appropriate for a single use. There is always the ability to further elucidate the correlates of a test, eliciting both its strengths and weaknesses. This ongoing evaluation provides one of the basic strengths of standardized tests: the ability to use continuing scientific evaluation to refine and improve our methods, something not possible with intuitive or non-scoreable methods.

It is expected that the tendency toward continual refinement of tests will increase as computers come in to greater use for scoring and storage purposes, making large data bases of patients available for this work. The use of computer scoring systems will also allow for scoring procedures to be changed easily (by modifying programs), as well as allowing us to retroactively rescore older protocols to see if an alternative method will provide better results. Such data bases will also allow for quick cross-validation of such studies as instruments are refined.

REFERENCES

Allen, M.J., & Yen, W.M. (1979). *Introduction to measurement theory.* Monterey, CA: Brooks/Cole Publishing.

Anastasi, A. (1982). *Psychological testing.* New York: Macmillan.

Baker, F.B. (1977). Advance in item analysis. *Review of Educational Research, 47,* 151–178.

Bem, S.L. (1974). The measurement of psychological androgyny. *Journal of Consulting and Clinical Psychology, 42,* 155–162.

Bem, S.L. (1977). On the utility of alternative procedures for assessing psychological androgyny. *Journal of Consulting and Clinical Psychology, 45,* 196–205.

Bender, L. (1938). A visual motor Gestalt test and its clinical use. *American Orthopsychiatric Association. Research Monographs,* (No. 3).

Bentler, P.M. (1975). A lower bound method for the dimension free measurement of internal consistency. *Social Science Research, 60,* 1–9.

Campbell, D.T., & Fiske, D.W. (1959). Convergent and discriminant validation by the multitrait-multimethod matrix. *Psychological Bulletin, 56,* 81–105.

Carroll, B.J., Fielding, J.M., & Blashki, T.G. (1973). Depression rating scales: A critical review. *Archives of General Psychiatry, 28,* 361–366.

Cronbach, L.J. (1951). Coefficient alpha and the internal structure of tests. *Psychometrika, 16,* 297–334.

Cronbach, L.J., & Meehl, P.E. (1955). Construct validity in psychological tests. *Psychological Bulletin, 52,* 281-302.
Ebel, R.L. (1965). *Measuring educational achievement.* Englewood Cliffs, NJ: Prentice-Hall.
Exner, J.E. (1974). *The Rorschach: A comprehensive system.* New York: John Wiley & Sons.
Fiske, D.W. (1978). *Strategies for personality research.* San Francisco: Jossey-Bass.
Gaito, J. (1970). Scale classification and statistics. In E.F. Heermann, & L.A. Braskamp (Eds.), *Readings in statistics for the behavioral sciences.* Englewood Cliffs, NJ: Prentice-Hall.
Galassi, J.P., Delo, J.S., Galassi, M.D., & Bastien, S. (1974). The college self-expression scale: A measure of assertiveness. *Behavior Therapy, 5,* 165–171.
Golden, C.J., Hammeke, T.A., Purisch, A.D., Berg, R.A., Moses, J.A., Jr., Newlin, D.B., Wilkening, G.N., & Puente, A.E. (1982). *Item Interpretation of the Luria-Nebraska Neuropsychological Battery.* Lincoln, NE: University of Nebraska Press.
Hays, W.L. (1973). *Statistics for the social sciences.* New York: Holt, Rinehart, & Winston.
Hopkins, C.D., & Antes, R.L. (1978). *Classroom measurement and evaluation.* Itasca, IL: F.E. Peacock Publishers.
Jackson, D.N. (1969). Multimethod factor analysis in the evaluation of convergent and discriminant validity. *Psychological Bulletin, 72,* 30–49.
Jackson, D.N. (1970). A sequential system for personality scale development. In C.D. Spielberger (Ed.), *Current topics in clinical and community psychology.* New York: Academic Press.
Jackson, D.N. (1975). Multimethod factor analysis: A reformulation. *Multivariate Behavioral Research, 19,* 259–275.
Jensen, A.R. (1980). *Bias in mental testing.* New York: The Free Press.
Jurgensen, C.E. (1947). Table for determining phi coefficients. *Psychometrika, 12,* 17–29.
Kaiser, H.F., & Michael, W.B. (1975). Domain validity and generalizability. *Educational and Psychological Measurement, 35,* 31–35.
Kallenberg, A.L., & Kluegel, J.R. (1975). Analysis of the multitrait multimethod matrix: Some limitations and an alternative. *Journal of Applied Psychology, 60,* 1–9.
Kerlinger, F.N. (1973). *Foundations of behavioral research.* New York: Holt, Rinehart, & Winston.
Kuder, G.F., & Richardson, M.W. (1937). The theory of estimation of test reliability. *Psychometrika, 2,* 151–160.
Rasch, G. (1966). An individualistic approach to item analysis. In P.F. Lazarsfeld & N.W. Henry (Eds.), *Readings in mathematical social sciences.* Cambridge, MA: MIT Press.
Weiss, D.J., & Davison, M.L. (1981). Test theory and methods. *Annual Review of Psychology, 32,* 629–658.
Wiggins, J.S. (1973). *Personality and prediction: Principles of personality assessment.* Reading, MA: Addison-Wesley.
Wright, B.D., & Stone, M.H. (1979). *Best test design: Rasch measurement.* Chicago: Mesa Press.

10

Epidemiology

Evelyn J. Bromet

INTRODUCTION

Epidemiology is the study of the distribution of illness in the population and the characteristics that influence that distribution (Lilienfeld, 1976). Epidemiology originally concentrated on acute infectious diseases. As these diseases came under public health control, epidemiologists began to focus on chronic diseases, including mental illness. Thus, psychiatric epidemiology refers to the study of psychiatric conditions and symptoms in the population and the factors associated with their distribution. Psychiatric epidemiologists are concerned with the extent and type of psychological disorder in a defined population and the risk factors which influence their origin and course. Epidemiologic research is conducted on three levels: descriptive, analytic, and experimental.

DEFINITIONS OF THE FIELD

Descriptive Epidemiology

Descriptive epidemiology aims at ascertaining the occurrence of disease by time, place, and person. The basic measurement tool of descriptive epidemiology is the rate; that is, the proportion of cases during a specific time period in a defined population. The rate may be a prevalence rate (i.e, the ratio of all existing cases at a given point in time to the defined population) or an incidence rate (i.e., the ratio of all new cases occurring during a period of time to the population at risk). Prevalence rates are typically used for planning of treatment facilities and services; that is, estimating manpower needs, number of hospital beds, number of clinic visits, and so on. Incidence rates are important for examining etiologic hypotheses about risk of illness.

To accurately calculate the incidence or prevalence rate of a disorder, three factors must be defined: the population at risk (i.e., the denominator), the illness, and, particularly in the case of incidence, the time of onset. The major sources of error in epidemiologic research derive from biases in the population studied and inadequacies in the measurement tools used for case identification. The latter has been an especially significant issue in psychiatric epidemiology, and will be explored in the next section on the field's evolution.

The Midtown Manhattan Study is a classic example of descriptive psychiatric epidemiology (Srole, Langner, Michael, Opler, & Rennie, 1962). Its aim was to determine the rate of psychological impairment in adults in a targeted area of New York City. A random sample of white midtown Manhattan residents aged 20–60 were administered a structured interview schedule containing an extensive symptom inventory. The interview data were systematically examined by two psychiatrists, and each subject was rated on a 6-point impairment scale. The point prevalence rate (i.e., the proportion of people designated as impaired at the time of interview) was 23.4%. The rate of impairment was higher in older respondents, unmarried individuals, immigrants and first-generation Americans, and people with lower socioeconomic status. These "person" characteristics have been confirmed as risk factors in other community studies using similar morbidity measures (Dohrenwend & Dohrenwend, 1969; Schwab & Schwab, 1978).

Investigators of the Midtown Manhattan Study used their 6-point impairment scale rather than clinical diagnosis in large part because of recognized unreliability in diagnosis at the time the study was conducted. Recent U.S. studies have taken advantage of advances in reliability of diagnosis and the development of structured diagnostic interview schedules, such as the Schedule for Affective Disorders and Schizophrenia (SADS) (Endicott & Spitzer, 1978) and the Diagnostic Interview Schedule (DIS) (Robins, Helzer, Croughan, & Ratcliff, 1981). Thus, in contrast to earlier work on global impairment, current descriptive research is aimed at establishing the life-time and current (point) prevalence rates and 1-year incidence rates of diagnosable episodes of mental disorder (Eaton, Regier, Locke, & Taube, 1981). Recent data from a community survey using the life-time version of the SADS indicated the life-time prevalence rate of major depression to be 18%–12% in men; 26% in women; and the point prevalence rate to be 4%–3% in men; 5% in women (Boyd & Weissman, 1981).

In addition to estimating rates by person characteristics, descriptive epidemiology is used to compare rates in different geographic areas and to study secular trends. For example, rates of hospitalization for schizophrenia have been found to be higher in inner-city areas and to decrease progressively toward the city's periphery where socioeconomic conditions were better (i.e., Faris & Dunham, 1939). These studies were interpreted as indicating that the stressful environmental conditions found in poor inner-city areas were causal agents which precipitated schizophrenic episodes. Subsequent studies have shown that downward drift of premorbidly vulnerable individuals may account for some of the variance in the geographic pattern (Lapouse, Monk, & Terris, 1956; Turner & Wagenfeld, 1967). One of the most elegant investigations of downward drift was conducted by Goldberg and Morrison (1963), who showed that schizophrenic patients failed to achieve the socioeconomic level of their fathers at the same stage of life.

The documentation of secular trends is a major use of descriptive epidemiology. Some mental disorders have been shown to be decreasing, such as conversion hysteria, general paresis, and pellagra psychosis. Other disorders are causes of concern because of their apparent increase in recent years, such as suicide rates in adolescents, tardive dyskinesia (an iatrogenic effect of long-term phenothiazine use), and senile dementia (Gruenberg, 1980). With regard to the latter, it is the *prevalence* rate which has increased. Prevalence is the product of incidence times duration. In this particular example, the *incidence rate* has remained constant, but the duration has increased with better medical care.

The findings from descriptive epidemiology are the foundation for developing hypotheses to be tested using analytic methodologies. The associations observed in descriptive studies may or may not prove to be of causal significance (Cooper & Morgan, 1973). To establish causality, which is the ultimate goal of epidemiology, analytic research strategies must be implemented.

Analytic Epidemiology

Analytic epidemiology attempts to determine *why* a rate is high or low in a particular group (Mausner & Bahn, 1974). Three approaches are used in analytic epidemiology: retrospective, prospective, and a combined prospective-retrospective design.

The most common type of retrospective study is the case-control design in which individuals with the disorder under investigation are compared with one or more control groups with respect to antecedent risk factors. For example, Paykel, Prusoff, and Myers (1975) were interested in assessing the role of life events in relation to suicide attempts. They collected retrospective information on life events experienced in the past 6 months from 53 suicide attempters, 53 depressed patients, and 53 normal community controls. The latter two groups were demographically matched to the suicide attempters. The suicide attempters reported four times as many life events as the normal controls during the 6-month period and 1.5 times as many life events as the depressed controls, with a peak number of events occurring during the month prior to the attempt.

A prospective study starts with a group of people (a cohort), all of whom are free of the disease, and follows them over time. At the beginning of the study, the cohort is classified according to the presence of the risk factor or exposure being assessed. The analysis attempts to link the risk factor to the *development* of disease. The most elegant prospective study in psychiatric epidemiology was conducted in Lundby, a small town in Sweden. In 1947, four psychiatrists interviewed 99% of the 25,550 inhabitants of Lundby, including adults and children (Essen-Möller, 1956). The life-time prevalence rate of psychiatric disorder was about 9%. Ten years later Hagnell (1966), also a psychiatrist, reexamined the original residents of Lundby, regardless of their current address, and interviewed the new residents as well. By this method, Hagnell was able to calculate the 10-year incidence rate and the risk of disorder based on the subject's marital and occupational status in 1947, and whether they had moved out of Lundby. The 10-year incidence rate for "impairment" was 11% for men and 20% for women. By contrast, the 10-year incidence rate for psychosis was .6% for men and women. The 10-year incidence rate was higher in married women than unmarried women, for both sexes in the highest occupational status positions, and for people aged 20–40. In addition, people who moved from Lundby into urban areas had a higher risk of developing a psychiatric disorder than those who either remained or moved into similar rural communities.

The third strategy is the mixed prospective-retrospective design, sometimes referred to as anterospective, in which a population is identified after exposure to a risk factor, along with a control group, and the rate of disease occurring since exposure is determined retrospectively. A highly significant anterospective study was that conducted by Robins (1966), in which 30-year-old child guidance records were used to identify a high risk group who were then intensively followed up and compared with matched controls. Valuable data on the natural history of childhood disorder and the relationship between childhood disorder and antisocial behavior were obtained.

Another more recent example of a mixed-design analytic study was conducted by Bromet, Parkinson, Schulberg, Dunn, and Gondek (1982) on the mental health effects of the accident at the Three Mile Island (TMI) nuclear plant in central Pennsylvania. Three cohorts were identified: mothers with small children who lived within 10 miles of the plant at the time of the accident, psychiatric outpatients who lived within 10 miles and were in treatment at the time of the accident, and union workers employed at the plant when the accident occurred. Their mental health before and after the accident was assessed by retrospective interview 1-year later and compared with control groups living near or working at a nuclear plant in western Pennsylvania. The risk of affective disorder in the TMI mother cohort during the year following the accident was 15% compared to 8% in the controls. No mental health differences were observed when the workers and psychiatric patients were compared with their controls.

A final example of a mixed design study entails follow-up of a cohort which had undergone a battery of psychological tests. Specifically, a questionnaire dealing with personality and psychological symptomatology was administered to students at the University of Pennsylvania from 1931–1940 (Paffenbarger & Asnes, 1966). The responses of 50 students who subsequently committed suicide were compared with those of 100 randomly selected controls. The suicide victims were found to differ on several premorbid variables, including sleeplessness, worrying, feeling self-conscious, seclusiveness, and an anxiety-depression index.

Experimental Epidemiology

Experimental epidemiology typically involves manipulating persons by randomly assigning them either to treatment or placebo groups in the case of a clinical trial or to exposure or non-exposure to an environmental agent. Apart from drug trials, the most common experimental design used in psychiatric epidemiology is the "natural experiment," in which groups exposed to a specific environmental agent are compared with people similar in every respect except for the exposure. The natural experiment differs from a true experiment in that subjects are not randomly assigned to exposure. Unlike the design described earlier for the Three Mile Island study, measurements are taken at the time of exposure and subjects are followed forward through time. Kasl's classic study of men terminated from their jobs by a plant closing is an example of a natural experiment in which the affected men and their controls were assessed monthly from the time the plant closed down until they were reemployed (Kasl, 1979a). Another example is Spitz's (1968) study of children evacuated from London during the bombing raids of World War II. Those placed in non-nuturant environments had higher morbidity and mortality rates than children placed in settings where attendants were more nurturant.

In summary, the ultimate goal of epidemiology is to identify causes of disease so as to provide information useful in disease prevention. Because we rarely are in a position to test hypotheses with a true experimental design, five criteria are used to judge whether a causal relationship between a risk factor and a disease exists: the strength of the association, consistency across studies, temporal sequence, specificity of the risk factor in relation to the disease, and congruence of the finding with existing knowledge. In the next section we consider the substantive and methodological development of psychiatric epidemiology in the United States and the key issues under consideration in the 1980s.

DEVELOPMENT OF PSYCHIATRIC EPIDEMIOLOGY

The development of psychiatric epidemiology has revolved primarily around attempts to identify agents in the social environment which might be conceptualized as promoting or preventing the occurrence of psychiatric disorder. The history of such research is typically divided into pre- and post-World War II accomplishments. In this section we will trace the development of research on mental health effects of stress in the social environment and show how methodological advancements in psychiatric epidemiology have influenced approaches to this issue.

In 1939, Faris and Dunham published their pioneering volume, *Mental Disorders in Urban Areas.* This study represented the first application of the ecological approach to documenting the geographic distribution of mentally ill patients. Between 1922–1931, 7,253 patients from Chicago were admitted to state hospitals for the first time and given a diagnosis of schizophrenia. Using these data, they then calculated the rate per 100,000 adult population for different sections of Chicago and found the highest rate in the center of the city with low rates in the city's periphery. In interpreting their findings, they argued that the social environment of the high rate subcommunities fostered isolation and seclusiveness, factors thought to influence the development of schizophrenia. Their argument was further strengthened by two additional findings. First, the geographic pattern was the same for young and old patients, indicating that it was unlikely that the distribution occurred because older people drifted into these areas and inflated the rates (i.e., a person rather than environmental explanation). Second, another source of data which supported the environmental hypothesis was the finding of higher rates among blacks living in predominantly white areas compared to blacks living in predominantly black areas. Similarly, the rates for whites were higher in areas in which they were in the minority.

There have been many replications and confirmations of the Faris and Dunham findings (e.g., Bloom, 1963; Klee, Spiro, Bahn, & Gorwitz, 1967; Schroeder, 1942), including a restudy of admissions from Chicago (Levy & Rowitz, 1973). These studies extended the findings by examining outpatients as well as inpatients, and public as well as private facilities. Although ecological studies continue to be useful for mental health planners, their research utility is limited to generating hypotheses rather than testing hypotheses. Without direct information from patients, it is difficult to draw inferences about which environmental variables, among an array of interrelated variables such as crowding, poverty, and mobility, are causally related to the observed high rate. Another significant problem is the ecology fallacy, in which inferences about individuals are made from correlations based on aggregated data (i.e., a correlation between census tract characteristics and rate of hospitalization for schizophrenia). Often the relationships observed in ecological studies (i.e., low social class areas have high rates of treated schizophrenia) are also found in studies using individual data. However, this need not always be the case (Kasl, 1979b, 1980; Robinson, 1950).

In the Faris and Dunham study, medical records were used to identify cases of mental illness. The other method of data collection often employed before World War II was an interview with key informants in which community leaders and knowledgeable residents identified mentally ill members of the community. However, both methods underestimate the true prevalence of mental disorder in the community.

The extent to which these methods underestimated the true prevalence became apparent during World War II for two reasons. First, the Army developed a psychological symptom screen, and thousands of presumably healthy recruits were rejected from the armed forces for psychiatric reasons. Second, combat stress reactions occurred in young men who had no identifiable predisposing vulnerability characteristics. Thus the role of stress as a precipitating variable became "a major unifying concept in the post-World War II studies in civilian settings" (Weissman & Klerman, 1978, p. 706). Both person variables, such as social class, and environmental variables, such as urban-rural setting, were to be conceptualized as stress-provoking agents.

The other activity that occurred in World War II which had an impact on subsequent research was the development of the Neuropsychiatric Screening Adjunct questionnaire, a symptom inventory which served as the basis for similar questionnaires used in the 1950s.

In the 1950s, several large-scale community surveys were conducted, such as the Midtown Manhattan Study described earlier, a national mental health survey conducted by the University of Michigan (Gurin, Veroff, & Feld, 1960), and a survey of a rural county in Canada by the Leightons (1963). All of these studies used representative samples and rated respondents on impairment scales based on a count of their symptomatology (primarily psychophysiologic and affective) rather than attempting to make diagnostic judgments. All of these studies reported that at least one-fifth of community residents suffered significant psychological impairment based on evaluations of the symptom inventories. In addition, they consistently found that higher rates of impairment were associated with being female, unmarried, or of lower social class.

Researchers in the 1960s conducted community surveys using short symptom scales. The scales were developed psychometrically from the extensive item pools used in the earlier studies. Thus, briefer instruments, such as Langner's (1962) 22-item screening questionnaire allowed more time in the interview to obtain other psychosocial data and eliminated the need to have psychiatrists review the protocols. In the 1960s considerable attention was given to the role of stressful life events in precipitating psychological morbidity. Specifically, these studies attempted to demonstrate a temporal association between the onset of symptoms and a recent increase in life events that required an adaptive response. Many investigators studying stressful life events adopted in original or modified form a 43-item checklist developed by Holmes and Rahe (1967). These items were intended to represent fairly common situations arising from family, personal, occupational, or financial events. One of the best-known studies of life events and psychological well-being was conducted by Myers, Lindenthal and Pepper at Yale (1972). A representative sample of more than 900 respondents was interviewed in 1967 and more than 700 were reinterviewed in 1969. The purpose of the study was to look cross-sectionally and longitudinally at the effects of stressful life events on mental health, and the anticipated significant relationships were found.

In recent years, both the life event and symptom measures used by many researchers in the 1960s and early 1970s have been sharply criticized. The life events inventories were seen as incomplete and unreliable, since they depended on the subject's memory. In addition, by including health-rated items among the life events, they overlapped in content with the outcome measure, thus artificially inflating the correlation. Although life events researchers consider life events as *environmental* risk factors, Kasl (in press) has argued convincingly that "life events are intimately bound up with a person's life style and reflect, furthermore, the person's stage in the life cycle." Even more important, the strength of the relationship between life events and symptoms has been surprisingly weak.

The use of short symptom inventories was based in part on findings that the scales discriminated between psychiatric patients and non-patients. The pitfalls of instruments developed in this way were cogently described by Seiler (1973). One serious problem he described was the flawed logic inherent in the psychometric method. Because psychiatric patients scored in a certain range, it did not necessarily follow that non-patients with similar scores were psychiatrically disturbed. Seiler also pointed out other problems, such as the failure of items to tap symptoms relevant for men, such as alcohol and aggression and the lack of concern with social role functioning. Recently, Dohrenwend has postulated that these types of symptom inventories measure demoralization rather than clinical psychiatric disorder, and only 50% of subjects rated as demoralized on these inventories might be clinically impaired (Dohrenwend, Dohrenwend, Gould, Link, Neugebauer, & Wunsch-Hitzig, 1980).

Two bodies of research emanated from concerns about the methodology and results of the stress-related research of the '60s and early '70s. One line of research was on social support as a stress-buffering factor. The second line of research was on the development and implementation of more clinically sensitive mental health questionnaires to be used in community surveys.

The epidemiological significance of social support stems from the belief that it may directly influence the occurrence of psychiatric disorder or buffer the impact of stressful life events. Early thinking about social support stemmed in part from the generally modest association between life events and symptoms. It was thought that social support might be mediating the effect. That is, among people with positive social support, stress might have little effect. However, among people with poor support, stress effects might be magnified. There were several sources of data that served as springboards for this line of research. One was the finding by Myers and his colleagues that people who developed symptoms in the absence of life event stressors were less well socially integrated than those with many events and few symptoms

(Myers, Lindenthal, & Pepper, 1975). The second was an often-cited (but probably rarely read) study by Nuckolls, Cassel and Kaplan (1972) showing that life events affected the outcome of pregnancy in women with poor psychosocial resources but not in women with positive resources. The third was a community survey of 200+ women in London which found that among working class women, stressful events had their most adverse impact on women with predisposing vulnerability, including lack of a confiding relationship with a member of the opposite sex (Brown, Bhrolchain, & Harris, 1975).

Since the mid-1970s, many studies have been designed to examine the interrelationships among life stress, social support, and mental health. Many studies have found a direct effect of social support on illness (e.g., Aneshensel & Stone, 1982; Lin, Simeone, Ensel & Kuo, 1979; Williams, Ware & Donald, 1981). In our own work in Three Mile Island, for example, social support was assessed by asking respondents about instrumental and emotional support provided by and given to the subject's social network of friends and relatives (Bromet et al., 1982). The perceived quality of the relationships was significantly correlated with symptomatology. However, the mediating effect of social support has received mixed findings, with some longitudinal studies finding evidence in support and others failing to confirm the buffering model. In the Three Mile Island data, social network support did not serve to mediate the relationship between stress and symptoms, regardless of how stress was operationalized (proximity to TMI, intensity of stressful life events, perception of TMI as dangerous), who was studied (mothers, workers, psychiatric outpatients), or whether instrumental or emotional aspects of social support were evaluated. In spite of the mixed results on social support as a stress buffer, it continues to be an important area of research.

The other direction is the development and implementation of clinically sophisticated interview schedules which can provide better estimates of the rates and correlates of psychiatric morbidity in the community. In 1969, Robins commented that:

> Failure to discriminate clinically meaningful symptoms from such universal complaints as headaches, worries, and fears has produced inflated rates in epidemiological surveys of psychiatric disorders in non-patient populations. (p. 100)

Indeed, one of the charges of the National Institute of Mental Health (NIMH) is to provide accurate data on the mental health status of the nation (Eaton et al., 1981). In 1977, the President's Commission on Mental Health highlighted the dearth of epidemiologic data on the incidence and prevalence of mental illness and recommended that reliable data be gathered. Thus, in the late 1970s, the NIMH funded a collaborative endeavor, the Epidemiologic Catchment Area (ECA) project, in which global measures of impairment were replaced by specific diagnoses.

It is important to identify the other antecedents of this change in approach to defining psychological morbidity in the community in the United States. One of the primary forces was the cross-national study of the diagnosis of depression and schizophrenia, often referred to as the U.S.-U.K. (United Kingdom) project (Kramer & Zubin, 1969). This study was undertaken to determine why the rate of affective disorders in hospitalized patients was higher in England than in the U.S., while the reverse was true for schizophrenia. Were the base rates actually different in the two countries, or were the differences due to diagnostic practices? For the first time, psychiatrists in the two countries were trained to use a structured diagnostic interview, the Present State Examination, which could be computer scored. The results of the study indicated that the differences were a function of diagnostic practices rather than true differences. When the same interview and diagnostic criteria were applied in the two countries, the differences disappeared.

Another antecedent of the ECA were studies which demonstrated the feasibility of collecting clinical data from untreated community residents. The Dohrenwends and their colleagues were among the first U.S. investigators to use a standardized clinical interview in the community (Dohrenwend, Egri, & Mendelsohn, 1971). In the mid-1970s, the lifetime version of the SADS was used in a feasibility study in New Haven (Weissman & Myers, 1978). Two non-psychiatrists with clinical experience were trained to administer the interview schedule, and in 1975, the cohort from Myers' 1967–69 life events study noted above was reinterviewed. The results showed that it was reasonable to train lay interviewers to conduct clinical interviews and that community residents were willing to participate in a diagnostic interview. However, the problem remained that semi-structured clinical interview schedules could only be administered by people with considerable clinical experience, which from a financial and pragmatic point of view made them less than desirable for field studies.

Thus, the first step of the ECA program was the development of a fully structured clinical interview schedule which could be administered by lay interviewers and yield reliable DSM-III diagnoses. The instrument designed for these purposes was the Diagnostic Interview Schedule (Robins et al., 1981). In order to show that the instrument was reliable in the hands of a lay interviewer, a study was designed in which patients were interviewed twice, once by a trained lay interviewer and once by a clinical psychiatrist. The psychiatrist had the option of asking additional questions after completing the entire structured interview if he/she needed more information in order to reach a diagnosis. Thus, three diagnoses were obtained: one based on the lay interviewer's protocol, a second based on the structured DIS given by the psychiatrist, and a third based on the DIS and additional information obtained by the psychiatrist. High inter-rater agreement was obtained for most of the diagnoses. This study is being replicated with non-patients as respondents.

One goal of the ECA program is to establish the incidence and prevalence of diagnosable mental disorder in the community and to identify etiological risk factors or correlates. Interviews are being conducted with 3,000 community residents and 500 institutionalized residents in each of five catchment areas: New Haven, Connecticut; Baltimore, Maryland; St. Louis, Missouri, Los Angeles, California; and Durham, North Carolina. In order to approximate a representative U.S. sample, the study sites included urban and rural areas, sites with high and low proportions of blacks and Mexican-Americans, poor and middle class areas, and sites with high and low concentrations of psychiatric treatment facilities (since supply has an effect on rates of illness under treatment).

In order to assess *incidence,* the entire sample of approximately 17,500 people is being reinterviewed 1 year after the initial interview. To date, preliminary reports indicate that the three disorders with the highest life-time prevalence rates are alcohol abuse and dependence, drug abuse and dependence, and major depression.

Thus, psychiatric epidemiology encompasses a broad range of research strategies on a wide variety of issues. As the field has evolved, measurement tools to test hypotheses have become more refined. Although the field appears to have moved through three stages—defining a case on the basis of treatment seeking, global symptom scales, and diagnostic categorization—all three approaches continue to be widely used. For example, current research on the epidemiology of affective disorders is assessing the impact of different coping styles among individuals exposed to stress. Studies are being conducted with treated samples (e.g., Felton, Brown, Lehmann, & Liberatos, 1980), community residents with depressive symptomatology (e.g., Pearlin, Liberman, Menaghan, & Mullan, 1981), and untreated community residents who meet diagnostic criteria for depression (e.g., Wheaton, 1983).

In the past 40 years, considerable progress has occurred in the development of design and assessment methodologies. Many correlates of mental illness have been identified. In pursuing further research, epidemiologists will be attempting to develop causal models, linking socio-environmental factors to mental illness, which will hopefully have implications for disease prevention.

RESEARCH EXAMPLE

One of the most influential contributors to the field of psychiatric epidemiology is George Brown, a British sociologist. Among his many accomplishments was a classic study of depression in women (Brown, Bhrolchain, & Harris, 1975; Brown & Harris, 1978). Because this study has stimulated a great deal of discussion and research, it is presented below, followed by a methodological critique.

The purpose of the study was to determine whether stressful life events were causally linked to the onset of clinical depression in working class and middle class women and whether certain social factors made women who experienced life events more vulnerable to depression. Stressful life events were conceptualized as "provoking agents." A detailed schedule of life events was administered which took into account the circumstances under which the event occurred, its meaning to the respondent, and the degree of threat inherent in the event. In addition to severe life events, long-term difficulties were ascertained, including problems with housing, money, children, and marriage, that had gone on for a month or more. The women were then classified into a group experiencing a severe event or a major difficulty, and those reporting neither one.

Four vulnerability, or intervening variables, were examined: lack of intimacy with husband, having 3 + children at home under 14 years of age, not being gainfully employed, and loss of own mother in childhood before age 11. Depression was determined from the Present State Examination, a semi-structured diagnostic interview. Of the 220 women selected randomly from a borough of London, 35, or 16%, were judged to have suffered from a psychiatric disorder within 3 months prior to interview. Of the 35, 21 had an onset during the year prior to interview, and 14 had been disturbed for over a year.

The results with respect to social class were striking. In the middle class group ($N=99$), 5% were rated as psychiatrically disturbed. Among the working class mothers ($N=121$), 25% were evaluated as disturbed. Among women with a child under 6 years of age, the discrepancy was even more marked, with 5% of the 22 middle class mothers who had a child under 6, and 42% of the 27 working class mothers with young children, being clinically depressed.

The authors then went on to test the effect of the four previously identified vulnerability factors. The results showed that among women who experienced a severe event or difficulty, presence of each of the vulnerability factors increased the risk of disorder. That is, 38% of women with low spouse intimacy, 67% of women with 3 + children under 14, 44% of mothers not employed, and 80% of women who lost their mothers in childhood were disturbed compared to 4%, 17%, 14% and 23%, respectively. Among women not experiencing a severe event or difficulty, no differences were found between those with and without the vulnerability characteristics.

Critique

The Brown study is an appealing piece of research for a variety of reasons. First, it presented an intriguing conceptual model consisting of provoking agents, protective factors, and their interrelationship in the illness process. Second, it used a sophisticated approach to defining clinical disturbance in the community, rather than relying on a scale assessing global impairment.

Third, the authors attempted to carefully date the onset of illness as well as the timing of the stressful event so as to offer a cause-effect analysis of the issue. However, this study also illustrates some of the limitations inherent in retrospective research.

No matter how carefully an investigator works at understanding the temporal sequence, data collected retrospectively are only as reliable as the respondent's memory. Bias in recall is well known. Although it might be possible with adequate prompting to date the occurrence of a life event, such a study would miss life events and difficulties which the respondent failed to remember. Failure to remember events may be significant in and of itself. Even more difficult is the timing of the onset of symptoms. Most psychiatric disorders have gradual onsets, which is one of the major difficulties in conducting chronic disease epidemiology. How a respondent times the onset may in fact be a direct effect of the stressful life event itself. George Brown himself has written eloquently about recall problems (1974), and a prospective study is currently underway in England to test conceptualization using this more rigorous design.

Another methodological problem is the confounding of measures. Confounding refers to conceptual overlap among categories of variables. In this case, the dimension of life events and major life difficulties was confounded with the vulnerability factors. For example, major life difficulties in the area of employment (provoking agent) may be directly linked to being unemployed (vulnerability characteristic). Another example would be a major difficulty in the marriage (provoking agent) and lack of intimacy with husband (vulnerability measure). Thus, the distinction between the provoking agents and vulnerability factors may be more artificial than real.

Another problem concerned the sample size. While the percentages reported in the paper were impressive, the actual number of women included in the denominator for those percentages was very small. Thus, any small increment in the numerator would have a major impact on the percentages calculated.

Finally, when a conceptual model emanates from pre-existing data, its efficacy cannot be evaluated using the same data base. In Brown's work, the vulnerability factors were identified empirically. As Brown and Harris (1978) stated:

> It was clear that other factors, also related to social class, must be at work, and we therefore looked for the vulnerability factors of our model. (p. 278)

The only way to explore the efficacy of the model is to test the interrelationships with a new sample.

Thus, the Brown study illustrates several important methodological concerns in epidemiologic research. These concerns are: (a) level of inference from retrospective data, (b) confounding, (c) adequacy of sample size for testing hypotheses, and (d) the need to test empirically based hypotheses on newly collected samples. Most of these concerns are being addressed in the current prospective study of depression in women by Brown and his colleagues.

SUMMARY

In this chapter, the basic principles of epidemiology and an overview of the development of psychiatric epidemiology were presented. At the beginning of the chapter, it was noted that the two major sources of error in epidemiologic research derive from using unrepresentative populations and inaccurate case identification techniques. Considerable progress has been made in both of these areas. Special attention is currently being given to formulating clinically relevant definitions for case identification in untreated populations, and clear operational criteria for classification in treatment populations. This work is being conducted in both child and adult psychiatry. Sophisticated statistical approaches have also allowed investigators to assess main effects of socio-environmental variables as well as interaction effects. As we learn more about the epidemiology of psychiatric disorders, the potential areas for preventive public health trials will expand. To date there have been successful interventions around toxic environmental agents, such as lead poisoning in children. Prospective studies of social stress and support should also yield results that will be useful in the design of primary intervention strategies.

REFERENCES

Aneshensel, C., & Stone, J. (1982). Stress and depression: A test of the buffering model of social support. *Archives of General Psychiatry, 39*, 1392–1396.

Bloom, B. (1963). An ecological analysis of psychiatric hospitalizations. *Multivariate Behavioral Research, 3*, 423–463.

Boyd, J., & Weissman, M. (1981) Epidemiology of affective disorders: A reexamination and future directions. *Archives of General Psychiatry 38*, 1039–1046.

Bromet, E., Parkinson, D., Schulberg, H., Dunn, L., & Gondek, P. (1982). Mental health of residents near the Three Mile Island reactor. *Journal of Preventive Psychiatry, 1*, 225–276.

Brown, G. (1974). Meaning, measurement, and stress of life events. In B.S. Dohrenwend & B.P. Dohrenwend (Eds.), *Stressful life events: Their nature and effects.* New York: John Wiley & Sons.

Brown, G., Bhrolchain, M., & Harris, T. (1975). Social class and psychiatric disturbance in urban population. *Sociology, 9*, 225–254.

Brown, G., & Harris, T. (1978). *The social origins of depression: A study of psychiatric disorder in women.* London: Tavistock.

Cooper, B., & Morgan, H.G. (1973). *Epidemiological psychiatry.* Springfield, IL: Charles Thomas.

Dohrenwend, B.P., & Dohrenwend, B.S. (1969). *Social status and psychological disorder.* New York: John Wiley & Sons.

Dohrenwend, B.P., Dohrenwend, B.S., Gould, M.S., Link, B., Neugebauer, R., & Wunsch-Hitzig, R. (1980). *Mental illness in the United States.* New York: Praeger.

Dohrenwend, B.P., Egri, G., & Mendelsohn, F.S. (1971). Psychiatric disorder in general populations. *American Journal of Psychiatry, 127*, 1304–1312.

Eaton, W., Regier, D., Locke, B., & Taube, C. (1981). The Epidemiologic Catchment Area program of the National Institute of Mental Health. *Public Health Reports, 96*, 319–325.

Endicott, J., & Spitzer, R. (1978). A diagnostic interview: The Schedule for Affective Disorders and Schizophrenia. *Archives of General Psychiatry, 35*, 837–844.

Essen-Möller, E. (1956). Individual traits and morbidity in a Swedish rural population. *Acta Psychiatrica Scandinavica* (Suppl. 100). Copenhagen: Ejnar Munksgaard.

Faris, R. & Dunham, H. (1939). *Mental disorders in urban areas: An ecological study of schizophrenia and other psychoses.* Chicago: University of Chicago Press.

Felton, B., Brown, P., Lehmann, S., & Liberatos, P. (1980). The coping function of sex-role attitudes during marital disruption. *Journal of Health and Social Behavior, 21*, 240–248.

Goldberg, E.M., & Morrison, S.Z. (1963). Schizophrenia and social class. *British Journal of Psychiatry, 109,* 785–802.

Gruenberg, E. (1980). Epidemiology. In H. Kaplan, A. Freedman, & B. Sadock (Eds.), *Comprehensive textbook of psychiatry* (3rd ed.). Baltimore: Williams & Wilkins.

Gurin, G., Veroff, J., & Feld, S. (1960). *Americans view their mental health: A nationwide interview survey.* New York: Basic Books, Inc.

Hagnell, O. (1966). *A prospective study of the incidence of mental disorder.* Lund, Sweden: Scandinavian University Books.

Holmes, T.H., & Rahe, R.H. (1967). The social readjustment rating scale. *Journal of Psychosomatic Research, 11,* 213–218.

Kasl, S. (1979a). Changes in mental health status associated with job loss and retirement. In J. Barrett, R. Rose, & G. Klerman (Eds.), *Stress and mental disorder.* New York: Raven Press.

Kasl, S. (1979b). Mortality and the business cycle: Some questions about research strategies when utilizing macro-social and ecological data. *American Journal of Public Health, 69*, 784–788.

Kasl, S. (1980). Problems in the analysis and interpretation of ecological data. *American Journal of Public Health, 70*, 413–414.

Kasl, S. (in press). Pursuing the link between stressful life experiences and disease: A time for reappraisal. In C. Cooper (Ed.), *Stress research: Where do we go from here?* Chichester, U.K.: John Wiley & Sons.

Klee, G., Spiro, E., Bahn, A., & Gorwitz, K. (1967). An ecological analysis of diagnosed mental illness in Baltimore. In R. Monroe, G. Klee, & E. Brody (Eds.), *Psychiatric epidemiology and mental health planning.* Washington, DC: American Psychiatric Association.

Kramer, M., & Zubin, J. (1969). Cross-national study of diagnosis of the mental disorders. *American Journal of Psychiatry, 125* (Suppl.), 1–46.

Langner, T.S. (1962). A twenty-two item screening score of psychiatric symptoms indicating impairment. *Journal of Health and Social Behavior, 3*, 269–276.

Lapouse, R., Monk, M., & Terris, M. (1956). The "drift" hypothesis in socioeconomic differentials in schizophrenia. *American Journal of Public Health, 46*, 978-986.

Leighton, D.C., Harding, J.S., Macklin, D.B., Macmillan, A., & Leighton, A. (1963). *The character of danger.* New York: Basic Books, Inc.

Levy, L., & Rowitz, L. (1973). *The ecology of mental disorders.* New York: Behavioral Publications.

Lilienfeld, A. (1976). *Foundations of epidemiology.* New York: Oxford University Press.

Lin, N., Simeone, R., Ensel, W. & Kuo, W. (1979). Social support, stressful life events, and illness: A model and an empirical test. *Journal of Health and Social Behavior, 20*, 108-119.

Mausner, J. & Bahn, A. (1974). *Epidemiology.* Philadelphia: W.B. Saunders Company.

Myers, J.K., Lindenthal, J.J., & Pepper, M.D. (1972). Life events and mental status: A longitudinal study. *Journal of Health and Social Behavior, 13*, 398-406.

Myers, J., Lindenthal, J., & Pepper, M. (1975). Life events, social integration and psychiatric symptomatology. *Journal of Health and Social Behavior, 16*, 421-427.

Nuckolls, K., Cassel, J., & Kaplan, B. (1972). Psychosocial assets, life crisis and the prognosis of pregnancy. *American Journal of Epidemiology, 95*, 431-441.

Paffenbarger, R.S., & Asnes, D.P. (1966). Chronic disease in former college students. III. Precursors of suicide in early and middle life. *American Journal of Public Health, 56,* 1026-1036.

Paykel, E., Prusoff, B., & Myers, J. (1975). Suicide attempts and recent life events. *Archives of General Psychiatry, 32*, 327-333.

Pearlin, L., Lieberman, M., Menaghan, E., & Mullan, J. (1981). The stress process. *Journal of Health and Social Behavior, 22,* 337-356.

Robins, L. (1966). *Deviant children grown up.* Baltimore: The Williams & Wilkins Company.

Robins, L. (1969). Social correlates of psychiatric disorders: Can we tell causes from consequences? *Journal of Health and Social Behavior, 10*, 95-104.

Robins, L., Helzer, J., Croughan, J., & Ratcliff, K. (1981). National Institute of Mental Health Diagnostic Interview Schedule: Its history, characteristics and validity. *Archives of General Psychiatry, 38*, 381-389.

Robinson, W.S. (1950). Ecological correlations and the behavior of individuals. *American Sociological Review, 15*, 351-357.

Schroeder, C. (1942). Mental disorders in cities. *American Journal of Sociology, 48,* 40-47.

Schwab, J., & Schwab, M. (1978). *Sociocultural roots of mental illness: An epidemiologic survey.* New York: Plenum Medical Book Company.

Seiler, L. (1973). The 22-item scale used in field studies of mental illness: A question of method, a question of substance, a question of theory. *Journal of Health and Social Behavior, 14*, 252-264.

Spitz, R.A. (1968). Anaclitic depression: An inquiry into the genesis of psychiatric conditions in early childhood. In W. Gaylin (Ed.), *The meaning of despair.* New York: Science House.

Srole, L., Langner, T., Michael, S., Opler, M., & Rennie, T. (1962). *Mental health in the metropolis: The Midtown Manhattan Study.* New York: McGraw Hill.

Turner, R.J., & Wagenfeld, M.O. (1967). Occupational mobility and schizophrenia: An assessment of the social causation and social selection hypotheses. *American Sociological Review, 32*, 104–113.

Weissman, M., & Klerman, G. (1978). Epidemiology of mental disorders. *Archives of General Psychiatry, 35*, 705–712.

Weissman, M., & Myers, J. (1978). Affective disorders in a U.S. urban community: The use of Research Diagnostic Criteria in an epidemiological survey. *Archives of General Psychiatry, 35,* 1304–1311.

Wheaton, B. (1983). Stress, personal coping resources, and psychiatric symptoms. *Journal of Health and Social Behavior, 24*, 208–229.

Williams, A., Ware, J., & Donald, C. (1981). A model of mental health, life events, and social supports applicable to general populations. *Journal of Health and Social Behavior, 22*, 324–336.

11

Research Methods in Behavioral Medicine

Francis J. Keefe

INTRODUCTION

Behavioral medicine is a relatively new, but important area of research activity for clinical psychologists. The defining characteristics of behavioral medicine were identified by a distinguished group of biomedical and behavioral scientists at the Yale Conference in 1976:

> Behavioral medicine is the field concerned with the development of behavioral science knowledge and techniques relevant to the understanding of physical health and illness and the application of this knowledge and these techniques to prevention, diagnosis, treatment, and rehabilitation. (Schwartz & Weiss, 1978, p. 7)

Three important features of this definition deserve comment. First, the definition stresses the multidisciplinary aspects of behavioral medicine. Active collaboration between biomedical and behavioral scientists is the sine qua non of this field. Second, behavioral medicine is a research-oriented field. The collection of information about how health and illness are related to behavioral and physiological responses is strongly emphasized. Third, this definition underscores the importance of practical applications of behavioral science concepts. Indeed, much of the behavioral medicine literature consists of evaluations of the clinical efficacy of methods such as operant conditioning, biofeedback training, and relaxation training.

This chapter provides an introduction to research methods in behavioral medicine. The chapter consists of brief reviews of a number of important research areas including: epilepsy, Raynaud's disease, chronic pain, Type A behavior, fecal incontinence, hypertension, asthma, and headaches. Each review includes a brief description of the disorder, an overview of the types of behavioral research studies conducted, and a critical commentary on the current status and future research directions. The chapter concludes with a detailed examination of a recently published research paper that deals with the behavioral treatment of headache (Blanchard et al., 1982). A methodological critique of this paper is carried out to illustrate how critical issues in behavioral medicine research are being practically addressed by investigators.

MAJOR RESEARCH AREAS

Epilepsy

Epilepsy is a symptom of central nervous system dysfunction. In epileptics, abnormal electrical discharges of brain cells produce recurrent and sudden seizures. The seizures involve changes in the state of consciousness, motor activity, or sensory phenomena. Convulsions in which the patient suddenly falls and displays violent, involuntary tonic and clonic contractions of the arms and legs may occur frequently.

Clinical manifestations of seizures vary and several types of seizures can be distinguished: grand mal, petit mal, psychomotor, infantile spasms, and epileptic equivalents. Grand mal seizures are the most frequent and occur in approximately 90% of patients. Psychomotor attacks affect 18% of patients; 6% of these patients having only psychomotor seizures and 12% experiencing psychomotor attacks combined with another seizure type.

Epilepsy is a common disorder affecting 1 to 2% of the population (Epilepsy Foundation of America, 1975). Epilepsy is also a costly problem, with annual costs to the government and to the individual estimated at 4.37 billion dollars (Epilepsy Foundation of America, 1975). Medical treatments for epileptic disorders are generally effective. Anticonvulsant agents such as Phenobarbital or Diphenylhydantoin (Dilantin) are often used alone or in combination. Pharmacologic approaches are effective in controlling seizures for 80% of epileptics (Masland, 1976). Surgical approaches to correct a lesion (such as an arteriovenous malformation) are rarely utilized because of possible iatrogenic problems (e.g., impairment of motor and cognitive functions).

While medical approaches are effective for most epileptics, there still remains a large population of individuals who cannot tolerate medications (because of side effects) or who find the medications ineffective. The possibility that behavioral methods might be useful in treating this segment of the population has stimulated research. Two major research topics have received attention: (1) contingency management of seizure and non-seizure behaviors, and (2) electroencephalographic (EEG) biofeedback.

The efficacy of contingency management programs for epileptic patients has been investigated in a number of research studies (see Lubar & Deering, 1981, and Mostofsky & Balaschak, 1977, for reviews of this area). These programs are based on the assumption that socioenvironmental consequences of seizure and non-seizure behaviors (such as increased attention or family concern) may exert some control over epileptic attacks. Treatment involves systematic manipulation of these consequences and careful observation of associated seizure activity.

Balaschak (1976) examined the effects of manipulating positive consequences (overt reward of non-seizure activity) in an 11-year-old epileptic patient. The child's teacher instituted an operant conditioning program in which verbal praise and candy were used as rewards for seizure-free periods in the classroom. Prior to the start of this program, the child had seizures on approximately 60% of school days. During the time the operant program was in effect, seizure frequency dropped to 21.2%. When the program was later stopped, seizure frequency increased to 62.5%. Case studies by Flannery and Cautela (1973) and Zlutnick, Mayville, and Moffat (1975) also indicate that reinforcement of non-seizure activity decreases seizure frequency.

Systematic management of aversive contingencies has also been used to control seizures. Wright (1976) delivered a mild electrical shock to a 14-year-old boy whenever seizures were observed. Within 3 days, seizure frequency decreased 75%. Zlutnick (1972) and Zlutnick et al. (1975) found that punishment (shouting "No" and grabbing and shaking the child vigorously) significantly decreased the rate of minor motor seizures in four school age children. Seizures were totally eliminated after 7 weeks of the punishment program. When the punishment program was withdrawn during part of the day, seizures once again began occurring. Aversive stimuli have also been utilized in an avoidance paradigm. Ounsted, Lee, and Hutt (1966) trained a child to significantly decrease spike and wave paroxysms in her EEG by delivering unpleasant photic stimulation when paroxysms appeared in her EEG record. If the child altered her EEG pattern by decreasing paroxysms within a 5 second time period, photic stimulation could be avoided.

EEG biofeedback training has also been used as a behavioral method for control of seizure activity. Sterman and Wyricka (1967) were among the first to study the sensory motor rhythm (SMR), a particular EEG pattern recorded from the sensory motor cortex. This pattern involves activity in the 12–16 Hz band. Sterman and Wyricka (1967) found that cats trained to increase the level of SMR activity tended to remain very still and alert. Sterman hypothesized that increased SMR activity might have an anticonvulsant effect because: (1) seizures involve motor activity, and (2) motor activity during seizures is related to paroxysmal discharges in the sensory motor cortex. Cats who learned to increase SMR activity, in fact, were quite resistant to seizure-inducing medications (Sterman, Wyricka, & Roth, 1969).

Sterman and his colleagues examined the efficacy of EEG biofeedback training to increase SMR activity in several studies. A 23-year-old woman having a long history of seizures reduced seizure frequency from an average of one to four times per month to zero following SMR, EEG biofeedback training. Sterman, MacDonald, and Stone (1974) carefully studied a sample of four epileptics given similar training and not only found significant decreases in seizures (60–70% reductions) but also found that the patient's clinical EEGs became more normal in appearance over treatment. Finley (1976, 1977) examined the efficacy of SMR training using an A-B-A-B single-blind design. In both studies, epileptic patients were given EEG biofeedback of SMR during the A phases. During the B phases, sham biofeedback that was unrelated to EEG activity was given. The patients were blind as to the type of feedback (SMR or sham) provided. In every case, the introduction of SMR training led to improvement in seizure frequency. Lubar (1981) conducted a similar study but also used a double-blind procedure to ensure that neither the patients nor the technicians knew when SMR feedback was introduced. Improvements in seizure frequency and clinical EEGs were observed only during SMR feedback training phases.

Comment. Behavioral scientists find that contingency management methods and EEG biofeedback training can reduce seizure frequency in certain epileptic patients. These methods are clearly promising. There are several important features of this research that deserve comment. First, a strong reliance on single case experimental designs is evident. In all of the studies cited above, each subject served as his own control. This research strategy is particularly appropriate for epilepsy investigations because the frequency, duration, and intensity of seizures varies so greatly from one patient to the next. Second, outcome research has examined the effects of intensive treatment. Typically, treatment sessions are given daily and brief interruptions of treatment are associated with relapse. The EEG biofeedback training approaches involve costly equipment, trained technician time, and many hours of direct patient contact. Such intensive treatment regimens cannot be practically applied to large groups of patients. Thus, their clinical utility may be limited. Third, evidence for specificity of training effects is impressive. In many areas of behavioral medicine research, arguments are made that effects ascribed to a particular technique (e.g., relaxation training) are due to nonspecific factors such as attention from a therapist or high expectations for improvement. Compelling evidence for the specificity of EEG biofeedback training comes from studies using a double-blind design. It should be noted that EEG responses are well suited to double-blind designs because subjects are normally unaware of the overt behavioral referents of EEG patterns. This is not the case when working with other physiological responses, such as muscle activity or skin temperature, which can be monitored more easily by a vigilant subject.

Future research efforts in the area are likely to focus on two topics: identifying patients who are likely to respond to treatment and evaluating the efficacy of combined behavioral and pharmacologic approaches. Lubar and Deering (1981) point out that contingency management methods are most likely to help patients having hysterical seizures or a mixture of hysterical and real seizures. In contrast to most epileptic seizures, hysterical or pseudoseizures are *not* associated with paroxysmal EEG activity. These seizures are more likely to be maintained by an operant mechanism. Minimizing attention given to seizure behaviors or programming-in rewards for non-seizure behavior may be effective in reducing the frequency of pseudoseizures. These methods are less likely to reduce the frequency of other types of seizures. Matching treatment methods to patient characteristics is important because some behavior therapy techniques may increase seizure frequency in epileptics. For example, in some patients relaxation training or hypnosis may increase seizure frequency by increasing slow wave activity (Lubar & Deering, 1981). In other patients (e.g., those whose seizures are associated with hyperactive behavior) relaxation training may be useful. It seems unlikely that any one behavioral treatment approach will benefit the heterogeneous population of epileptics. A detailed description of seizure type, frequency, intensity, and duration as well as clinical EEG findings needs to be provided in research reports to help researchers identify patients who are likely to respond to particular treatment methods.

Behavioral approaches for epilepsy are currently considered only in cases that fail to respond to pharmacologic interventions. Behavioral treatment may also function as an adjunctive approach to enhance the efficacy of drugs. With treatment, patients may be able to decrease anticonvulsant intake and thereby lessen side effects associated with long-term use. Single case experimental methodologies already employed in behavioral epilepsy research are well suited to study the efficacy of behavioral vs. medical vs. combined behavioral-medical treatment regimens. Future research on this topic may greatly expand the range of behavioral treatment applications in epilepsy.

Raynaud's Syndrome

Raynaud's disease is a peripheral vascular disorder characterized by bilateral vasospasms in the digits of the hands and feet. The vasospasms are accompanied by a sequence in which the digits first blanch, then turn blue because of cyanosis, and finally turn red as reactive hyperemia sets in. Exposure to cold or emotional stress can trigger vasospasms. Raynaud's disease was first described by the French physician Maurice Raynaud in 1863. The symptom complex he described is now termed Raynaud's syndrome, and it is known to occur in a number of peripheral vascular diseases. The diagnosis *Raynaud's disease* is currently used to classify patients whose vasospasms are idiopathic. The diagnosis *Raynaud's phenomenon* is used when the vasospasms occur secondary to trauma, neurologic conditions (e.g., carpal tunnel syndrome) or collagen vascular diseases (e.g., scleroderma or lupus erthematosus).

The triphasic color changes occurring in the digits during vasospasms are a reflection of blood flow changes. Significant reductions in peripheral blood flow occur during vasospasms. While the pathophysiology of Raynaud's syndrome is not completely known, two major theories have been advanced. Raynaud hypothesized that the attacks are a result of increased sympathetic nervous system (SNS) activity, and he felt the attacks only occur in individuals who have excessive SNS sensitivity. Lewis (1949) maintained that vasospasms are more likely related to abnormalities in the digits that make them more sensitive to cold.

Medical and surgical treatments for Raynaud's syndrome are not particularly effective. Medications that increase peripheral blood flow, such as Reserpine, Quinethadine, and Methyldopa, are only recommended in severe cases and are usually prescribed for a brief time. Side effects such as severe depression, extrapyramidal signs, gastrointestinal complications, and tachycardia make long term reliance on these agents risky. Surgical sympathectomy is sometimes advocated for severe cases. Unfortunately, most patients relapse after surgery, probably because the sympathetic intervention of the digits is so diffuse.

The possibility that central and corticol processes can control peripheral vascular responses has fascinated behavioral scientists for years (Lisina, 1958; Sokolov, 1963). DiCara and Miller (1968) demonstrated that through a process of operant conditioning, rats could learn to produce vasodilation in one ear or the other. Lisina (1958) found that humans could increase forearm blood flow if allowed to watch a polygraph display of this response. Numerous other studies demonstrated that small, but reliable changes in peripheral skin temperature could be obtained in normal humans through temperature biofeedback training (Keefe, 1975, 1978; Lynch,Hanna,Kohn, & Miller, 1976; Surwit, Shapiro, & Feld, 1976). These animal and human studies were important for two reasons. First, they raised questions about distinctions drawn by learning theorists as to the types of physiological responses that could be modified through instrumental vs. classical conditioning. Second, they indicated that learned control of peripheral blood flow was feasible and their results suggested that this learned control might be applied to clinical problems such as Raynaud's disease.

Early behavioral studies of Raynaud's disease examined the effects of intensive training in single cases. Surwit (1973) trained a 21-year-old woman suffering from Raynaud's disease to control peripheral blood flow through the use of temperature biofeedback, autogenic training, and progressive relaxation. A total of 52 laboratory sessions were carried out. Training was done in the winter months in a cold climate (Montreal, Canada). Over training, basal hand temperature increased from 23.3°C to 26.6°C. The patient also reported a significant decrease in vasospasms. Blanchard and Haynes (1975) had similar findings in a case treated with temperature biofeedback. These early case studies were interesting but had two major faults. First, their experimental designs did not allow one to compare the efficacy of different training or treatment procedures. Second, evaluations of outcome were primarily based upon patient reports rather than on observed physiological changes.

Surwit and I carried out a series of controlled studies at Harvard Medical School designed to investigate the efficacy of behavioral therapy methods for Raynaud's disease. In the first study (Surwit, Pilon, & Fenton 1978), 30 patients diagnosed as having idiopathic Raynaud's disease were trained to increase peripheral blood flow by means of temperature feedback, autogenic training, or a combination of both methods. Outcome was evaluated through self-report (daily recording of vasospasm frequency and intensity) and an objective laboratory procedure (the cold stress test). The cold stress test measured patients' digital temperatures as they sat in a temperature-controlled chamber that was slowly dropped in temperature from 26°C to 17°C. Following behavioral training, all patients reported improvements in vasospasms with an average daily decrease in frequency of 40%. A significant increase in digital temperature was observed in a cold stress test carried out following training. Improvements in cold stress performance could not be attributed to habituation since patients who did not receive training had a decrease in digital temperature when given a second cold stress test. No differences in the efficacy of the three behavioral treatment approaches were found. Keefe, Surwit, and Pilon (1980) used a similar research strategy to evaluate the effects of autogenic training vs. relaxation training vs. autogenic training combined with home temperature biofeedback training. Cold stress tests were repeated at weeks 1, 3, and 5 of training to objectively evaluate changes in digital temperature control occurring over time. Once again, no significant differences among the different behavioral training conditions occurred. All three training approaches resulted in a decrease in reported vasospasm frequency. Average digital temperature during the cold stress test increased gradually and significantly over the course of treatment. It should be noted that both the Surwit et al. (1978) and Keefe et al. (1980) studies were carried out during the winter months in Boston, Massachusetts. Cold temperatures typical of winter in that area of the United States would tend to increase the severity of Raynaud's symptoms. Keefe et al. (1980) examined daily outdoor temperatures and found that clinical improvements occurred with behavioral treatment despite the fact that the average outdoor temperature dropped during training.

Long-term maintenance of behavioral treatment effects has been studied by Keefe, Surwit, and Pilon (1979). Nineteen patients who had participated in earlier research were contacted 1-year later and asked to return for a repeat cold-stress test and to keep a record of vasospasm frequency. Vasospasm frequency at 1-year was found to be identical to that reported at the end of treatment. Ability to maintain temperature control, however, had reverted to pretreatment levels. Freedman, Lynn, and Ianni (in press) recently reported enhanced maintenance of treatment effects in Raynaud's patients trained in temperature biofeedback methods. Patients who were trained to increase blood flow while simultaneously having a cold stimulus applied to their digits had excellent long-term outcomes. These patients had decreases in vasospasms of 90% or more and displayed excellent temperature control up to 1-year posttreatment.

Recent studies have also examined patient characteristics related to good vs. poor outcome to behavioral treatments for Raynaud's disease. Surwit, Bradner, Fenton, and Pilon (1979) reported that improvements in cold stress performance could be predicted by scores on the Alienation scale of Lanyon's (1973) Psychological Screening Inventory. Freedman, Lynn, and Ianni (1982) suggest that temperature changes in response to stressful imagery also may be useful in differentiating those patients having stress-related symptoms.

Another recent research topic in the Raynaud's area is the combined effect of behavioral and medical treatments. Surwit, Allen, Gilgor, Schanberg, and Duvic (1982) compared the effects of Prazosin (a peripheral vasodilator) to autogenic training to a Prazosin-autogenic-training combined treatment program. Patients in the combined treatment group had a significantly elevated finger temperature response to cold stress (16°C). Neither the Prazosin nor autogenic group showed improvement. This report is significant in that it appears to be the first published investigation demonstrating a synergistic effect of behavioral treatment and medical treatment for a sympathetically mediated physiological response.

A final important topic that is attracting research attention is the application of behavioral methods to patients having Raynaud's phenomenon. Keefe, Surwit, and Pilon (1981) described results achieved in a patient having Raynaud's phenomenon secondary to mixed connective tissue disease. This patient was quite limited functionally because of frequent (6 to 8 per day) and painful vasospasms affecting her hands. During the winter months, ulcerations typically affected her fingertips and these ulcerations could not be treated effectively because of diminished blood flow to the fingers. Following the onset of a combined autogenic-temperature biofeedback program, a reduction of vasospasms and improvement in cold stress performance was noted. Two year follow-up data revealed maintenance of these gains. The patient had also been free of ulcerations. Freedman, Lynn, Ianni, and Hale (1981) reported reductions in vasospasms of greater than 90% in four Raynaud's phenomenon patients. One year follow-up data supported the stability of improvements noted. Taken together, these two reports suggest the potential for behavioral methods in Raynaud's phenomenon. Further controlled research is obviously needed to determine whether the results of these successful case reports are generalizable to the larger population of Raynaud's phenomenon sufferers.

Comment. In many ways, Raynaud's syndrome is a disorder that is well suited to behavioral medicine research. First, Raynaud's patients have clearly observable symptoms that are triggered by exposure to a specific stimulus (cold temperatures). Second, vasospastic attacks are accompanied by pronounced hysiological changes that can be accurately recorded. Third, peripheral blood flow is an autonomically mediated response long believed to be involuntary. Investigations of Raynaud's disease provide an opportunity to study the clinical benefits of learned voluntary control of an autonomic reponse. Fourth, effective medical and surgical treatments for this disorder do not exist. While Raynaud's syndrome may not be a common physical disorder, it does provide a good model with which to evaluate certain treatment methods widely used in behavioral medicine.

The existent research literature supports the efficacy of temperature biofeedback and autogenic training for the management of idiopathic Raynaud's disease (cf. Freedman et al., 1982; Keefe, 1982a; Surwit, 1982). These techniques are increasingly being incorporated into the routine medical management of patients. Current evidence also suggests that both of these methods may be helpful in the treatment of Raynaud's phenomenon.

Methods developed and evaluated in behavioral research studies on Raynaud's disease are being extended to other more common medical conditions. Patients suffering from rheumatoid arthritis are being trained to increase peripheral blood flow to affected joints by means of temperature biofeedback. Achterburg, McGraw, and Lawlis (1981) and DeBacher (1979) have reported decreases in pain, joint stiffness and Erythrocyte Sedimentation Rate (ESR) in arthritics who have undergone temperature feedback training. Varni (1981) has had success using similar methods in hemophiliacs having joint pain.

Several important issues remain to be addressed by behavioral researchers. First, methods to enhance compliance with treatment instructions need further investigation. Raynaud's patients often become symptom-free during the warmer seasons of the year. At these times of the year, motivation to practice behavioral methods may greatly decrease. Keefe, Surwit, and Pilon (1981) found that frequency of practice generally fell to near zero levels during the summer. Patients who practiced frequently, however, were better able to maintain improvements on both self-report and physiological measures at 1 year. Shelton and Levy (1981) describe a number of compliance enhancement methods which could easily be applied to Raynaud's patients. Evaluation of the efficacy of these methods with Raynaud's patients is needed. Second, the effects of different types of generalization training needs to be examined. Freedman et al. (1982) offered some intriguing possibilities in this area. They found that training patients to warm finger temperature while their fingers were being cooled by a thermoelectric device was quite useful. They have also used telemetric recording devices to measure peripheral blood flow changes that occur during vasospasms in the natural environment. Finally, behavioral researchers need to examine whether systematic training enhances the effects of a number of "palliative" measures typically recommended to the Raynaud's patient. Physicians instruct Raynaud's sufferers to avoid cold drafts or to wear warm socks and gloves. No one has investigated whether behavioral methods such as self-monitoring or reinforcement may enhance the patient's compliance with such instructions.

Behavioral scientists are now turning their attention to understanding the basic mechanisms by which behavioral strategies work for Raynaud's disease. Surwit, Allen, Gilgor, Schanberg, Kuhn, and Duvic (1982) have examined neuroendocrine responses to cold stress in patients having Raynaud's syndrome. They exposed 11 patients to a cold stress test and continuously sampled venous blood by means of a pump. Patients who fit the diagnostic criteria for idiopathic Raynaud's disease had higher plasma cortisol levels than patients having Raynaud's phenomenon (A variety of relaxation methods are known to reduce plasma cortisol levels. Thus, this result may explain why a specific training approach designed to alter blood [temperature biofeedback] is as effective as a variety of generalized relaxation methods [e.g., autogenic and relaxation training] in reducing vasospasms in idiopathic Raynaud's disease patients.)

Chronic Pain

Chronic pain is one of the most common problems primary care physicians treat. Chronic low back pain alone incapacitates almost seven million Americans (Hendler, Derogatis, Avella, & Long, 1977). The costs of chronic pain in terms of physician office visits, hospitalization, and disability payments are staggering (Nagi, Riley, & Newby, 1973). The federal government has recently recognized chronic pain as a major health problem (Holden, 1978).

Medical and surgical approaches to chronic pain are of limited benefit. Most chronic pain patients, in fact, can be characterized as failures of extensive medical and surgical treatment. Drug treatments, such as narcotics, are inappropriate for management of chronic pain because of side effects such as habituation, constipation, and addiction. Surgical treatments that help most acute pain sufferers rarely help chronic pain patients (Aitken, 1959; White, 1966). Even the innovative neurosurgical approaches that have recently been developed offer little hope to the vast majority of chronic pain sufferers (Urban, 1982). Neurodestructive and neuroaugmentation procedures help only a small fraction of patients and are usually used only as a last resort because they can produce permanent neurologic and motor defects (loss of bladder/bowel control, muscle weakness).

Behavioral and psychological factors are increasingly viewed as important in the development and maintenance of chronic pain syndromes (Bonica, 1977). There is also growing interest in incorporating behavioral procedures into the routine evaluation and treatment of chronic pain.

Two major topics have been addressed by behavioral researchers working in the chronic pain area: (1) evaluating the outcome of treatment programs that use behavioral methods, and (2) developing better behavioral assessment methods.

In the past decade there have been numerous reports coming from multidisciplinary behaviorally- oriented chronic pain treatment programs documenting clinical outcome. In each of these studies, results achieved in a consecutive series of patients are described. Fordyce et al. (1973) carried out a classic study investigating the utility of operant conditioning methods in altering the behavior of 36 patients having protracted pain histories. Most of the patients had multiple surgeries (mean = 2.7) and were extremely inactive (mean time out of bed daily = 8 hours). Many of them were addicted to habit-forming pain medications. All patients were hospitalized for treatment in a rehabilitation unit. Nursing staff in the unit were trained to use their attention and praise as a form of social reinforcement. Patients were praised by nursing staff for engaging in "well behaviors" such as exercise or spending time out of bed. When patients engaged in "pain behaviors" such as complaining of pain or limping, they were given minimal attention. Spouses or family members were also trained in these social reinforcement methods. To break the association between pain complaint and pain medication, all medications were delivered to patients in a "pain cocktail." The "cocktail" consisted of a mix of narcotic medication and a cherry syrup base. This medication was delivered on a time-contingent basis (every 4 hours) rather than PRN (as needed). The amount of narcotic was gradually reduced over time. Outcome data collected over treatment indicated that significant increases in activity level and exercise tolerance were obtained. Intake of analgesic and narcotic medications had also decreased significantly. Improvements in physical functioning were maintained at 22-month follow up.

Several studies have described results obtained when chronic pain patients are trained in self-control methods such as relaxation training, assertive training and self-paced exercise, or medication reduction methods. These programs are based on the assumption that with training, chronic pain patients can assume responsibility for managing their pain and pain behavior. Results have been as good, if not better, than results obtained with the operant conditioning approach. Gottlieb et al. (1977), for example, obtained significant increases in functional activity and decreases in pain behavior in 50 of 72 patients having severe and very chronic problems with low back pain. A 6-month follow-up revealed that 19 of 23 patients contacted had returned to work or were in vocational retraining programs. Keefe, Block, Williams, and Surwit (1981) employed self-control methods to treat 111 chronic low back pain patients. Significant decreases in muscle tension (EMG), subjective tension, pain, and medication intake occurred over the span of 2 to 3 weeks of inpatient treatment. Two behaviorally-oriented multidisciplinary programs have used a combination of operant conditioning and self-management strategies to treat chronic pain patients (Painter, Seres, & Newman, 1980; Swanson, Swenson, Maruta, & McPhee, 1976). Impressive results have been obtained in both programs.

The results reported in the outcome studies reviewed are fairly consistent.

First, most programs are successful in reducing pain medication intake and in increasing activity level. Second, while decreases in pain intensity are obtained, the size of these decreases is generally in the range of 20 to 40%. Third, most studies report that there is considerable variability in treatment outcome. Patients having the best outcomes typically are not receiving disability or financial compensation payments, have had fewer operations for pain, and have shorter histories of pain (Keefe, Block, Williams & Surwit, 1981). Fourth, maintenance of treatment gains has been noted in 40% or more of patients over time periods ranging from 6 months to 5 years. These results are very impressive when one considers that they were achieved with a group of patients who had repeatedly failed to respond to prior treatment. Obvious methodological problems are evident. The lack of control procedures makes it difficult to conclude that changes obtained were due to treatment. While a long history of pain problems provides some baseline against which to compare the results reported, controlled outcome research is needed.

Recently, investigators have attempted to use more stringent control procedures to evaluate the efficacy of behavioral treatment methods for chronic pain. Single case experimental designs have been used in several studies. Cairns and Pasino (1977) examined the effects of different reinforcement methods for increasing exercise in chronic pain patients. Walking and bicycle riding were monitored daily in a small group of patients. Verbal reinforcement, either alone or in combination with a publicly posted graph, was effective in increasing exercise levels. Decrease in exercise occurred when verbal reinforcement was given non-contingently or when verbal reinforcement was withheld. Wolf, Nacht, and Kelly (1982) evaluated paraspinal EMG biofeedback training for low back pain using a reversal design. A low back pain patient was provided with EMG feedback and learned to decrease abnormal EMG activity associated with dynamic movement. When feedback was subsequently withdrawn, low back muscle activity once again became abnormal. When feedback was re-introduced, appropriate use of the musculature was again displayed. Improvements in pain level paralleled those in muscle activity.

Controlled group outcome studies have also recently been carried out. Rybstein-Blinchick (1979) studied the effects of training patients in different cognitive pain coping methods. Chronic pain patients hospitalized in a rehabilitation center were randomly assigned to four different training groups. Group I was trained to reinterpret pain signals (i.e., attempt to make pain feel like another sensation). Group II was trained to divert their attention from pain to other activities or thoughts. Group III was trained to focus their attention on pain signals. Group IV served as an attention placebo control. Patients trained in reinterpretation strategies (Group I) had substantial decreases in pain and pain behavior relative to the other groups. Turner (1982) recently compared relaxation training to a cognitive-behavioral pain coping skills package (Meichenbaum & Turk, 1976) and a waiting list control. Patients receiving either behavioral treatment had improvements in pain, anxiety, and function relative to the wait list control group. This study, however, was carried out with a rather atypical group of pain patients in that only three patients had had prior surgery.

A second major topic in behavioral research on chronic pain is assessment. Research efforts have been hindered by a lack of objective and reliable outcome measures. More advanced methods to assess the overt motor, cognitive/affective, and psychophysiologic responses of chronic pain patients have recently been developed (e.g., Keefe, Brown, Scott, & Ziesat, 1982).

Research by Sanders (1979) and Kremer, Block, and Gaylor (1981) suggested that chronic pain patients tend to distort their reports of activity in a negative direction. Electromechanical devices, such as the "uptime clock" (Cairns, Thomas, Mooney, & Pace, 1975) and a microswitch-activated clock to monitor standing time (Sanders, 1980), have recently been introduced. These devices permit automatic recording of important indices of general activity.

Keefe and Block (1982) described an observation method to record nonverbal pain behaviors (guarded movement, bracing, rubbing the painful area, grimacing, sighing) in low back pain patients. Kremer et al. (1981) and Cinciripini and Floreen (1982) have incorporated such direct observation methods into an ongoing behavioral treatment program.

While the tendency toward cognitive distortion and the cognitive coping skills of pain patients are presumed to be very important, methods of assessing these variables have only recently been investigated. Lefebvre (1981) developed a questionnaire to measure cognitive errors and distortions that are related to depression in low back pain patients. Rosenstiel and Keefe (in press) also recently devised a questionnaire to evaluate patients' use of pain coping strategies (distortions, reinterpretation of pain, positive self statements, ignoring pain sensations, praying/hoping, and catastrophizing) and to assess the efficacy of coping strategies.

Significant advances have been made in measures of pain perception and report. In the past, patients have usually rated pain using numerical scales (0 to 10). These scales measure only the intensity dimension of pain and are also psychometrically unsound (Tursky, Jamner, & Friedman, 1982). The McGill Pain Questionnaire (MPQ) (Melzack & Torgerson, 1971) has recently become widely used in pain research because it allows for a multidimensional assessment of pain and possesses adequate reliability and validity. The MPQ consists of 20 sets of adjective descriptors that classify pain into three dimensions: sensory, affective, and evaluative. Advanced psychophysical methods also are beginning to be used in clinical situations for pain assessment. Tursky, Jamner, and Friedman (1982) have presented a four-part pain profile that employs controlled nociceptive stimuli and psychophysical scaling methods. This profile measures pain threshold and tolerance, tests the ability of the patient to judge painful stimuli, and individually calibrates patient's use of pain word descriptors. Gracely, McGrath, and Dubner (1978, 1979) have used similar methods to study the differential effects of drugs on pain perception.

Comment. Research on chronic pain is in a preliminary state of development compared to other behavioral medicine research areas. The lack of controlled outcome studies is an apparent weakness. While more objective assessment methods are being developed, these methods are not yet fully incorporated into clinical practice.

A number of obstacles to treatment outcome research on chronic pain can be identified. First, patients and their referring physicians are reluctant to agree to wait list or attention placebo control procedures. Withholding treatment from a patient who experiences constant daily pain is a difficult proposition, at best. Second, the effects obtained from behavioral treatment take some time to achieve and are not easily reversible. It may take 2 to 3 weeks of physical therapy to build up muscles weakened by disuse or to taper narcotic medications to zero levels. Third, time periods of 6 months or longer are needed to definitively assess treatment outcomes. It is already known that many patients who improve in specialized inpatient programs relapse when they return to their home environment. Fourth, the type of comparative research studies carried out in many areas of behavioral medicine are not likely to be applicable to the chronic pain area. The vast bulk of the behavioral medicine literature consists of comparisons of one behavioral treatment (e.g., relaxation training) to another (e.g., biofeedback) to a control condition. Chronic pain patients have entrenched and severe problems that are unlikely to change as a result of a single behavioral treatment procedure. Along these lines, it is interesting to note that the few comparative treatment studies (e.g., Nouwen & Solinger, 1979; Turner, 1982) that have been carried out had samples of patients who had relatively brief histories of pain and who had no or very few operations for pain.

Recently, there has been a call for more research on the efficacy of behavioral methods for chronic pain. Proponents of this line of research inquiry (Keefe, 1982b; Sanders, 1980; Turner & Chapman, 1982a, 1982b) have maintained that initial studies should examine the outcome of "treatment packages." These packages would combine a variety of behavioral treatment methods (e.g., relaxation, cognitive strategies, biofeedback, operant conditioning) and be delivered to the patient on an intensive basis. Presumably, a broad spectrum of treatments is more likely to address the multiple and complex problems of chronic pain patients. While this approach has merit, it may be premature.

Chronic pain patients are a heterogeneous group and have a heterogeneous set of behavioral problems. The variability on many outcome measures is so great that in order for statistically significant outcome effects to be obtained, the vast majority of patients would need to report *complete* pain relief, *complete* withdrawal from medications, *full* return to work, and so on. Behavioral researchers need to recognize the inherent heterogeneity of the chronic pain population and begin to do research focused on identifying commonalities in symptom presentation. Behavioral assessment research that attempts to identify homogeneous subgroups of patients on the basis of their behavior is sorely needed.

An overriding concern is the lack of basic information on how patients who have pain behave. A systematic inquiry into the behavior of pain patients is likely to be a fruitful area for research. A sequence of studies is needed, beginning with the development of behavioral measures, progressing to the study of how these measures are influenced by socio-environmental variables, and terminating in the development of specific treatments designed to alter maladaptive behavioral-environmental relationships. Our own investigations of non-verbal pain behavior are designed along these lines (Keefe & Block, 1982). More sophistication in terms of how physical factors affect pain behavior patterns is also needed. Closer collaboration with other pain specialists, (e.g, neurosurgeons, orthopedists, anesthesiologists, and neurologists) will enable behavioral scientists to more fully understand the tissue pathology basis for observed patterns of behavior.

Type A Behavior

Friedman and Rosenman (1974) were the first to describe the Type A behavior pattern and to discuss the relationship of Type A behavior to coronary heart disease. The Type A individual is one who is characterized by competitive drive, a sense of time urgency and hostility. Research on the Type A behavior pattern has been prolific. Three research topics have received a great deal of attention: (1) the relationship between Type A behavior and acute coronary heart disease events and coronary artery disease, (2) physiologic and neuroendocrine mechanisms of Type A behavior, and (3) interventions to modify the Type A behavior pattern.

Several large-scale studies have examined Type A behavior and coronary heart disease relationships. The Western Collaborative Group Study (Rosenman, Brand, Jenkins, Friedman, Strauss & Wurm, 1975) evaluated coronary heart disease (CHD) risk in over 3,000 middle-aged men. This study examined the relationship between a number of risk factors (smoking, obesity, diet, exercise, and Type A behavior) and the frequency of CHD events. The results of this study indicate that Type A males had twice as many acute CHD events (e.g., myocardial infarction, angina pectoris, recurrent myocardial infarction, and death) as Type B males. The increased risk for Type A individuals was clearly apparent even when other risk factors were controlled for statistically. A Type A behavior scale was also constructed from interview records kept as part of the longitudinal Framingham Study (Haynes, Feinleib, Levine, Scotch, & Kannel, 1978). Individuals scoring high on this scale were also found to be much more likely to experience CHD events. Taken together, the results of these and similar studies have established the Type A behavior pattern as a major risk factor for CHD.

The relationship between Type A behavior and coronary artery disease (CAD) has also been studied intensively. Each of these studies has assessed coronary artherosclerosis by means of coronary arteriography. This method is commonly utilized to study patients who are candidates for coronary bypass surgery, thus a large population of patients are available for study. Zyzanski, Jenkins, Ryan, Flessas, and Everist (1976) studied 94 men who had undergone arteriography. The men also completed the Jenkins Activity Survey (JAS), a measure of Type A behavior. High scores on the JAS Type A scale were strongly associated with narrowing of coronary arteries. Frank, Heller, Kornfeld, Sporn, and Weiss (1978) found similar results using a structured interview to assess Type A in a larger sample that included both males and females. In addition, Frank et al. found that Type A behavior was an independent risk factor comparable in impact to other risk factors. Similar results have been reported by Blumenthal, Williams, Kong, Schanberg and Thompson (1978). Williams, Haney, Lee, Kong, Blumenthal, and Whalen (1980) have studied the largest sample ($n = 424$) to date and found a highly significant relationship between CAD disease and Type A behavior. Over 70% of 319 Type A patients had at least one artery significantly occluded by CAD, whereas only 56% of the Type B patients had significant occlusion. This study also found that scores on the Hostility subscale of the MMPI were highly related to coronary occlusion.

Research on the physiologic and neuroendocrine mechanisms of Type A behavior has examined the role of cardiovascular and catecholamine hyperresponsivity to stress. The basic design of these studies involves assessment of various cardiovascular responses and catecholamine responses under baseline and stressful conditions (e.g., mental arithmetic, reaction time, solving difficult puzzles). Williams et al. (1982) studied a sample of Type A and Type B college students. Type As had forearm blood flow rates in response to mental arithmetic that were significantly greater than those of Type Bs. Type As also showed much larger increases in neuroendocrine response to mental arithmetic with substantial changes in norepinephrine, epinephrine, and cortisol. Examination of data collected during a reaction time task revealed a very interesting finding. Type As showed hyperresponsivity in cortisol and blood pressure response relative to Type Bs only if they had a positive family history of cardiovascular disease. Studies of this kind are important in that they help elucidate mechanisms that may be responsible for the increased CHD and

CAD risk observed in Type A individuals. The identification of such mechanisms may help practitioners more rationally match pharmacologic and behavioral treatments to the needs of the individual patient who exhibits the Type A behavior pattern.

Intervention studies attempting to alter the Type A behavior pattern began by investigating the efficacy of broad-spectrum approaches to treatment. For example, Suinn and Bloom (1978) used a multimodal stress management approach called Anxiety Management Training (Suinn, 1977) to modify Type A behaviors in normal volunteers. This training involves a combination of self-monitoring, relaxation, and cognitive behavioral techniques. Type As exposed to this training had lower scores on the Jenkins Activity Scale. Suinn (1975) also reported success in using this stress management approach in 10 patients treated immediately after myocardial infarction (MI).

Comparative studies of Type A interventions have more recently been carried out. Jenni and Wollersheim (1979) compared a stress management approach to cognitive behavior therapy to a no-treatment control. Outcome was evaluated on a sample of 42 subjects, seven of whom were post-MI. Cholesterol levels increased in the stress management group. Decreases in state anxiety, as measured by Spielberger's Static-Trait Anxiety Inventory, were obtained for both treatment groups. Roskies, Sperack, Surkis, Cohen, and Gilman, (1978) have also compared a stress management approach to brief psychotherapy. Significant improvements in psychological measures (satisfaction and time pressure) and physiological measures (blood pressure and cholesterol) were found for both treatments, with no significant differences between the two groups.

Recent studies have examined the effects of behavioral interventions other than stress management. Blumenthal and his colleagues (Blumenthal, Williams, Williams, & Wallace, 1980) studied the effects of a 10-week supervised exercise program on Type A behavior and physiologic measures in healthy adults. Twenty-one subjects were classified as Type A and 25 as Type B. All subjects showed improvements in physical fitness as demonstrated by significant decreases in blood pressure and weight, and increases in treadmill performance and plasminogen activator release. Type A behavior (as measured by the JAS) decreased significantly in the Type A subjects. Friedman (1980) also has a major project in progress to study the effects of a combined medical information and behavior therapy program in reducing coronary mortality in post-MI patients. A sample of over 1,000 Type A individuals are being studied over a 5-year period.

Comment. Research on Type A behavior differs from most other behavioral medicine research in two important ways. First, there is greater attention to understanding pathophysiologic mechanisms evident in the Type A literature. Neuroendocrine and physiologic correlates of the Type A pattern already have been tentatively identified. Research on mechanisms is likely to continue and may well contribute to the development of more effective treatments for individuals at risk for heart disease. Second, large scale epidemiologic studies have been conducted on the Type A behavior pattern. The fact that these studies demonstrate that Type A behavior is predictive of coronary artery disease, coronary heart disease, and higher mortality levels lends strong support to the validity of the Type A concept.

Additional research needs to be carried to develop a better understanding of how measures of Type A behavior taken from structured interviews or questionnaires (JAS) relate to overt behavioral measures (Blumenthal, 1982). Type A behavior is generally considered a reflection of a personality trait. Thus, we might expect Type As to show consistent behavior across settings and time. This assumption, however, has never been empirically tested. Behavioral observations may well indicate that variability in Type A behavior does occur and that socioenvironmental events may either elicit or serve to reinforce these behavior patterns. Behavioral observations may help researchers pinpoint target behaviors that could be modified through treatment. Present treatments for Type A behavior tend to be non-specific, and for many patients are only minimally effective.

Fecal Incontinence

Fecal incontinence is a symptom associated with a variety of physical disorders, including: congenital problems such as spina bifida, endocrine disorders such as diabetes mellitus, and neurologic disorders such as multiple sclerosis. Incontinence also can be a sequela of rectal or spinal surgery or can be brought about by long-term use of anti-cholinergic medications. Incontinence is estimated to effect 1 out of every 1,000 individuals (Milne, 1976), with higher incidence rates occurring in the elderly.

The physiology of continence is well understood. Fecal matter entering the rectum normally elicits a reflex relaxation of the internal anal sphincter. Relaxation of the internal sphincter is associated with a brief contraction of the external anal sphincter leading to evacuation of fecal material. A number of behavioral training methods have been employed to teach incontinent patients to control their symptoms. Certain methods are better suited to treating certain types of fecal incontinence (Engel, 1982).

Overflow incontinence is a problem in patients who retain stool material and are chronically constipated. Young (1973) used a classical conditioning strategy to modify this problem. Children who had symptoms of overflow fecal incontinence were trained to toilet themselves within one-half hour after eating. This is a time period when increased bowel motility normally occurs reflexively. Repeated toileting trials at this time interval significantly reduced incontinence. Incontinence secondary to memory or cognitive deficits has been found to respond well to contingency management approaches. Foxx and Azrin (1973), for example, have trained mentally retarded patients to decrease incontinence using a habit training procedure that involves structured prompts and reinforcement.

Engel, Nikoomanesh, and Schuster (1974) developed an operant conditioning procedure that can be applied to rectrosphincteric responses to assess and treat fecal incontinence. A set of balloons is inserted into the rectum. Distention of a balloon placed in the rectum produces reflex contraction in a balloon located at the internal sphincter and (in continent subjects) a brief contraction in a balloon placed at the external anal sphincter. Patients with fecal incontinence often fail to show the appropriate external sphincter response. These patients are provided visual feedback of a polygraph display of internal and external sphincter responses and then trained to produce contractions of the external sphincter. A discrimination training paradigm is used to teach patients to produce external sphincter contractions only when rectal distension approaches the threshold that elicits a reflex internal sphincter response. After this task is mastered, visual feedback is gradually faded out.

Cerulli, Nikoomanesh, and Schuster (1979) reported results achieved with 25 patients who had been incontinent following rectal surgery. Twenty-four of 25 patients became fully continent after 1 to 2 hours of training. Engel et al. (1974) and Cerulli et al. (1979) have also reported on results achieved in patients incontinent because of peripheral nerve dysfunction. Success rates varied from 30% (in peripheral neuropathy cases) to 80% (in post-laminectomy patients). Engel (1982) reports that a patient's ability to detect large rectal distensions was related to outcome. Patients who could not discriminate rectal distensions greater than 15 ml had a poor response to treatment. Whitehead, Parker, Masek, Cataldo, and Freeman (in press) used a variation of the operant conditioning method described above to teach spina bifida children to become continent. This report found that the children did have an ability to discriminate rectal distensions, but that their reflex response to distension was abnormal. These patients showed reflex relaxation of both internal and external sphincters. A shaping procedure was therefore employed to teach the children first to produce external sphincter contractions spontaneously, and then to emit this response following rectal distensions.

Comment. The behavioral research literature on fecal incontinence is interesting for several reasons. First, the methods appear to be quite effective. The operant conditioning methods described by Engel et al. (1974) are now considered the treatment of choice for patients having incontinence following rectal surgery. Second, this research has emphasized the importance of psychophysiological analysis in planning rational treatment. Only after observing the functioning of external and internal sphincters can one rationally select from the various treatments. Third, the approaches used are simple and straightforward. The promising results obtained by Engel and others need to be confirmed by other investigators. If these results are supported, we may expect that behavioral methods for treating incontinence will become incorporated in the routine medical management of many patients within the next decade.

Recently, Engel and Whitehead have begun extending their treatment program to patients having urinary incontinence. Training patients to inrease the activity of muscles controlling urinary flow appears to be effective in reducing longstanding stress incontinence. Given the prevalence of stress incontinence, this research is potentially a very important development.

Hypertension

Hypertension, or high blood pressure, is a disorder that affects almost 15% of adults in the United States. Hypertension significantly increases an individual's risk for developing serious renal dysfunction and cardiovascular problems (e.g., cerebrovascular accidents, peripheral vascular disease, angina pectoris, myocardial infarction, congestive heart failure). Pharmacologic approaches to hypertension are commonly utilized and are effective for many patients. Long-term use of these medications may be contraindicated in some patients because of side effects such as hypercholerolemia, hyperglycemia, and hyperuricemia. Behavioral interventions for hypertension are advantageous because they avoid these side effects and may also modify basic causative factors such as smoking, body weight, exercise, or stress.

A thorough review of behavioral approaches to hypertension is beyond the scope of this chapter but the interested reader may wish to read excellent recent articles by Reeves and Victor (1982), Shapiro (1982), and Shapiro and Goldstein (1982). Two major groups of behavioral treatment methods can be delineated: (1) those that attempt to change physiological responses, and (2) those that attempt to alter behavioral factors affecting blood pressure.

Early attempts to modify blood pressure in hypertensives involved the use of biofeedback. Blood pressure biofeedback only became feasible after the development of the "constant cuff" recording method in the late 1960s (Shapiro, Tursky, Gershon, & Stern, 1969). The inherent variabilities of blood pressure make intermittent readings of blood pressure minimally useful. The "constant cuff" method permits continuous beat-by-beat measurement and feedback of blood pressure changes. Benson, Shapiro, Tursky, and Schwartz (1971) were the first to employ the constant-cuff method to train hypertensives to lower blood pressure. Five patients diagnosed as having essential hypertension underwent intensive and systematic training following a baseline recording phase. Reductions in systolic blood pressure were marked, and averaged 17 mm HG from baseline. Subsequent studies (Goldman, Kleinman, Snow et al., 1975; Kristt & Engel, 1975) showed that the effects of blood pressure biofeedback training generalized to the patient's home setting. Elder, Ruiz, Deabler, et al. (1973) have also reported that substantial reductions in diastolic blood pressure can be obtained in hypertensives using the constant-cuff feedback procedures.

Recent investigations of blood pressure biofeedback have attempted to compare the efficacy of biofeedback to other behavioral and conventional pharmacologic approaches. A good example of this more recent work is a study by Goldstein, Shapiro, Thananopavarn, and Sambhi (1982). In this study, 36 mild hypertensives were assigned randomly to one of four conditions: blood pressure biofeedback, relaxation (Benson's meditation procedure), a standard drug regimen, or a self-monitoring control group. Blood pressures were recorded repeatedly over the study both in laboratory and home settings. The drug regimen was found to be significantly more effective than all other treatments in reducing blood pressure recorded at home. However, the biofeedback group showed reduced blood pressures that were of the same magnitude as that for the drug regimen group in the laboratory.

Relaxation approaches for reducing blood pressure in hypertensives have also been investigated widely. Benson, Beary, and Carol (1974) examined the effects of a meditation method in 36 hypertensive patients. Significant reductions in systolic and diastolic pressures were observed after 3–4 months of daily practice. Taylor, Farquhar, Nelson, and Agras (1977) also have found a tape recorded relaxation training program effective for hypertensives.

The largest reductions in blood pressure in hypertensives reported in the behavioral research literature have been obtained by Patel (1977). Patel's (1977) treatment program attempts to alter excessive sympathetic nervous system activity. She uses a combination of skin resistance biofeedback, yoga relaxation exercises, and meditation. Patel (1973) studied 20 hypertensives who had undergone 36 treatment sessions over 3 months. Blood pressure dropped from 160/120 mm Hg pre-treatment to 134/86 mm Hg post-treatment. Decreases in medication of over 40% were also obtained. Subsequent studies utilizing more rigorous control procedures, such as an age and sex matched control group (Patel, 1975) and randomized assignment to treatment conditions (Patel & North, 1975), found similar results.

Behavioral interventions are also now being used to modify risk factors that influence hypertension, such as diet and exercise. Recent studies suggest that modifying salt, caffeine, and alcohol intake can significantly influence blood pressure in hypertensives. Parijs, Joosseens, Van der Linden et al. (1973) found that simple instructions to patients to avoid salty foods and salt shakers produced a drop in blood pressure of 8/4 mm Hg. Caffeine appears to have potent effects on blood pressure. The level of caffeine in two to three cups of coffee is enough to raise blood pressure 14/10 mm Hg in normals (Robertson, Frolick, Carr et al. 1978). It is also well known that heavy drinkers of alcohol are much more likely to suffer from hypertension.

Increases in exercise have been associated with decreased blood pressure in most studies of hypertensives. Walking and jogging programs of 12 to 24 weeks duration have consistently produced decreases in blood pressure of approximately 14/10 mm Hg (Boyer & Kasch, 1970; Johnson & Grover, 1976). These studies generally find that the largest reduction in blood pressure occurs in patients having the highest initial blood pressure (see Reeves & Victor, 1982).

Comment. The research literature demonstrates that a variety of behavioral techniques (biofeedback, relaxation, or meditation) can be used to teach hypertensive patients to directly decrease blood pressure. The magnitude of blood pressure reductions, however, is typically small, and the clinical significance of these methods remains to be determined. It is not clear, for example, whether the modest blood pressure decreases achieved through biofeedback can reduce patients' risk of developing coronary heart and coronary artery disease. Alternative training methods designed to enhance treatment effects and facilitate transfer of learned blood pressure control from laboratory to natural settings need to be investigated. The effects of biofeedback may be heightened if training is carried out under stressful conditions. Reeves, Shapiro, and Cobb (1979) reported that biofeedback does help normal subjects control their cardiovascular responses to laboratory stressors. Adapting such training to patient populations may prove useful.

The fact that behavioral research has moved beyond attempts to modify blood pressure to a consideration of lifestyle factors that influence blood pressure is an encouraging development. Behavioral interventions designed to alter risk factors such as diet, exercise, and non-compliance with pharmacologic therapy may ultimately prove more effective than biofeedback. The results of initial studies in this area are promising and further research appears warranted.

The recent development of ambulatory blood pressure monitors is an important technological advance for researchers interested in behavioral assessment of the hypertensive patient. These devices permit investigators to examine blood pressure as a continuous variable. Blood pressure changes occurring over the patient's day and in response to particular environmental events can be easily measured and analyzed. These devices may also permit investigators to better evaluate the effects of pharmacologic and behavioral interventions in the natural environment.

Asthma

Asthma is a disorder characterized by intermittent attacks of shortness of breath and difficulty breathing. Asthmatic attacks involve obstructions of the small and large airways due to smooth muscle spasm, excessive mucous production, or the swelling of tissue. The attacks vary in severity from mild to life threatening (status asthmaticus). A 1960 survey estimated that two million children in the United States suffer from asthma. There are no commonly accepted criteria that can be used to distinguish asthma from bronchitis and other pulmonary diseases. Improved diagnostic procedures such as bronchial challenges, lung-function tests, and exercise testing are promising and may provide a much-needed standardized approach to the diagnosis of asthma (Chai, 1975; Creer, 1982). Medical management of the asthmatic entails symptomatic treatment of the acute attack through the use of bronchodilators and medications, avoidance of allergens that serve to trigger attacks, and avoidance of respiratory infections. Asthma is a chronic disease that requires medical supervision over a long time period.

Asthma has long been considered a psychosomatic disorder (French & Alexander, 1941) that might be amenable to psychotherapy. In a recent review, Creer (1982) concludes "there is no data to support the contention that there is a unique personality of those with asthma. . . . [also] there is no evidence that traditional methods of psychotherapy alleviate asthma" (p. 916).

Asthma has been approached by behavioral researchers by means of biofeedback training and behavioral management strategies. One biofeedback training approach has been to give patients feedback regarding changes in respiratory function. Khan, Staerk, and Bonk (1973) induced bronchospasm in asthmatic children and then trained them with visual and verbal feedback to increase the volume of air expired in one second (FEV_1). Children who had undergone this biofeedback training had significant reductions in asthmatic attacks, emergency room visits, number of hospitalizations, and medication intake when compared to controls. Vachon and Rich (1976) found that asthmatic adults could learn to lower total respiratory resistance through biofeedback of this parameter. Several studies have also examined the efficacy of biofeedback in altering peak expiratory flow rates in asthmatics (cf. Alexander, 1981). The magnitude of changes achieved through feedback training of respiratory parameters has been small, and these studies are primarily of theoretical rather than practical significance.

Kotses and Glaus (1981) have found frontalis EMG biofeedback training to be effective in reducing asthmatic symptoms in children. In the first of a series of studies, Kotses, Glaus, Crawford, Edwards, and Scherr (1976) randomly assigned 36 asthmatic children to three groups: true frontalis EMG feedback, bogus EMG feedback, or no feedback. Children receiving true feedback showed marked improvements in peak expiratory flow rates. A subsequent study by Kotses, Glaus, Bricel, Edwards, and Crawford (1978) replicated the original results and also showed that EMG feedback from another muscle group had no effect on respiratory parameters.

Research on behavioral management strategies has been caried out primarily by a group of researchers at the National Asthma Center in Denver (Creer,

Renne, & Christian, 1976). At this center, children with chronic asthma have been trained to become more aware of the onset of asthmatic attacks through several procedures. First, peak expiratory flow rate values were calculated twice daily, and children were taught that flow rates below a critical value were likely to be associated with an attack (Taplin & Creer, 1978). Second, parents were trained to closely attend to their child's asthmatic attack behavior to learn to recognize the early warnings signs of an acute episode. Early recognition enhanced the efficacy of medical management. Third, training parents in behavioral management methods of controlling problem behavior occurring during asthmatic attacks has been found useful. Research indicates that when parents learn to handle attacks in a calm systematic manner, panic behavior, medication intake, and emergency medical visits can be minimized (Creer, 1974; Renne & Creer, 1976).

Comment. Behavioral approaches to managing asthma are interesting. The literature reviewed above suggests that behavioral methods may have a role in helping patients and their families to better cope with asthmatic attacks. Initial results obtained by Creer (1982) and others are promising, and this area is likely to be a fruitful one for further research. The potential contribution of biofeedback approaches to asthma is more controversial. While frontalis EMG feedback and feedback regarding respiratory functioning does tend to improve performance on certain respiratory parameters, questions remain as to the clinical significance of the changes obtained (Alexander, 1981). It is generally known that changes of 15% or more in FEV_1 are needed to produce a clinically significant effect in asthmatics. Biofeedback methods however, usually produce changes in FEV_1 of approximately 3%. At this point, it seems fair to conclude that biofeedback methods are interesting but may have limited clinical utility.

The development and evaluation of behavioral treatment strategies is one of the most interesting recent developments in asthma research. Further research on this important topic is likely to have important implications for a wide range of respiratory disorders.

Muscle Contraction and Vascular Headache

Tension (muscle contraction) and migraine (vascular) headaches are among the most frequent medical complaints experienced by the general population. Chronic contraction of the muscles of the face, scalp, neck, and shoulders is believed to be the major cause of muscle contraction or tension headaches. A variety of over-the-counter medications are used by muscle contraction headache sufferers. Some patients become reliant on sedative-hypnotic agents and narcotics for pain relief. Migraine or vascular headaches are believed to be due to a disturbance of extra and intracranial blood flow. Migraine headaches are intermittent and usually are located unilaterally. These headaches are often preceded by prodromal symptoms (e.g., flashes of light, paresthesias) and often accompanied by nausea and vomiting. Medical management typically involves the use of aspirin or codeine for mild headaches and ergot derivatives for more severe headaches.

Headache management has been one of the most active areas of behavioral medicine research, and several excellent reviews of this literature are available (e.g., Adams, Feuerstein & Fowler, 1980; Blanchard & Andrasik, 1982). A number of effective behavioral treatments have been identified for both muscle contraction and vascular headaches.

Numerous studies have examined the efficacy of muscle relaxation methods for treating muscle contraction headaches. Interest in this topic was first generated by a report (Budzynski, Stoyva, & Adler, 1970) on frontalis EMG biofeedback training. Muscle contraction headache patients were given EMG biofeedback from large surface electrodes placed symmetrically over the frontal region. Both visual (a meter panel) and auditory feedback (a tone) was provided. Clinically significant improvements in headaches occurred after several weeks of training. Subsequent controlled group studies have generally supported these findings. Budzynski, Stoyva, Adler, and Mullaney, (1973), for example, compared frontalis EMG feedback training to a non-contingent feedback control and a no-treatment control condition. Patients in the true EMG feedback condition had marked reductions in daily headache activity over an 8-week training period and were able to maintain improvements at 3- and 18-month follow-up. Patients in the control conditions showed no change in headache activity.

The efficacy of frontalis EMG feedback training has been compared to general muscle relaxation methods in several studies. Cox, Freundlich, and Meyer (1975) assigned 27 muscle contraction headache sufferers to one of three groups: frontalis EMG feedback, progressive relaxation training, and placebo medication. Patients in the biofeedback and relaxation group had fewer headaches, lower frontalis EMG levels, and decreased medication intake compared to placebo controls. The magnitude of treatment effects was roughly equal for patients in the biofeedback and relaxation training conditions. Similar results have been obtained by Haynes, Griffin, Mooney, and Parise (1975) and Chesney and Shelton (1976).

Stress management methods have also been found useful for muscle contraction headache. Holroyd, Andrasik, and Westbrook (1977) compared the effects of a cognitive therapy program in which patients were taught to alter maladaptive cognitive responses to head pain to the effects of frontalis EMG feedback and a waiting-list control. Results showed that EMG activity decreased in both treatment groups. Decreases in EMG were greater for patients in the biofeedback group than for patients in the cognitive therapy group.

Patients in the cognitive therapy condition, however, reduced daily headache activity by 75% whereas those in the frontalis EMG condition had reductions of 25%. Frontalis EMG biofeedback was *not* found effective in reducing headache activity when compared to a control group. This study is important because it clearly shows that behavior therapy methods other than relaxation training may be effective for muscle contraction headache patients.

Behavioral treatments for vascular headache primarily attempt to alter headache by modifying peripheral blood flow. Sargent, Green, and Walters (1973) were the first to investigate the utility of temperature biofeedback as a treatment for vascular headache. Seventy-five patients were given feedback regarding the difference between forehead and finger temperature and instructed to warm their hands relative to their foreheads. Patients were also instructed in autogenic training methods focusing on hand heaviness and warmth. Fifty-one of 75 patients were rated by the investigators as showing moderate to very good improvement. Subsequent studies employing more objective outcome measures and more rigorous control procedures have generally supported the initial positive results of Sargent et al. (1973). Training patients to increase their level of peripheral blood flow control either through temperature biofeedback, autogenic training, or cephalic vasomotor biofeedback has been found useful in alleviation of vascular headaches (Olton & Noonberg, 1980).

Research topics currently under investigation by headache researchers include the treatment of headache in children, the efficacy of self-administered behavioral treatments, the prediction of treatment outcome, and long-term maintenance. Andrasik (Andrasik, Blanchard, Edlund, & Rosenblum, in press) has recently begun a series of studies with children having chronic headache complaints. Initial reports usng single case designs indicate that a combined autogenic-temperature feedback as well as frontalis EMG feedback is effective in reducing headaches in this population. Kohlenberg and Cahn (1981) have recently examined the efficacy of a self-help manual for migraine sufferers. Patients who received the self-help manual had fewer headaches than a control group who read a book that provided general information on headache. This study, like others on self-administered treatments, however, had a very high drop-out rate. Blanchard and his colleagues have carried several recent studies that have examined the extent to which psychological test scores (Blanchard et al., 1982), and psychophysiological response patterns (Blanchard et al., in press) are predictive of response to behavioral treatment. We will examine one of these studies in detail in the next section of this chapter. Studies of maintenance of treatment gains have generally supported the efficacy of biofeedback and behavioral treatments for headache. Most studies have been retrospective however. Research is currently being conducted by Blanchard's research group to examine the relative efficacy of different maintenance enhancement strategies on a prospective basis (Blanchard & Andrasik, 1982).

Comment. The research we have reviewed indicates that behavioral strategies are a viable treatment alternative for many headache patients. The consistency of positive findings across studies in impressive. Behavioral research in this area is fairly well advanced. Standardized methods for recording and quantifying headache data are now used. Comparative treatment studies with adequate controls have been carried out. Predictors of treatment outcome are being identified and long-term maintenance issues are being investigated. A solid foundation for further research has been established.

Several topic areas are likely to attract research attention in the future. First, recent studies have begun to identify factors that are predictive of treatment outcome. Cross validation studies on these predictors need to be carried out. Second, the efficacy of combined pharmacologic and behavioral treatment approaches needs to be studied. In spite of the demonstrated efficacy of behavioral approaches, the vast majority of patients having tension and migraine headaches continue to be treated with drugs. Studies comparing behavioral, drug, and combined behavioral-drug treatments may provide more compelling evidence of behavioral treatment efficacy that may shift current medical practice trends. Third, the mechanisms by which behavioral methods work need to be elucidated (Blanchard & Andrasik, 1982). The physiological and behavioral changes brought about by successful relaxation or biofeedback training are not fully understood. Changes in pain behavior patterns (e.g., medication intake, activity level, and non-verbal pain behaviors) that occur in successfully vs. non-successfully treated headache patients have not been studied.

METHODOLOGICAL CRITIQUE OF A RESEARCH STUDY

This section provides an extended critique of a behavioral medicine research study. In the process of this critique, methodological issues of importance to a broad range of behavioral medicine research areas will be identified and discussed.

The study selected for consideration is a recent one conducted by Blanchard et al. (1982) entitled "Biofeedback and Relaxation Training with Three Kinds of Headache: Treatment Effects and Their Prediction" that was published in the *Journal of Consulting and Clinical Psychology.* The critique of the study will examine important sections of this paper, including the introduction, the experimental design, the subject sample, measurement methods, statistical methods, and the discussion.

Introduction

The significance of a study must be clearly established in introductory comments that review previous research. Blanchard et al. (1982) do a good job of providing the reader with a perspective on their work. Previous headache studies examined outcome in relatively small numbers of patients and failed to identify factors essential with differential outcome. The study by Blanchard et al., in contrast, reports results with a large number of patients having either muscle contraction, vascular, or combined muscle-contraction/vascular headaches. This study also evaluates whether psychological test results are predictive of treatment outcome.

An important question in evaluating any piece of research is the degree to which it makes a contribution to the literature. Does this study appear to add anything to the literature beyond what has previously been published? As we noted in the previous section on headache, research does indeed support the efficacy of behavioral treatment methods. Blanchard et al. (1982) are correct, however, in pointing out that prior research has used relatively small sample sizes. This weakness is common in behavioral medicine research. Many studies that compare various treatment methods are based on small samples of 6–10 subjects per condition. Replication with large numbers of patients certainly provides more compelling evidence for the clinical significance of behavioral treatment methods. When objective assessments of predictor and outcome variables are also employed, patients who can expect to attain a certain criterion of success can potentially be identified. Thus, in this study, Blanchard et al. address issues that are important not only for the headache area but for the entire field of behavioral medicine.

Experimental Design

In a study by Blanchard et al. (1982), sequential treatment design is used in which all patients first undergo relaxation training. Patients who fail to respond to relaxation are then offered an opportunity to undergo further biofeedback training. This design does not allow direct comparisons to be made between various types of biofeedback training and relaxation methods. In addition, predictors of biofeedback treatment outcome can only be made for patients who have already failed to make progress with relaxation methods. This group of "treatment failures" is probably not representative of the broad range of headache patients. Thus, the sequential treatment design has some inherent limitations. Blanchard et al.'s (1982) decision to use this design is essentially based on two points: (1) relaxation is simpler than biofeedback and thus should be given first, and (2) giving all patients the same treatment initially provides a large pool for examination of predictors of outcome. The first point is a weak one. Relaxation and biofeedback treatments are fairly comparable in terms of their complexity. Point number two is the more compelling. If the main purpose of this study is to examine the response of a large number of patients to a specified treatment, then starting as many patients as possible with an identical treatment makes sense.

A second problem with the study design is the lack of an attention placebo, no treatment, or routine medical management control group. This would be a serious design flaw if this study had been one of the first on the efficacy of behavioral methods for headache. Many studies, however, have already demonstrated that relaxation and biofeedback methods are more effective than control procedures for headache patients.

Subjects

The subjects in this study were 91 patients who completed a pretreatment neurological assessment. The attention given to specification of patient diagnosis is especially noteworthy. Headache type was diagnosed independently by a neurologist and one of the researchers using standard criteria. Percentage agreement calculated between the diagnosticians was high (86.4% exact agreement). As one reviews the behavioral literature, it is relatively rare that such careful diagnostic screening is carried out or described in detail. In many studies, patients are simply described as having "chronic pain," "epilepsy," or "asthma," and no information on physical diagnosis is provided at all. Biomedical researchers consider physical diagnosis to be extremely important, and they are likely to ignore psychological and behavioral studies that fail to attend to diagnostic classification.

The recruiting procedure used in this study deserves comment. Half of the patients were referred by their physician and the other half volunteered after hearing of the project through the media. While such a sampling procedure is commonly used in behavioral medicine studies, it does have certain limitations. Patients who volunteer for a research study may be atypical of the general headache population. The expectations of these patients and their level of motivation are likely to be higher than in a randomly sampled group of headache patients.

Measures

Two sets of measures were utilized in this study: (1) outcome measures, and (2) measures of predictor variables. One concern in evaluationg a study of this type is the reliability and validity of methods used to obtain these measures.

Treatment outcome was assessed by means of a headache diary. This diary was developed in an earlier study (Blanchard, Theobald, Williamson, Silver, & Brown, 1978). The diary provides measures of headache intensity and duration as well as medication intake. A study by Blanchard, Andrasik, Neff, Jurish, and O'Keefe (1981) supported the social validity of the diary. In that study, patients' ratings of improvement correlated well with general ratings of improvement obtained from significant others. The headache diary has been found to be a reliable measure and is currently employed by many headache researchers (Blanchard & Andrasik, 1982). The headache diary, in fact, is one of the better developed outcome measures currently employed in behavioral medicine research. In many treatment studies, outcome measures are devised for a study and little or no information is given on their reliability or validity.

The predictor variables examined in this study were measured by means of psychological test instruments. These instruments included the MMPI, Beck Depression Inventory, State-Trait Anxiety Inventory, Rathus Assertiveness Survey, Psychosomatic Symptom Checklist, Social Readjustment Rating Scale, and the Autonomic Perception Questionnaire. These tests are all psychometrically sound, and their reliability and validity have been examined in numerous studies.

In summary, the measurement methods used in this study are generally sound. The study is strengthened by incorporation of these methods.

Training Methods

Three training approaches are described in this paper: relaxation, frontalis EMG, and thermal biofeedback.

The relaxation training program was the same one described in a previously published training manual (Bernstein & Borkovec, 1973). In the present paper the schedule of training sessions is described and an outline of topics covered in these sessions is provided. This relaxation training method is very commonly used in clinical and research applications. The frontalis EMG and thermal biofeedback training approaches used in the study are similar to that used in prior headache research studies. Thus, this paper contains a fairly thorough description of training methods. There is enough information and reference material presented to permit replication of the study.

Two important issues regarding training procedures are not addressed in this paper. First, no information is provided regarding the patient's compliance with training instructions. The training methods evaluated in this study must be applied by the patient if they are to be effective. Failure to practice the training methods means that the adequacy of the training cannot be evaluated. One flaw of this study is that no independent check was made to verify that patients actually practiced. Thus, it is difficult to determine whether patients who failed to respond to relaxation did so because the treatment was ineffective or because they had not complied with training instructions. This methodological flaw is important because it is so commonly encountered in behavioral treatment studies.

A second problem is that no information is given as to differences in type and dosage of medications used by patients during training. In the present study, medication intake is considered a dependent variable and decreases in intake are considered a sign of improvement. Patients having migraine vs.

tension headaches, however, are likely to be on very different medications. Migraineurs often take ergot derivatives such as Fiorinal or Caffergot. Tension headache patients often take analgesics or narcotics. As the reader will recall, in this study, tension and migraine headache patients who failed to respond to relaxation were subsequently assigned to one of two biofeedback training methods (frontalis EMG and thermal feedback respectively). In fact, tension and migraine patients received a combination of biofeedback and whatever pharmacologic treatments they had been taking. The two groups thus differed not only in the biofeedback training they received but also in the type of medications that they took concurrently. If the purpose of this study was to compare the efficacy of the two treatments, this flaw would be a critical one. Given that this is not the purpose of the study, the flaw is simply a limitation that the reader needs to keep in mind.

Statistical Methods

The statistical approaches used in this study are more sophisticated than those generally employed in behavioral medicine research. To evaluate headache and medication intake changes occurring over the treatment, a multivariate analysis of variance (MANOVA) was employed. This data analysis strategy is particularly appropriate because pain measures constituted three of the four outcome variables. These measures are likely to be closely related to one another. When multiple statistical tests are carried out on such related dependent variables, alpha level is often contaminated, leading to spurious results. To identify potential predictors of post-treatment headache activity, a hierarchical multiple regression analysis was used. This type of analysis examines a pool of predictor variables and selects the predictor having the best relationship to outcome and enters that into the next step of the regression analysis. One limitation of this approach is that the predictors so identified are not always those that are the most theoretically meaningful. Interpretation of the findings can be difficult. In the present studies, six different psychological test scores predicted post-relaxation headache levels. Many different sets of psychological test scores predicted post-biofeedback headache level. In fact different grouping of predictors were identified for each of the headache groups treated. The findings are thus varied and difficult to describe or interpret.

Discussion

The discussion section of this paper does an excellent job of summarizing the findings and highlighting some of the limitations of the study. In fact, many of the methodological problems we have discussed are candidly described by the authors. The need for replication is strongly emphasized by the authors.

Given the wide variety of predictors of post-headache activity, identified cross-validation studies are particularly important.

When we consider this paper as a whole, certain conclusions can be made. First, the study is significant in that it addresses some major weaknesses in the headache literature in particular, and the behavioral medicine literature in general. These weaknesses include a reliance on small sample sizes, a failure to attend to physical diagnosis, and lack of information on predictors of treatment response. Second, while the design of the study does have certain weaknesses, the design also has some inherent strengths that are well suited to the authors' purposes. Third, the attention given to diagnostic classification and incorporation of reliable and valid measurement methods are impressive. Fourth, the training methods and statistical techniques used are clearly specified. Replication of the study can thus be more easily attempted by subsequent investigators.

The study by Blanchard et al. (1982) is important not only because of its findings but because it illustrates how problems encountered in many areas of behavioral medicine research are being addressed on a practical level by experienced investigators.

SUMMARY

The brief reviews provided in this chapter illustrate how diverse the field of behavioral medicine is. A wide range of research topics are actively being investigated, and the research strategies utilized are equally broad-ranging. The reviews provided cover only a portion of the important research areas currently being addressed. Readers interested in other topics or an expanded discussion of the topics we have briefly addressed are referred to several recent publications (Blanchard, 1982; Keefe & Blumenthal, 1982; Surwitt, Williams, Steptoe, & Biersner, 1982).

One of the most appealing aspects of behavioral medicine research is that the assessment and the treatment strategies investigated are potentially quite useful clinically. While further research is needed before the utility of behavioral approaches can be fully realized, fundamental issues regarding the research process have already been addressed in many areas. Behavioral medicine researchers appear to be committed to the development of objective methodologies (Keefe & Blumenthal, 1982) and to the application of controlled experimental designs in their respective areas of research. It is this commitment to research that makes the field of behavioral medicine one of the most promising areas of psychological investigation.

REFERENCES

Achterberg, J., McGraw, P., & Lawlis, G.F. (1981). Rheumatoid arthritis: A study of relaxation and temperature biofeedback as an adjunctive therapy. *Biofeedback and Self-Regulation, 6*, 207–233.

Adams, H.E., Feuerstein, M., & Fowler, J.L. (1980). Migraine headache: Review of parameters, etiology, and intervention. *Psychological Bulletin, 87*, 217-237.

Aitken, A.T. (1959). The present status of invertebrae disc surgery. *Michigan State Medical Society, 58*, 1121-1127.

Alexander, A.B. (1981). Behavioral approaches in the treatment of bronchial asthma. In C.K. Prokop & L.A. Bradley (Eds.), *Medical Psychology: Contributions to behavioral medicine.* New York: Academic Press.

Andrasik, F., Blanchard, E.B., Edlund, S.R., & Rosenblum, E.L. (in press). Autogenic feedback in the treatment of two children with migraine headache. *Child and Family Behavior Therapy.*

Balaschak, B.A. (1976). Teacher-implemented behavior modification in a case of organically based epilepsy. *Journal of Consulting and Clinical Psychology, 44*, 218-223.

Benson, H., Beary, J.F., & Carol, M.P. (1974). The relaxation response. *Psychiatry 37*, 37-46.

Benson, H., Shapiro, D., Tursky, B., & Schwartz, G.E. (1971). Decreased systolic blood pressure through operant conditioning techniques in patients with essential hypertension. *Science, 173*, 740-742.

Bernstein, D.A., & Borkovec, T.D. (1973). *Progressive relaxation training: A manual for the helping professions.* Champaign, IL: Research Press.

Blanchard, E.B. (1982). Behavioral medicine: Past, present, and future. *Journal of Consulting and Clinical Psychology, 50*, 795-796.

Blanchard, E.B., & Andrasik, F. (1982). Psychological assessment and treatment of headache: Recent developments and emerging issues. *Journal of Consulting and Clinical Psychology, 50*, 859-879.

Blanchard, E.G., Andrasik, F., Neff, D.F., Arena, J.G., Ahles, T.A., Jurish, S.E., Pallmeyer, T.P., Saunders, N.L., Teders, S.J., Baron, K.D., & Rodlichak, L.D. (1982). Biofeedback and relaxation training with three kinds of headache: Treatment effects and their prediction. *Journal of Consulting and Clinical Psychology, 50*, 562-575.

Blanchard, E.B., Andrasik, F., Neff, D.F., Jurish, S.E., & O'Keefe, D.M. (1981). Social validation of the headache diary. *Behavior Therapy, 12*, 711-715.

Blanchard, E.B., & Haynes, M.R. (1975). Biofeedback treatment of a case of Raynaud's disease. *Journal of Behavior Therapy and Experimental Psychiatry, 6*, 230-234.

Blanchard, E.B., Theobald, D.E., Williamson, D.A., Silver, B.V., & Brown, D.A. (1978). Temperature biofeedback in the treatment of migraine headaches. *Archives of General Psychiatry, 35*, 581-588.

Blanchard, E.B., Andrasik, F., Arena, J.G., Neff, D.F., Saunders, N.L., Jurish, S.E., Teders, S.J., & Rodichok, L.D. (in press). Psychophysiological responses of headache patients as predictors of behavioral treatment outcome. *Behavioral Therapy.*

Blumenthal, J.A. (1982) Assessment of patients with coronary heart disease. In F.J. Keefe & J.A. Blumenthal (Eds.), *Assessment Strategies in behavioral medicine.* New York: Grune and Stratton, Inc.

Blumenthal, J.A., Williams, R.B., Kong, Y., Schanberg, S.M., & Thompson, L.W. (1978). Type A behavior pattern and coronary atherosclerosis. *Circulation, 58*, 634-639.

Blumenthal, J.A., Williams, R.S., Williams, R.B., & Wallace, A.G. (1980). Effects of exercise on the Type A (coronary-prone) behavior pattern. *Psychosomatic Medicine, 42,* 289–296.

Bonica, J.J. (1977). Neurophysiological and pathologic aspects of acute and chronic pain. *Archives of Surgery, 112,* 750–761.

Boyer, J.L., & Kasch, F.W. (1970). Exercise therapy in hypertensive men. *Journal of the American Medical Association, 211,* 1668.

Budzynski, T.H., Stoyva, J.M., & Adler, C.S. (1970). Feedback induced muscle relaxation: Application to tension headache. *Journal of Behavior Therapy and Experimental Psychiatry, 1,* 205–211.

Budzynski, T.H., Stoyva, J.M., Adler, C.S., & Mullaney, D.J. (1973). EMG biofeedback and tension headache: A controlled outcome study. *Psychosomatic Medicine, 35,* 484–496.

Cairns, D., & Pasino, J. (1977). Comparison of verbal reinforcement and feedback in the operant treatment of disability due to chronic low back pain. *Behavior Therapy, 8,* 621–630.

Cairns, D., Thomas, L., Mooney, V., & Pace, J.B. (1975). A comprehensive treatment approach to chronic low back pain. *Pain, 2,* 301–308.

Cerulli, M.A., Nikoomanesh, P., & Schuster, M.M. (1979). Progress in biofeedback conditioning for fecal incontinence. *Gastroenterology, 76,* 742–749.

Chai, H. (1975). Management of severe chronic perennial asthma in children. *Advances in Asthma and Allergy, 2,* 1–12.

Chesney, M.A., & Shelton, J.L. (1976). A comparison of muscle relaxation and electromyogram biofeedback experiments for muscle contraction headache. *Journal of Behavior Therapy and Experimental Psychiatry, 7,* 221–225.

Cinciripini, P.M., & Floreen, A. (1982). An evaluation of a behavioral program for chronic pain. *Journal of Behavioral Medicine, 5,* 375–390.

Cox, D.J., Freundlich, A., & Meyer, R.A. (1975). Differential effectiveness of electromyographic feedback, verbal relaxation instructions, and medication placebo with tension headaches. *Journal of Consulting and Clinical Psychology, 43,* 892–898.

Creer, T.L. (1974). Biofeedback and asthma. *Advances in Asthma and Allergy, 1,* 6–11.

Creer, T.L. (1982). Asthma. *Journal of Consulting and Clinical Psychology, 50,* 912, 921.

Creer, T.L., Renne, C.M., & Christian, W.P. (1976). Behavioral contributions to rehabilitation and childhood asthma. *Rehabilitation Literature, 37,* 226–232.

DeBacher, A. (1979). *Vasomotor response training in the arthritis patient* (Project report R-58). Atlanta, GA: Emory University School of Medicine, Regional Research and Training Center.

DiCara, L.V., & Miller, N. (1968). Instrumental learning of vasomotor response by rats: Learning to respond differentially in the two ears. *Science, 159,* 1485–1486.

Elder, S.T., Ruiz, Z.R., Deabler, H.L. and Dillenkoffer, R.L. (1973). Instrumental conditioning of diastolic blood pressure in essential hypertensive patients. *Journal of Applied Behavior Analysis, 6,* 377–382.

Engel, B.T. (1982). Behavioral treatment of fecal incontinence. In R.S. Surwit, R.B. Williams, Jr., A. Steptoe, & R. Biersner (Eds.), *Behavioral treatment of disease: Proceedings of a NATO Symposium on Behavioral Medicine*. New York:

Plenum Press.

Engel, B.T., Nikoomanesh, P., & Schuster, M.M. (1974). Operant conditioning of rectrosphincteric responses in the treatment of fecal incontinence. *New England Journal of Medicine, 240*, 646–649.

Epilepsy Foundation of America. (1975). *Basic statistics on the epilepsies.* Philadelphia: F.A. Davis.

Finley, W.W. (1976). Effects of sham feedback following successful SMR training in an epileptic. Follow-up study. *Biofeedback and self-regulation, 1*, 227–236.

Finley, W.W. (1977). Operant conditioning of the EEG in two patients with epilepsy: Methodological and clinical considerations. *Pavlovian Journal of Biological Science, 12*, 93–111.

Flannery, R.B., Jr., & Cautela, J.R. (1973). Seizures: Controlling the uncontrollable. *Journal of Rehabilitation, 39*, 34–36.

Fordyce, W.E., Fowler, R.S., Lehman, J.R., DeLateur, B.J., Sand, P.L., & Trieschmann, R.B. (1973). Operant conditioning in the treatment of chronic pain. *Archives of Physical Medicine and Rehabilitation, 54*, 399–408.

Foxx, R.M., & Azrin, N.H. (1973). *Toilet training in the retarded.* Champaign, IL: Research Press.

Frank, K.A., Heller, S.S., Kornfeld, D.S., Sporn, A.A., & Weiss, M.D. (1978). Type A behavior pattern and coronary atherosclerosis. *Journal of the American Medical Association, 240*, 761–763.

Freedman, R.R., Lynn, S.J., & Ianni, P. (1982). Behavioral assessment of Raynaud's Disease. In F.J. Keefe & J.A. Blumenthal (Eds.), *Assessment strategies in behavioral medicine.* New York: Grune and Stratton.

Freedman, R.R., Lynn, S.J., & Ianni, P. (in press). Behavioral treatment of Raynaud's Disease. *Journal of Consulting and Clinical Psychology.*

Freedman, R., Lynn, S., Ianni, P., & Hale, P. (1981). Biofeedback treatment of Raynaud's disease and phenomenon. *Biofeedback and Self-Regulation, 6*, 355–364.

French, T.M., & Alexander, F. (1941). Psychogenic factors in bronchial asthma. *Psychosomatic Medicine Monograph. 1*, No. 4.

Friedman, M. (1980). [Progress report on the recurrent coronary prevention project]. Unpublished raw data.

Friedman, M., & Rosenman, R.H. (1974). *Type A behavior and your heart.* Greenwich, CT: Fawcett.

Goldman, H., Kleinman, K., Snow, M., Bidus, D.R., & Korol. (1975). Relationship between essential hypertension and cognitive function: Effects of biofeedback. *Psychophysiology, 12*, 569–573.

Goldstein, I.B., Shapiro, D., Thananopavarn, C., & Sambhi, M.P. (1982). Comparison of drug and behavioral treatments of essential hypertension. *Health Psychology, 1*, 7–26.

Gottlieb, H., Laban, C.S., Koller, R., Madorskey, A., Hackersmith, V., Kleeman, M., & Wagner, J. (1977). Comprehensive rehabilitation of patients having chronic low back pain. *Archives of Physical Medicine and Rehabilitation, 58*, 101–108.

Gracely, R.H., McGrath, P., & Dubner, R. (1978). Validity and sensitivity of ratio scales of sensory and affective verbal pain descriptors: Manipulation of affect by Diazepam. *Pain, 5*, 19–29.

Gracely, R.H., McGrath, R., & Dubner, R. (1979). Narcotic analgesic: Fentanyl reduces the intensity but not the unpleasantness of painful tooth pulp sensations. *Science, 203,* 1261–1263.

Haynes, S.G., Feinleib, M., Levine, S., Scotch, N., & Kannel, W. (1978). The relationship of psychosocial factors to coronary heart disease in The Framingham Study. *American Journal of Epidemiology, 107,* 384.

Haynes, S.N., Griffin, P., Mooney, D., & Parise, M. (1975). Electromyographic biofeedback and relaxation instructions in the treatment of muscle contraction headaches. *Behavior Therapy, 6,* 672–678.

Hendler, N., Derogatis, L., Avella, J., & Long, D. (1977). EMG biofeedback in patients with chronic pain. *Diseases of the Nervous System, 38,* 505–509.

Holden, C. (1978). Pain, dying and the health care system. *Science, 203,* 984–985.

Holroyd, K.A., Andrasik, F., & Westbrook, T. (1977). Cognitive control of tension headache. *Cognitive Therapy and Research, 1,* 121–133.

Jenni, M.A., & Wollersheim, J.P. (1979). Cognitive therapy, stress management training, and the Type A behavior pattern. *Cognitive Therapy and Research, 3,* 61–75.

Johnson, W.P., & Grover, J.A. (1976). Hemodynamic and metabolic effects of physical training in four patients with essential hypertension. *Canadian Medical Association Journal, 96,* 842.

Keefe, F.J. (1975). Conditioning changes in differential skin temperature. *Perceptual and Motor Skills, 40,* 283–288.

Keefe, F.J. (1978). Biofeedback vs. instructional control of skin temperature. *Journal of Behavioral Medicine, 1,* 383–390.

Keefe, F.J. (1982a). Behavioral treatment of Raynaud's disease. In P.A. Boudewyns & F.J. Keefe (Eds.), *Behavioral medicine in general medical practice.* Menlo Park, CA: Addison Wesley Publishing Company.

Keefe, F.J. (1982b). Behavioral assessment and treatment of chronic pain: Current status and future directions. *Journal of Consulting and Clinical Psychology, 50,* 896–911.

Keefe, F.J., & Block, A.R. (1982). Development of an observation method for assessing pain behavior in chronic low back pain patients. *Behavior Therapy, 13,* 363–375.

Keefe, F.J., Block, A.R., Williams, R.B., & Surwit, R.S. (1981). Behavioral treatment of chronic pain: Clinical outcome and individual differences in pain relief. *Pain, 11,* 221–231.

Keefe, F.J., & Blumenthal, J.A. (Eds.). (1982). *Assessment strategies in behavioral medicine.* New York: Grune and Stratton.

Keefe, F.J., Brown, C., Scott, D.S., & Ziesat, H. (1982). Behavioral assessment of chronic pain. In F.J. Keefe & J.A. Blumenthal (Eds.), *Assessment strategies in behavioral medicine.* New York: Grune and Stratton.

Keefe, F.J., Surwit, R.S., & Pilon, R.N. (1979). A one-year follow-up of Raynaud's patients treated with behavioral therapy techniques. *Journal of Behavioral Medicine, 2,* 385–391.

Keefe, F.J., Surwitt, R.S., & Pilon, R.N. (1980). Biofeedback autogenic training and progressive relaxation in the treatment of Raynaud's disease. *Journal of Applied Behavior Analysis, 13,* 3–11.

Keefe, F.J., Surwit, R.S., & Pilon, R.N. (1981). Collagen vascular disease: Can behavior therapy help? *Journal of Behavior Therapy and Experimental Psychiatry, 12*, 171–175.

Khan, A.V., Staerk, M., & Bonk, C. (1973). Role of counterconditioning in the treatment of asthma. *Journal of Psychosomatic Research, 17*, 389–392.

Kohlenberg, R.J., & Cahn, T. (1981). Self-help treatment for migraine headaches: A controlled outcome study. *Headache*, 196–200.

Kotses, H., & Glaus, K.D. (1981). Applications of biofeedback to the treatment of asthma: A critical review. *Biofeedback and Self-Regulation, 6*, 573–593.

Kotses, H., Glaus, K.D., Bricel, S.K., Edwards, J.E., & Crawford, P.L. (1978). Operant muscular relaxation and peak expiratory flow rate in asthmatic children. *Journal of Psychosomatic Research, 22*, 17–23.

Kotses, H., Glaus, K.D., Crawford, P.L., Edwards, J.E., & Scherr, M.S. (1976). Operant reduction of frontalis EMG activity in the treatment of asthma in children. *Journal of Psychosomatic Research, 20*, 453–459.

Kremer, E., Block, A., & Gaylor, M. (1981). Behavioral approaches to chronic pain: The inaccuracy of patient self-report measures. *Archives of Physical Medicine and Rehabilitation, 62*, 188–191.

Kristt, D.A., & Engel, B.T. (1975). Learned control of blood pressure in patients with high blood pressure. *Circulation, 51*, 370–378.

Lanyon, R.I. (1973). *Psychological Screening Inventory: Manual.* Goshen, NY: Research Psychologists' Press.

Lefebvre, M.F. (1981). Cognitive distortion and cognitive errors in depressed psychiatric and low back pain patients. *Journal of Consulting and Clinical Psychology, 49*, 517–525.

Lewis, T. (1949). *Vascular disorders of the limbs: Described for practitioners and students.* London: Macmillan.

Lisina, M.I. (1958). The role of orientation in the transformation of involuntary reactions into voluntary ones. In L. Voronin, A. Leontien, & A. Luria (Eds.), *Orienting reflex and exploratory behavior.* Washington, DC: American Institute of Biological Sciences.

Lubar, J.F. (1981). EEG operant conditioning in intractable epileptics: Controlled multidimensional studies. In L. White & B. Tursky (Eds.), *Clinical biofeedback: Efficacy and mechanisms.* New York: Guilford Press.

Lubar, F., & Deering, W.M. (1981). *Behavioral approaches to neurology.* New York: Academic Press.

Lynch, W.C., Hanna, H., Kohn, S., & Miller, N. (1976). Instrumental control of peripheral vasomotor responses in children. *Psychophysiology, 13*, 219–221.

Masland, R.L. (1976). Epidemiology and basic statistics on the epilepsies: Where are we? Paper presented at the Fifth National Conference on the Epilepsies, Washington, DC.

Meichenbaum, D., & Turk, D. (1976). The cognitive-behavioral management of anxiety, anger, and pain. In P.O. Davidson (Ed.), *Behavioral management of anxiety, depression, and pain.* New York: Brunner/Mazel.

Melzack, R., & Torgerson, W.S. (1971). On the language of pain. *Anesthesiology, 34*, 50–59.

Milne, J.S. (1976). Prevalence of incontinence in the elderly age groups. In E.L. Willington (Ed.), *Incontinence in the elderly.* London: Academic Press.

Mostofsky, D.J., & Balaschak, B. (1977). Psychobiological control of seizures. *Psychological Bulletin, 84*, 723–750.

Nagi, S.Z., Riley, L.E., & Newby, L.G. (1973). A social epidemiology of back pain in a general population. *Journal of Chronic Disease, 26*, 769–779.

Nouwen, A., & Solinger, J. (1979). The effectiveness of EMG biofeedback in low back pain. *Biofeedback and Self-Regulation, 4,* 103–112.

Olton, D.S. & Noonberg, A.R. (1980). *Biofeedback: Clinical applications in behavioral medicine.* Englewood Cliffs, NJ: Prentice-Hall, Inc.

Ounsted, C., Lee, D., & Hutt, S.J. (1966). Electroencephalographic and clinical changes in an epileptic child during repeated photic stimulation. *Electroencephalographic and Clinical Neurophysiology, 21*, 388–391.

Painter, J.R., Seres, J.L., & Newman, R.I. (1980). Assessing benefits of the pain center: Why some patients regress. *Pain, 8*, 101–113.

Parijs, J., Joossens, J.V., Van der Linden, L., Verstreken, G. & Amery, A.K. (1973). Moderate sodium restriction and diuretics in the treatment of hypertension. *American Heart Journal, 85*, 22.

Patel, C.H. (1973). Yoga and biofeedback in the management of hypertension. *Lancet, 2*, 1053–1055.

Patel, C.H. (1975). Yoga and biofeedback in the management of "stress" in hypertensive patients. *Clinical Science and Molecular Medicine, 48* (Suppl. 2,) 171–174.

Patel, C.H. (1977). Biofeedback-aided relaxation in the management of hypertension. *Biofeedback and Self-Regulation, 2*, 1–41.

Patel, C.H., & North, W.R.S. (1975). Randomized controlled trial of yoga and biofeedback in management of hypertension. *Lancet, 2*, 93–95.

Reeves, J.L., Shapiro, D., & Cobb, L.F. (1979). Relative influence of heart rate biofeedback and instructional set in the perception of cold pressor pain. In N. Birbaumer & H.D. Kimmel (Eds.), *Biofeedback and self-regulation.* Hillsdale, NJ: Erlbaum.

Reeves, J.L., & Victor, R.G. (1982). Behavioral strategies for treating hypertension. In P.A. Boudewyns & F.J. Keefe. (Eds.), *Behavioral medicine in general medical practice.* Menlo Park, CA: Addison-Wesley Publishing Company.

Renne, C.M., & Creer, T.L. (1976). The effects of training on the use of inhalation therapy equipment by children with asthma. *Journal of Applied Behavioral Analysis, 9*, 1–11.

Robertson, D., Frolick, J.C., Carr, R.K., Watson, J.T., Hollifield, J.W., Shand, D.G., & Oates, J.A. (1978). Effects of caffeine in plasma renin activity, catecholamines, and blood pressure. *New England Journal of Medicine, 298*, 181.

Rosenman, R.H., Brand, R.J., Jenkins, D., Friedman, M., Strauss, R., & Wurm, M. (1975). Coronary heart disease in the western collaborative group study: Final follow-up experience of 8½ years. *Journal of the American Medical Association, 233*, 872–877.

Rosenstiel, A.K., & Keefe, F.J. (in press). The use of coping strategies in chronic low back pain patients: Relationship to patient characteristics and current adjustment. *Pain.*

Roskies, E., Sperack, M., Surkis, A., Cohen, C., & Gilman, S. (1978). Changing the coronary prone (Type A) behavior pattern in a non-clinical population. *Jour-*

nal of Behavioral Medicine, 1, 201–216.

Rybstein-Blinchick, E. (1979). Effects of different cognitive strategies in the chronic pain experience. *Journal of Behavioral Medicine, 2*, 93–102.

Sanders, S. (1979). The behavioral assessment and treatment of chronic pain: Appraisal of current status. In M. Hersen, R. Eisler, & P. Miller (Eds.), *Progress in behavior modification* (Vol. 8). New York: Academic Press.

Sanders, S. (1980). Assessment of up-time in chronic low back pain patients: Comparison between self-report and automated measurement systems. Paper presented at the meeting of the Association for the Advancement of Behavior Therapy, New York, New York.

Sargent, J.D., Green, E.E., & Walters, E.D. (1973). Preliminary report on the use of autogenic feedback training in the treatment of migraine and tension headaches. *Psychosomatic Medicine, 35*, 129–135.

Schwartz, G.E., & Weiss, S.M. (1978). *Proceedings of the Yale Conference on Behavioral Medicine* (Publication No. [NIH] 78–1424). Washington, DC: Department of Health, Education and Welfare.

Shapiro, D. (1982). Hypertension from the standpoint of behavioral medicine. In R.S. Surwit, R.B. Williams, Jr., A. Steptoe, & R. Biersner (Eds.), *Behavioral treatment of disease: Proceedings of a NATO Symposium on Behavioral Medicine.* New York: Plenum Press.

Shapiro, D., & Goldstein, I.B. (1982). Biobehavioral perspectives on hypertension. *Journal of Consulting and Clinical Psychology, 50*, 841–858.

Shapiro, D., Tursky, B., Gershon, E., & Stern, M. (1969). Effects of feedback and reinforcement on the control of human systolic blood pressure. *Science, 163*, 588–590.

Shelton, J.L., & Levy, R.L. (1981). *Behavioral assignments and treatment compliance: A handbook of clinical strategies.* Champaign, IL: Research Press.

Sokolov, Y.N. (1963). *Perception and the conditioned reflex.* London: Pergamon Press.

Sterman, M.D., MacDonald, L.R., & Stone, R.K. (1974). Biofeedback training of the sensory motor electroencephalographic rhythm in man. Effects on epilepsy. *Epilepsia, 15*, 395–416.

Sterman, M.B., & Wyricka, W. (1967). EEG correlates of sleep: Evidence for separate forebrain substrates. *Brain Research, 6*, 143–163.

Sterman, M.B., Wyricka, W., & Roth, S.R. (1969). Electrophysiological correlates and neural substrates of alimentary behavior in the cat. *Annals of the New York Academy of Sciences, 157*, 723–739.

Suinn, R. (1975). The cardiac stress management programs for Type A patients. *Cardiac Rehabilitation, 5*, 13–15.

Suinn, R. (1977) *Manual: Anxiety management training.* Fort Collins, CO: Rocky Mountain Behavioral Science Institute.

Suinn, R., & Bloom, L. (1978). Anxiety management training of Pattern A behavior. *Journal of Behavioral Medicine, 1*, 25–35.

Surwit, R.S. (1973). Raynaud's disease. In L. Birk (Ed.), *Biofeedback: Behavioral Medicine.* New York: Grune and Stratton.

Surwit, R. S. (1982). Behavioral treatment of Raynaud's syndrome in peripheral vascular disease. *Journal of Consulting and Clinical Psychology, 6*, 922–932.

Surwit, R.S., Allen, L.M., III, Gilgor, R.S., Kuhn, Schanberg, S. & Duvic, M. (1982). The combined effect of prazosin and autogenic training on cold reactivity in Raynaud's phenomenon. *Biofeedback and Self-Regulation, 7*, 537–544.

Surwit, R.S., Bradner, M.N., Fenton, C.H., & Pilon, R.N. (1979). Individual differences in response to the behavioral treatment of Raynaud's disease. *Journal of Consulting and Clinical Psychology, 47*, 363–367.

Surwit, R.S., Pilon, R.N., & Fenton, C.H. (1978). Behavioral treatment of Raynaud's disease. *Journal of Behavioral Medicine, 1*, 323–335.

Surwit, R.S., Shapiro, D., & Feld, J.L. (1976). Digital temperature autoregulation and associated cardiovascular changes. *Psychophysiology, 13*, 242–248.

Surwit, R.S., Williams, R.B., Steptoe, A., & Biersner, R. (Eds.). (1982). *Behavioral treatment of disease: Proceedings of the NATO Symposium on Behavioral Medicine.* New York: Plenum Press.

Swanson, D.W., Swenson, M.W., Maruta, T., & McPhee, M.C. (1976). Program for managing chronic pain. I. Program description and characteristics of patients. *Mayo Clinic Proceedings, 51*, 401–408.

Taplin, P.S., & Creer, T.L. (1978). A procedure for using peak expiration flow rate data to increase the predictability of asthma episodes. *The Journal of Asthma Research, 16*, 15–19.

Taylor, C.B., Farquhar, J.W., Nelson, E., & Agras, S. (1977). Relaxation therapy and high blood pressure. *Archives of General Psychiatry, 34*, 339–342.

Turner, J.A. (1982). Comparison of group progressive-relaxation training and cognitive-behavioral group therapy for chronic low back pain. *Journal of Consulting and Clinical Psychology, 50*, 757–765.

Turner, J.A., & Chapman, C.R. (1982a). Psychological interventions for chronic pain: A critical review. I. Relaxation training and biofeedback. *Pain, 12*, 1–12.

Turner, J.A., & Chapman, C.R. (1982b). Psychological interventions for chronic pain: A critical review. II. Operant conditioning, hypnosis, and cognitive-behavioral therapy. *Pain, 12*, 23–46.

Tursky, B., Jamner, L., & Friedman, R. (1982). The pain perception profile: A psychophysical approach to the assessment of pain report. *Behavior Therapy, 13*, 376–394.

Urban, B.J. (1982). Therapeutic aspects in chronic pain: Modulation of nociception, alleviation of suffering, and behavioral analysis. *Behavior therapy, 13*, 430–437.

Vachon, L., & Rich, E.S. (1976). Visceral learning in asthma. *Psychosomatic Medicine, 38*, 122–130.

Varni, J.W. (1981). Self-regulation techniques in the management of chronic arthritic pain in hemophilia. *Behavior Therapy, 12*, 185–194.

White, A.W. (1966). Low back pain in men receiving workmen's compensation. *Canadian Medical Association Journal, 95*, 50–56.

Whitehead, W.E., Parker, L.H., Masek, B.J., Cataldo, M.F., & Freeman, J.M. (in press). Biofeedback treatment of fecal incontinence in meningomyocoele. *Developmental Medicine and Child Neurology.*

Williams, R.B., Haney, T.L., Lee, K.L., Kong, Y., Blumenthal, J.A., & Whalen, R.E. (1980). Type A behavior hostility and coronary atherosclerosis. *Psychosomatic Medicine, 42*, 539–549.

Williams, R.B., Lane, J.D., Kuhn, C.M., Melosh, W., White, A.D., & Schanberg,

S.M. (1982). Type A behavior and elevated physiological and neuroendocrine responses to cognitive tasks. *Science, 218*, 483–485.

Wolf, S.L., Nacht, M., & Kelly, J.L. (1982). EMG feedback training during dynamic movement for low back pain patients. *Behavior Therapy, 13*, 395–406.

Wright, L. (1976). Psychology as a health profession. *Clinical Psychologist, 29, 16*–19.

Young, G.C. (1973). The treatment of childhood encopresis by gastro-ileal reflex training. *Behaviour Research and Therapy, 11*, 499–503.

Zlutnick, S.I. (1972). The control of seizures by the modification of pre-seizure behavior: The punishment of behavioral chain components (Doctoral dissertation, Utah State College, 1972). *Dissertation Abstracts International, 33*, 63. (University Microfilms No. 72–31, 182)

Zlutnick, S.I., Mayville, W.J., & Moffat, S. (1975). Behavioral control of seizure disorders: The interruption of chained behavior. In R.C. Katz & S.I. Zlutnick (Eds.), *Behavior therapy and health care: Principles and applications.* Elmsford, NY: Pergamon Press.

Zyzanski, S.J., Jenkins, C.D., Ryan, T.J., Flessas, A., & Everist, M. (1976). Psychological correlates of coronary angiographic findings. *Archives of Internal Medicine, 136*, 1234–1237.

12

Research Issues in Clinical Child Psychology

Susan B. Campbell

INTRODUCTION

The field of clinical child psychology is growing rapidly, and has witnessed a remarkable increase in empirical research over the past decade. Historically, clinical child psychology has its roots in clinical theory and research on adults; much early work has been merely a downward extension of methodology, diagnostic categories, treatment approaches, and etiological models to younger populations. Unfortunately, this has meant that notions derived from work with adults are often applied to children whether appropriate or not, and there is not always adequate appreciation of developmental issues (see Campbell, 1983; Wenar, 1982). More recently, there has been a shift in perspective among *some* workers in the field and some attempt to examine childhood problems from a more developmental and contextual approach. Thus, the field of clinical child psychology in the 1980s is enriched by its roots in *both* clinical and developmental psychology; research questions and methodologies which take into account developmental processes and the consequences for both research and theory in dealing with an organism in a constant state of developmental change (see Overton & Reese, 1972) can only lead to more relevant and informed work on childhood problems.

The six preceding chapters on substantive areas in clinical psychology focus mainly, if not exclusively, on work with adults, but there is also considerable research in these and related areas with children. A review of publications devoted to child psychopathology and clinical child research reveals a number of areas which have attracted research attention and generated reasonable-to-excellent clinical research. Clinical child psychology is roughly 10 years behind the adult area in the delineation of widely accepted diagnostic categories, the development of moderately effective intervention strategies, and the construction of models to encompass a range of potential etiological factors. In my personal view, the field has progressed slowly partly because of its overdependence on methods and concepts derived from research with adults and the consequent absence of a truly developmental focus. Despite this, recent studies covering such diverse areas as diagnosis and classification, treatment efficacy and course of disorder, and family factors and childhood problems are beginning to bring some order into the field.

In this chapter I plan to briefly review several areas to provide a thumbnail sketch of recent trends in the clinical child field. I will cite several representative studies and, when applicable, recent review articles; an exhaustive review will not be attempted. Next, some theoretical and design issues which have particular relevance to child-oriented research will be addressed. This is meant to highlight methodological considerations which are of particular importance when studying a developing organism; these issues are rarely considered in the clinical literature, but derive from theoretical models which have dominated and shaped developmental psychology. Then, two research areas will be examined in more depth: (1) research on syndrome definition which stems from a relatively traditional clinical focus, and (2) research on family risk factors in the development of child psychopathology, some of which derives from a developmental model. Finally, a representative family risk study will be discussed in more detail.

RECENT RESEARCH TRENDS IN CLINICAL CHILD PSYCHOLOGY

In this section general trends in the field will be described. There will be no attempt at a critical appraisal of all areas since that would be beyond the scope of this chapter; a number of critical reviews already exist and are cited where appropriate. Research areas are listed in Table 12.1 to provide an overview of the field.

Epidemiological research in child psychopathology has focused on the prevalence of particular symptoms as reported by adults (parents or teachers) familiar with the child. Symptoms are examined as a function of age and sex in school-age samples using cross-sectional designs (e.g., Rutter, Tizard, & Whitmore, 1970; Shepherd, Oppenheim, & Mitchell, 1971; Werry & Quay, 1971). More recently attention has been paid to the prevalence of specific problems in children of preschool age and younger (e.g., Crowther, Bond, & Rolf, 1981; Earls, 1980; Richman, Stevenson, & Graham, 1982) and to rates of specific disorder, particularly hyperactivity-attention deficit disorder (e.g., Bosco & Robin, 1980; Trites, Dugas, Lynch, & Ferguson, 1979). In general, studies indicate higher rates of symptomatic behaviors in boys than in girls through early adolescence, particularly aggressive, defiant, and overactive behavior. Further, problem behaviors such as fears, worries, tantrums, and bedwetting are less common in older samples, suggesting age changes in the nature of common problems. Finally, studies indicate that while specific symptoms are common, rates of diagnosable disorder are relatively low (e.g., Rutter et al., 1970). However, the lack of clear diagnostic criteria makes the study of specific disorders rather difficult. Epidemiological studies which focus on the

Table 12.1. Representative Research Areas in Clinical Child Psychology

Research Areas
Epidemiology of childhood problems
Empirical classification of childhood disorders
Syndrome definition
childhood depression
attention deficit disorder-hyperactivity
Descriptive psychopathology
family correlates
cognitive correlates
social correlates
behavioral correlates
Assessment of childhood disorders
observational measures
psychological tests
diagnostic interviews
parent and teacher reports
self-reports
peer ratings
Treatment
behavioral and cognitive behavioral
psychopharmacology
Follow-up and outcome
Family risk-factors
family discord and dysfunction
pregnancy, birth, medical complications
parental psychopathology
environmental disadvantage

prevalence rates of common clusters of behavior known to interfere with functioning and to impede development are clearly the logical next step; further, studies must examine disorder not only within a developmental and social context, but over time, to determine the developmental significance of problem behaviors at different ages (Richman et al., 1982).

Closely related to work on perceived problems in childhood is the issue of diagnosis and classification. Although epidemiological studies may indicate relatively high rates of specific problem behaviors, frequencies of specific behaviors in isolation tell us little about actual disorder. Research examining clusters of problem behaviors which occur together and which may vary as a function of age, sex, and family factors is required to introduce some order into the classification area. Two main approaches to classification dominate the field: psychiatric description and empirical classification. The revised psychiatric nomenclature (DSM-III, American Psychiatric Association, 1980) includes more detailed descriptions of childhood disorders than were included in earlier editions. Further, these descriptive criteria have been derived from both research data and clinical experience; however, the usefulness of this classification system remains to be demonstrated empirically. Descriptions tend not to be developmental in nature (e.g., attention deficit disorder) and some diagnostic categories rely solely on adult criteria to diagnose childhood disorder (e.g., depression).

Within clinical child psychology, research on classification has taken a more empirical approach and literally hundreds of studies have examined clusters of adult-reported behavior problems in children. In general, empirical studies on classification subject parent or teacher ratings of a large number of symptomatic behaviors to factor analysis in order to derive clusters of symptoms which tend to occur together. After over 20 years of research on classification of childhood disorders (see recent reviews by Achenbach & Edelbrock, 1978, 1981; Quay, 1979), there is relatively wide agreement that children's problems can be characterized by two major or broad band factors: (1) externalizing or outer-directed behaviors high in annoyance value that sometimes interfere with the rights of others; and (2) internalizing or inner-directed problems reflected in quiet, withdrawn, and socially isolated behavior (Achenbach & Edelbrock, 1978). Within the framework of an empirical approach to classification, Achenbach and Edelbrock (1981) have recently developed and standardized a relatively comprehensive parent report measure, the Child Behavior Checklist, which provides normative data on symptom factors by age and sex and assesses both socially adaptive behavior and behavior problems.

There is good agreement on the existence of the two broad band factors of externalizing and internalizing behavior which appear repeatedly in factor analytic studies, but there is less agreement as to the specific subclassifications which constitute these broad band factors. Debate reflects a combination of the inconsistent factor structure obtained with different instruments (e.g., Achenbach & Edelbrock, 1981; Goyette, Conners, & Ulrich, 1978; Quay, 1977), varying theoretical viewpoints on the nature of childhood psychopathology (e.g., Lefkowitz & Burton, 1978; Petti, 1981), and the contradictory results obtained from empirical studies of syndrome definition (e.g., Milich, Loney, & Landau, 1982; Plomin & Foch, 1981). Recent debate has focused on the independence of hyperactivity and conduct problem diagnoses (Milich, Loney, & Landau, 1982; Sandberg, Rutter, & Taylor, 1978) and on whether or not childhood depression exists as a distinct diagnostic entity (e.g., Carlson & Cantwell, 1980; Lefkowitz & Burton, 1978).

It is obvious that a reliable diagnostic system which permits the selection of relatively homogeneous groups for research purposes is basic to the development of the field. Empirical study of behavioral and family correlates of disorder, developmental course, and the efficacy of particular therapeutic approaches all depend upon the researcher's ability to select a specific population for study. The field clearly has been hampered by this lack; erroneous conclusions have been drawn about etiology (e.g., see Rie & Rie, 1980, for a discussion of problems created by the diagnosis of "minimal brain dysfunction") and family correlates (e.g., Stewart, De Blois, & Cummings, 1980) because heterogeneous samples have been lumped together under misleading diagnostic labels.

Despite these diagnostic problems, there have been a number of studies which can be considered under the rubric of descriptive psychopathology. In particular, a large number of studies have begun to elucidate the cognitive, social, and familial correlates of childhood hyperactivity defined on the basis of parent and teacher ratings on standardized scales. There is surprisingly good consensus among studies indicating that hyperactive youngsters show specific deficits in sustained attention (Douglas & Peters, 1979) and impulse control (Douglas, 1980); that they do more poorly in the peer group since they are more aggressive and disruptive (Klein & Young, 1979; Pelham & Bender, 1982) and less popular than classroom controls (Klein & Young, 1979; Milich, Landau, Kilby & Whitten, 1982); that they perform more poorly in school (Barkley & Cunningham, 1978); and, that they engage in more negative and conflict-ridden interactions with parents (Cunningham & Barkley, 1979) and siblings (Mash & Mercer, 1979). Despite variations in sample definition and source, as well as methodology, findings have converged to indicate that hyperactive youngsters have difficulties that affect their day-to-day functioning at home, in school, and in the peer group and also interfere with optimal cognitive and social development (Ross & Ross, 1982). However, few studies have compared hyperactive youngsters to children with other types of disorder; therefore, it is not entirely clear which of these problems reflect psychopathology in general, which reflect externalizing problems, and which are specific to hyperactivity. Further, the relative role of family and child variables remains to be explored (Paternite & Loney, 1980).

Descriptive studies have also examined children labelled depressed (e.g., Leon, Kendall, & Garber, 1980), phobic (Hampe, Noble, Miller, & Barrett, 1973), learning disabled (Quay & Weld, 1980), conduct disordered (Thompson & Bernal, 1982), and autistic (Prior, 1979). Other researchers have taken a more conservative approach in view of diagnostic and definitional problems. Thus, for example, Forehand and his collaborators (e.g., Forehand & King, 1974; Peed, Roberts, & Forehand, 1977) have studied child non-compliance, while Patterson (1976, 1980) has defined his problem samples in terms of childhood aggression. Thus, these researchers have selected subjects who manifest a specific problem behavior in order to avoid the confusion inherent in diagnosing a more broadly defined disorder and on the apparent assumption that behaviors such as aggression and non-compliance serve as markers for more general problems reflecting externalizing symptomatology.

In order to accomplish the ardous task of diagnosis, we require an armamentarium of assessment instruments with adequate reliability and validity that are also appropriate for use with children of different developmental levels. While there has been renewed interest of late in the development of assessment measures, the majority of measures available are woefully inadequate. Assessment in the child psychopathology field can be divided into objective checklist/questionnaire measures which are either self-report or other report (parents, teachers, or peers), structured interview schedules for children and parents, standard psychological tests, and behavioral observations conducted in the laboratory or in the natural environment.

A good deal of recent research has emphasized the development of assessment measures, particularly parent and teacher checklists (e.g., Achenbach & Edelbrock, 1981), peer rating scales (e.g., Pekarik, Prinz, Liebert, Weintraub, & Neale, 1976), child self-report forms (e.g., Kovacs, 1980), and structured diagnostic interviews (e.g., Herjanic & Reich, 1982). The most progress has been made with structured adult rating scales and peer ratings, which appear to show surprisingly good reliability and validity relative to other assessment approaches. However, there is still a paucity of adequately designed child self-report forms and most do not provide age norms. It is unclear that self-report measures are appropriate for use with primary school-age children, although little attempt has been made to examine test reliability or validity as a function of age. Structured diagnostic interviews hold some promise, but they are a direct translation of adult interviews for use with children. While they may add to diagnostic information within a specific framework (i.e., DSM-III or Research Diagnostic Criteria), they fail to address the child's developmental history or take into account the child's developmental level. It is unlikely that questions appropriate for a 6 or 7-year-old are also appropriate for a 15-year-old, or that very young children can reliably report much of the information sought on these interviews. These measures are an improvement over unstructured clinical interviews, but they require further validation against other measures such as parent and teacher reports, behavioral observations, peer ratings, and independent clinician ratings.

Treatment outcome research has emphasized behavioral approaches including parent training (e.g., Peed et al., 1977), social skills training (e.g., La Greca & Santogrossi, 1980), and classroom management (e.g., Rosenbaum, O'Leary & Jacob, 1975). In addition, cognitive behavioral methods have been adapted for use with children. Hyperactive and aggressive children have been trained in attentional and self-control strategies (e.g., Camp, Blom, Herber, & van Doorninck, 1977; Kendall & Finch, 1978) and in social problem solving skills (Chandler, 1973). These studies were critically reviewed recently by Urbain and Kendall (1980), who concluded that cognitive techniques hold promise, but that problems with sample selection, and outcome measures, as well as lack of clear generalization and maintenance of treatment effects, problems which have also plagued more strictly behavioral approaches, have not been dealt with adequately.

Literally hundreds of treatment studies have examined the efficacy of stimulant medication with hyperactive children (see Barkley, 1977 for a review) and it is clear that roughly 70% of school-age hyperactive children show some symptomatic improvement with medication; however, debates continue on the ethical issues of drug treatment with children and on the long-term implications of medication use (see Whalen & Henker, 1980). Pharmacological studies abound with other groups as well (see Werry, 1978). More recently, studies have begun to examine the relative efficacy of drug treatment alone or in combination with parent training and/or cognitive behavioral approaches (e.g., Cohen, Sullivan, Minde, Novak, & Helwig, 1981; Gittelman-Klein, Klein, Abikoff, Katz, Gloisten, & Kates, 1976; O'Leary, 1980), with results consistently favoring medication over more psychological approaches, at least for short-term amelioration of symptoms.

Follow-up studies are particularly important when considering childhood problems since education and therapy decisions as well as public policy obviously must be influenced by factors such as whether problems in childhood persist or reflect a transient phase of development. Should scarce resources be provided for parent education? infant stimulation? child therapy? Will problems with early or late onset differ in their course, with some more likely than others to be outgrown? Results from a number of follow-up studies (e.g., Campbell, Breaux, Ewing, & Szumowski, in press; Loney, Kramer, & Milich, 1980; Richman et al., 1982; Robins, 1966; Weiss, Hechtman, & Perlman, 1978) converge to demonstrate that externalizing symptoms are likely to persist over time in preschoolers and school-age youngsters. Follow-up studies from school-age to young adulthood are particularly suggestive and indicate that environmental adversity, poor parenting, and aggressive behavior are associated with persistent problems.

As this brief overview indicates, there is a growing body of empirical research in clinical child psychology and a number of provocative research questions which remain to be resolved. However, much of this research is not conceptualized within a developmental framework and some important questions may, therefore, be overlooked.

RESEARCH ISSUES IN DEVELOPMENTAL PSYCHOPATHOLOGY

Inherent in models of development are several basic assumptions which necessarily shape research methodology (Overton & Reese, 1972). Developmental psychology has been influenced primarily by organismic and stage theories of ontogenetic change (e.g., Piaget, 1952; Werner & Kaplan, 1964) in which the child is construed as active rather than reactive, propelled by both internal and external forces toward growth and development. Organism-environment interactions are viewed as dynamic and transactional; that is, there is a continuous interplay of child-environment interaction which is reciprocal and constantly changing (McCall, 1977; Overton & Reese, 1972; Sameroff & Chandler, 1975). Since development is characterized by reorganization and transformation (e.g., Piaget's concepts of assimilation and accommodation), change is, by definition, neither linear nor quantitative. Rather, developmental transitions reflect reorganizations of the cognitive structures which underlie behavior and are characterized by shifts in focus from one developmental task to another (e.g., from a focus on mother-infant attachment to interest in peers or from object play to pretend play) (Garvey, 1977; Sroufe, 1979).

Clinical child psychology has been slow to integrate developmental thinking into conceptual formulations. Consequently, research questions have been primarily non-developmental in nature and age is rarely included as an independent variable in clinical research studies. For example, in studies of classification, symptoms are defined similarly across the age range from preschool to adolescence, and treatment approaches are often geared to target symptoms such as poor social skills or child non-compliance with little concern for the different meanings, manifestations, or implications of these problem behaviors at different ages.

There are several implications of a developmental viewpoint for clinical child research. First, problem behaviors must be defined in developmentally appropriate ways and measures must likewise be tailored to the child's developmental level. Second, if development is not linear, quantitative, or reactive, one can expect the manifestations of clinically significant problems to change over time; similarly, the nature of a particular behavior may change with age, though it may appear topographically similar. For example, aggression may be reflected in hitting, kicking, and yelling across the age range. However, with development there is a decrease in physical aggression and a concomitant increase in verbal aggression; further, the nature of aggressive encounters may also change (Feshbach & Feshbach, 1972; Hartup, 1974).

In preschoolers, aggressive encounters often ensue as a result of toy, space, or activity struggles; 3-year-olds Jimmy and Johnny both want to play with the same truck, ride the same tricycle, or dig in the same corner of the sandbox. Lacking the cognitive-developmental prerequisites to take the other child's perspective or to negotiate a fair exchange (e.g., sharing or turn-taking), a struggle is likely to ensue. What are the developmental implications of such an encounter in the preschool? Observations indicate that such toy struggles are relatively common (Smith & Green, 1975), although they show a dramatic decrease from toddlerhood through the early school years (e.g., Bakeman & Brownlee, 1982; Hartup, 1974). From a cognitive-developmental perspective, increased inability to see the other's point of view is reflected in a decrease in toy struggles and a concomitant increase in organized social exchanges involving sharing and turn-taking (Rubin, 1980).

With increased cognitive development, person-oriented aggression becomes more common than object-oriented aggression. Person-oriented aggression is often elicited by a threat to one's self-esteem (Hartup, 1974) and thus, is dependent upon a more advanced level of cognitive development which can accommodate a sense of self and the ability to perceive the behavior of another as threatening in a psychological sense. From this vantage point, changes in the antecedents of aggression are interpreted to reflect major transformations in the organization of social cognition and highlight the importance of studying both the sequence of observable behaviors and children's cognitive constructions of their social world. These findings come primarily from cross-sectional studies of non-clinical samples. We know little about the nature of aggressive behavior in problem children or whether problem children show similar developmental changes in the manifestations or antecedents of aggressive outbursts (Campbell & Cluss, 1982). Clinically significant aggression in school-age youngsters, however, appears to have prognostic implications (Milich & Loney, 1979; Robins, 1979).

This raises another important issue for clinical research with children. As McCall (1977) has noted, to be truly developmental, research must be longitudinal. Cross-sectional studies have allowed us to piece together data about age-related developmental change and to make inferences about differences among age groups. However, it is generally agreed that children do not all develop in a uniform manner and that individual differences in genes, environments, and gene-environment transactions insure that children do not follow the same developmental track (McCall, 1981; Sameroff & Chandler, 1975; Sroufe, 1979). Thus, to understand intraindividual transitions in development the same children must be studied longitudinally (e.g., McCall, Eichorn, & Hogarty, 1977).

For example, longitudinal studies may suggest that there are individual differences in the organization and timing of developmental transitions and in the degree of continuity or discontinuity observed in development. Environmental differences may likewise be associated with variations in development. For example, there is evidence that environmental factors such as family discord, poor economic circumstances, and parental psychopathology are associated with persistent symptoms in troubled children, while problem children living in more harmonious and supportive families are more likely to outgrow their difficulties with or without treatment (e.g., Paternite & Loney, 1980; Richman et al., 1982). That is, children from differing environments follow different developmental paths (McCall, 1981) and environmental factors are associated with differing degrees of developmental continuity. Other recent longitudinal studies suggest individual differences in children's initial reactions and their adaptations over time to stressful life events such as divorce, the birth of a sibling, and environmental instability (e.g., Dunn & Kendrick, 1980; Hetherington, Cox, & Cox, 1978; Rutter, 1981; Vaughn, Egeland, Sroufe, & Waters, 1979; Wallerstein & Kelly, 1980). Thus, many of the central questions in clinical child psychology require longitudinal designs and focus on the nature of change as a function of child and family characteristics, environmental events, and social circumstances.

The lack of longitudinal data and controls for developmental change have led to misconceptions about the nature of change in clinical populations. For example, 20 years ago, clinicians assumed that hyperactivity was outgrown in adolescence (e.g., Eisenberg, 1966). This conclusion was based on cross-sectional studies of non-clinical samples and on short-term follow-up studies which lacked non-clinical comparison groups to control for age changes in relevant behaviors. Better designed studies (e.g., Weiss et al., 1978) indicate that the manifestations of problem behavior change with development, but that hyperactive youngsters continue to have more cognitive and social difficulties in young adulthood than non-clinical controls.

Similarly, it is often assumed that children's fears and anxieties are transient developmental phenomena (see Campbell, in press). However, there is surprisingly little longitudinal research on the natural course of children's fears and worries across the life span. Cross-sectional evidence on age differences in the nature of specific fears indicates changes which reflect cognitive development (e.g., fear of concrete objects vs. imaginary creatures) and changes which mirror developmental tasks (e.g., separation distress in infancy, reluctance about entry into the peer group in toddlerhood, social and achievement concerns among school-age children). However, there is little evidence available to indicate whether an anxious and insecure infant develops into a fearful preschooler or a socially anxious fourth grader. The appropriate longitudinal studies have not been done, partly because the manifestations of children's anxieties would be expected to change with development, making definitional and measurement problems formidable. Furthermore, there is considerable debate within developmental psychology on the nature of behavioral continuity and whether the expectation of continuity is consistent with a transactional model of development (e.g., Brim & Kagan, 1980; McCall, 1977; Sameroff & Chandler, 1975; Sroufe, 1979). However, for the clinical child psychologist prognostic questions have both theoretical and practical importance, making longitudinal studies of clinical phenomena of particular relevance.

Thus, developmental models paired with a focus on clinically relevant issues have the potential to sensitize child psychopathology researchers to the complexities of developmental change, the difficulties of defining the behavioral manifestations of problems in appropriate developmental terms, the importance of longitudinal designs with appropriate comparison groups to control for developmental change, and the need to examine children's problems within a family and social context. Further, as Sroufe (1979) has cogently argued, we need not find continuities in specific behaviors in order to see coherence in development.

Representative Research Areas

As noted in the introduction to this chapter, there are a number of provocative issues in the clinical child field attracting considerable attention from researchers. Two will be selected for more detailed discussion because they highlight some important problems in clinical child research and because they derive more directly either from a clinical or from a developmental framework. First, some issues in syndrome definition will be examined using attention deficit disorder-hyperactivity as the example. Second, studies concerned with the identification of children at risk to develop psychopathology will be discussed.

Syndrome Definition. Studies indicate that broad factors of externalizing and internalizing symptomatology emerge consistently from factor analyses of ratings of childhood behavior problems (Achenbach & Edelbrock, 1978), but there is less consistency in findings on subclassifications within these broad problem areas. Thus, a body of research has examined the degree to which behaviors which theoretically define a clinically significant disorder co-vary. In particular, there has been considerable debate about whether hyperactivity is a distinct symptom complex, a syndrome in the more traditional sense, or a facet of a more generalized externalizing disorder which is characterized also by aggression and defiance (conduct disorder).

Factor analytic research indicates that a high activity level, attentional problems, and poor impulse control co-vary and that these behaviors can be seen as a distinct cluster of symptoms (e.g., Achenbach & Edelbrock, 1981; Loney, Langhorne, & Paternite, 1978). Further, children who are rated as hyperactive by parents and/or teachers differ from non-clinical comparison groups on a range of objective measures of sustained attention, impulsivity, restlessness, academic achievement, and social interaction. This very large body of findings has been reviewed in a number of recent articles and books (e.g., Barkley, 1981; Douglas & Peters, 1979; Milich & Landau, 1982; Ross & Ross, 1982; Whalen & Henker, 1980). Although there is still debate on whether or not objective measures of these behaviors co-vary as well (e.g., Sandberg et al., 1978; Schroeder, Milar, Wool, & Routh, 1980; Spring, Greenberg, & Yellin, 1977), this cluster of symptoms has been incorporated into DSM-III under the label "Attention Deficit Disorder with Hyperactivity" (APA, 1980).

In order to establish the validity of a diagnostic construct, it is necessary to demonstrate that children with the relevant target symptoms differ from comparison groups in meaningful ways. While studies do demonstrate that children labeled hyperactive differ from non-clinical control groups on a variety of measures of target symptoms, the constructs of activity level, attention deficit, and impulse control are themselves not clearly defined and different definitions and methods of measurement have led to confusing findings. For example, numerous studies have demonstrated that hyperactive youngsters have difficulty sustaining attention, but results are less consistent when the effects of distractors are examined. Thus, the definition of attention deficit (sustained attention, selective attention, distractibility, attentional focus, etc.) requires further refinement (Douglas & Peters, 1979; Rosenthal & Allen, 1978), although it is widely agreed that attentional problems are a core feature of the disorder (APA, 1980; Barkley, 1980).

Variations in methodology have also led to inconsistent findings and made it difficult to generalize across studies. For example, studies which focus primarily on activity level (Battle & Lacey, 1972) differ in their results from studies which have included a more broadly defined syndrome which includes attentional problems and poor impulse control (Cunningham & Barkley, 1979; Milich et al., 1982). Samples also differ in exclusion criteria such as level of IQ cut-off and the presence or absence of brain-injured children (e.g., Milich, Loney, & Landau, 1982; Schroeder et al., 1980). Further, some researchers have employed non-clinical samples of children rated on parent and/or teacher questionnaires (Lahey, Green, & Forehand, 1980; Sandberg, Weiselberg, & Shaffer, 1980); others have included only children seeking treatment in a clinical setting (Loney et al., 1978; Weiss et al., 1978). Referral and rating sources differ as well and there is often little overlap among children seen as problematic by parents, teachers, and pediatricians (Lambert, Sandoval, & Sassone, 1978; Plomin & Foch, 1981), prompting some investigators only to include children rated as a problem by both teachers and parents (Barkley, 1980).

Samples also differ in age and in age range. In view of developmental changes in symptom expression (Campbell, 1983; Ross & Ross, 1982), it is important to examine age differences which may otherwise obscure results. With this in mind, some investigators have preferred to study homogeneous age groups (Campbell, Szumowski, Ewing, Gluck, & Breaux, 1982; Prinz, Connor, & Wilson, 1981) or to include cross-sectional age comparisons (Paulauskas & Campbell, 1979). Further, some studies include both boys and girls in their samples (Lahey et al., 1980); others are restricted to boys only (Milich, Loney, & Landau, 1982) given the much higher ratio of hyperactive boys to hyperactive girls (Trites et al., 1979) and the consequent difficulty finding a large enough sample of girls to analyze sex differences.

In addition, hyperactive children are not in constant motion or continuously inattentive. Thus, inconsistent findings may reflect, in part, the erratic nature of hyperactivity, making test-retest reliability a problem and highlighting the importance of multidimensional, cross-situational assessments during which children are observed on more than one day (e.g., Campbell et al., 1982). Finally, ecological factors influence behavior. Hyperactive youngsters have more difficulty controlling their inappropriate behavior in highly structured situations and in responding to rules and regulations than they have dealing with less structured situations in which minimal demands are made (e.g., Cunningham & Barkley, 1979; Henker & Whalen, 1980). Further, ecological factors appear to interact with developmental level. Hyperactive preschoolers have a difficult time focusing on toys even during free play (Campbell et al., 1982), whereas school-age youngsters do not consistently differ from controls during an unstructured play observation (Plomin & Foch, 1981). Findings from one follow-up study (Weiss et al., 1978) suggest that hyperactive young adults fare better once they leave the sedentary environment of the classroom and seek employment in positions permitting more activity and stimulation. Thus, this is a complex area in which definitional problems are compounded by problems with sample composition, the selection and measurement of relevant behavioral variables, developmental changes, and situational factors. Indeed, given the variation across studies, and the many potential sources of error, it is surprising that findings converge as well as they do.

There is relatively wide agreement, then, that hyperactivity represents a diagnostically meaningful cluster of symptoms. However, there is less agreement about whether it constitutes a syndrome (Loney, 1980; Ross & Ross, 1982). Research on etiology, plagued by the methodological problems just noted as well as the difficulty of establishing causality in psychological studies, has been relatively inconclusive. Few people in the field assume that there is one identifiable cause of hyperactivity; rather, there is some consensus that more complex multifactor models which consider constitutional and environmental transactions must be employed (Loney, 1980; Ross & Ross, 1982). Studies of symptom course and outcome have been more consistent in indicating that problems persist in a large proportion of children and that antisocial difficulties become prominent in adolescence and early adulthood (e.g., Ackerman, Dykman, & Peters, 1977; Paternite & Loney, 1980; Weiss et al., 1978). These findings have intensified the debate on whether hyperactivity is a distinct disorder since follow-up studies indicate that course and outcome, as well as family correlates of poor outcome, parallel results from studies of conduct disordered youth (Robins, 1979; Rutter et al., 1970).

Studies have indicated some convergent validity among measures of target symptoms: attentional problems, high activity level, and poor impulse control groups, some findings may not be specific to hyperactivity, but may reflect psychopathology in general, or more particularly externalizing symptstrate. Since most studies in the field have not included other psychiatric control groups, some findings may not be specific to hyperactivity, but may reflect psychopathology in general, or more particularly externalizing symptoms. Other critics of the hyperactivity construct cite the high correlations between conduct disorder and hyperactivity factors (Lahey et al., 1980; Sandberg et al., 1978).

This issue has likewise generated research on both sides of the debate. Several researchers have attempted to demonstrate the similarity in behavioral correlates, family history, and potential etiological factors among children rated high on symptoms of conduct disorder and those rated high on hyperactivity measures (Lahey et al., 1980; Sandberg et al., 1978; Sandberg, Wieselberg & Shaffer, 1980; Stewart et al., 1980). However, these studies, too, are far from definitive. Both Lahey et al. (1980) and Sandberg et al. (1980) studied non-clinical samples and Lahey et al.'s sample was half female. In both studies rating scales alone were used to assess symptomatic behaviors. Sandberg et al. examined only parent-reported historical information and psychosocial stress, along with biological markers (minor physical anomalies) which are not specific to hyperactivity but characterize children with a range of behavior and learning problems (Krouse & Kauffman, 1982). Not surprisingly, children rated high on conduct disorder factors did not differ from hyperactive youngsters on most measures. No direct measures of child behavior or attention were included. Furthermore, since teachers and parents rated different children as disturbed, children were probably not severely impaired and, thus, the significance of these findings is questionable.

Lahey et al. (1980) found that teacher ratings of conduct disorder and hyperactivity did not contribute significant independent variance to criterion measures including peer ratings, classroom behavior, or achievement test performance. However, studies which attempt to define syndromes on the basis of inter-relationships among clinically significant measures in non-clinical samples are based on the implicit assumption that problem children differ from non-problem controls only quantitatively and that behaviors are organized similarly. From a developmental, transactional view, this assumption in itself would be questionable and open to empirical investigation. Furthermore, it is clear that there are sex differences in the organization and patterning of symptomatic behaviors (Achenbach & Edelbrock, 1981) and the inclusion of girls and boys in these analyses may have biased these results in unknown ways.

Stewart and his colleagues (Stewart et al., 1980; Stewart, Cummings, Singer, & De Blois, 1981) studied the family characteristics and psychiatric status of consecutive admissions to a child psychiatry clinic. Children and parents were diagnosed on the basis of independent psychiatric interviews. Unfortunately, DSM-III criteria were not used to diagnose hyperactive or aggressive disorders and the criteria which were employed were not entirely appropriate to the 3 to 16 year age range included. Despite these problems, some children were diagnosed as aggressive, some as hyperactive, and some as both hyperactive and aggressive. Children who were considered hyperactive only were, not surprisingly, less severely impaired than aggressive youngsters on several symptom scales derived from the clinical interviews, but they had more academic problems. Further, there was a slightly lower prevalence of alcoholism among fathers of hyperactive-only boys as compared to children who were aggressive (with or without hyperactivity).

Sandberg et al. (1978) also question the existence of hyperactivity as distinct from general conduct disorder. They studied 68 boys referred to a child psychiatry clinic; measures included behavioral observations and psychological tests along with interview and questionnaire data. Boys rated above a cutoff on the hyperactivity factor of the teacher or parent versions of the Conners questionnaire did not differ from the remaining subjects on most measures. However, children diagnosed as hyperactive by psychiatrists did differ from comparison subjects on measures of impulsivity and cognitive functioning. They were also likely to demonstrate neurological immaturities and their problems were of earlier onset.

These investigators have interpreted their data to indicate that most children rated as hyperactive by parents and teachers demonstrate externalizing symptoms including restlessness, attentional problems, and impulsivity characteristic of hyperactivity, and aggression and non-compliance characteristic of conduct disorder. In contrast, Loney and her colleagues (Loney & Milich, 1981; Milich, Loney, & Landau, 1982; Paternite & Loney, 1980) argue that hyperactivity and aggression are distinct problems with a different etiology, course, and outcome. Further, Loney contends that the confusion and contradiction in the field reflect the failure of researchers and clinicians to carefully discriminate these problems in research studies or clinical practice. Thus, conclusions are based on a heterogeneous group of hyperactive, aggressive, and hyperactive-aggressive youngsters.

In a series of empirical studies, Loney and her co-workers have demonstrated that hyperactivity and aggression contribute unique variance to concurrent measures of child behavior and to outcome. In a heterogeneous group of male clinic attenders, Milich, Loney, & Landau (1982) reported that independent chart ratings of hyperactivity and aggression contributed unique variance to maternal and teacher ratings of hyperactivity and inattention. Chart ratings of hyperactivity did not, however, contribute to ratings of conduct disorder. Hyperactivity scores likewise contributed unique variance to behavioral indices obtained during free play and structured tasks. Furthermore, in a series of replications, these investigators have found that among a sample of hyperactive boys treated with Ritalin, childhood aggression and environmental factors are associated with poor outcome in adolescence and that this prediction is independent of hyperactivity ratings at intake or follow-up (Paternite & Loney, 1980). While these outcome data are not inconsistent with the arguments of Sandberg and others, they highlight the importance of assessing these two symptom dimensions independently. Loney and others found that although hyperactivity and aggression are associated, not all hyperactive youngsters are aggressive and not all aggressive youngsters show attentional deficits (Loney et al., 1978; Prinz et al., 1981; Stewart et al., 1980). This debate is far from resolved, but it underlines the importance of studying clinical samples when clinically significant behaviors are at issue, of carefully defining the symptoms of interest, and of employing multiple measures from multiple sources including parent and teacher ratings, school information, and behavioral observations in a naturalistic setting (Whalen & Henker, 1980).

Identification of Children At Risk for Psychopathology. The search for risk factors which render children vulnerable to develop problems in childhood and/or adulthood has generated a good deal of recent research. In particular studies have examined pregnancy and birth complications, economic deprivation, marital discord, and parental pathology as possible precursors of later cognitive and social difficulties. In general, when these factors have been examined individually, results have been inconclusive and have underlined the importance of studying the combined impact of multiple risk factors. For example, Sameroff and Chandler (1975) reviewed studies of reproductive risk and concluded that pregnancy and birth complications were often correlates of psychosocial stress and disadvantage. However, the combined effect of a poorly functioning infant in a less than optimal caretaking environment was more likely to set up a cyclical pattern of poor infant functioning and unresponsive caretaking and to lead to continued difficulties than either birth complications or psychosocial stress alone.

Early work on parental psychopathology as a risk factor focused on the offspring of schizophrenic women and was geared to the study of the etiology of schizophrenia in a sample at higher risk to develop the disorder than children selected from the general population (e.g., Mednick & Schulsinger, 1968). Since roughly 10% of children of schizophrenic mothers themselves become schizophrenic and another 30 to 40% develop other disorders (Gottesman, 1978), the probability of finding early indicators of psychopathology is increased. However, most adult schizophrenics do not have a schizophrenic parent, suggesting that many relevant risk factors have not yet been identified. Further, study of a sample of children at risk for schizophrenia prior to the onset of disorder avoids the problem inherent in most studies of adult schizophrenics; that is, the inability to separate causal factors from correlates of disorder or from the effects of chronic mental illness. Since the majority of risk studies focus on children raised in a family with a schizophrenic parent, genetic factors and family interaction and communication patterns are still confounded, making it impossible to disentangle the relative contribution of genetic and environmental factors or to clarify specific aspects of the widely accepted diathesis-stress model (Garmezy, 1978; Gottesman, 1978; Sameroff,

Seifer, & Zax, 1982). In addition, differing selection criteria in early high risk research have led to the study of biased samples which in turn has resulted in inconsistent and spurious findings (Mednick, 1978; Sameroff et al., 1982).

One major problem with early high risk studies was the failure to include psychiatric control groups. Thus, it was difficult to determine whether differences between the offspring of schizophrenic mothers and offspring of nonclinical controls reflected vulnerabilities specific to schizophrenia or the effects of being raised by a disturbed parent. Therefore, more recent studies have included offspring of other disturbed groups to control for the effects of psychopathology per se. These studies almost uniformly suggest that the majority of group differences reflect severe and chronic psychopathology rather than a specific parental diagnosis and cast doubt upon conclusions drawn about schizophrenia from early high risk studies. For example, in several recent studies few differences have been found between offspring of schizophrenic parents and offspring of depressives on a variety of cognitive, attentional, and school-related measures, although both groups differed from controls (Emery, Weintraub, & Neale, 1982; Rolf, 1976; Weintraub, Prinz, & Neale, 1978; Winters, Stone, Weintraub, & Neale, 1981). Children of schizoprenics performed more poorly than children of depressives on language and cognitive measures designed to assess thought disorder (Harvey, Weintraub, & Neale, 1982; Oltmanns, Weintraub, Stone, & Neale, 1978). In addition, Garmezy (1974) reported that children of schizophrenic mothers showed attentional deficits which were less amenable to environmental manipulations than the attentional deficits of offspring of depressives and externalizing clinic children. Thus, impairment on a range of measures of social and cognitive functioning appear to be associated with having a severely disturbed parent. More subtle measures of attention deficit and thought disorder may be specific to schizophrenia and may identify school-age children at risk for later pathology (Oltmanns et al., 1978).

Studies which fail to pinpoint differences between offspring of schizophrenics and offspring of parents with other disorders are difficult to interpret. The most parsimonious explanation of these findings is that severe pathology is more relevant than specific symptoms in its impact on children. However, developmental issues may also be relevant here. Studies have found few differences between the social behavior and cognitive development of infants as a function of maternal diagnosis (Grunebaum, Cohler, Kauffman, & Gallant, 1978; Sameroff & Zax, 1978). Severe pathology may translate into less consistent, reciprocal, or predictable patterns of early maternal caretaking which over-ride more subtle distinctions in symptom expression when children are young, but may become more differentiated in older children. Similarly, peer and teacher ratings which tend not to differentiate among a number of school-age risk groups (Rolf, 1976; Weintraub, Neale, & Liebert, 1975; Weintraub et al., 1978) may indicate that naive raters are making global assessments of disordered behavior rather than the fine distinctions made by researchers. Observational studies of peer relations may indicate more subtle differences in communicative competence or friendship initiations. The specific cognitive and attentional differences noted by Garmezy (1974) and the Stony Brook group (Harvey et al., 1982; Oltmanns et al., 1978) may not be apparent until children reach a certain level of cognitive development, at which time more subtle aspects of "cognitive slippage" and attention deficit can be assessed. Given the difficulty in finding large samples of families in which a parent meets stringent diagnostic criteria, few researchers have been able to restrict their samples to children within a narrow age range. Therefore, the specific behavioral manifestations of risk status as a function of age have yet to be described in detail.

Recent studies have been conceptualized from a developmental perspective with an emphasis on the early development of children at risk, rather than on precursors of schizophrenia per se (Garmezy, 1978; Neale & Weintraub, 1975; Sameroff et al., 1982), and with an interest in prevention as well as onset and course of disorder (Rolf & Hasazi, 1977). Further, several of these studies have examined combinations of factors thought to place infants and children at risk. In general, they indicate that parental diagnosis per se is less predictive of child maladjustment than a range of variables which may interact with or correlate with parental psychopathology. For example, Sameroff and Zax (1973) examined the relationship among maternal diagnosis, severity of psychopathology, maternal anxiety, and obstetric and birth complications. They found that severity of disorder and maternal anxiety during pregnancy were associated with more obstetric and neonatal complications. Emery et al., (1982) found that a high level of marital discord characterized couples with a schizophrenic or a depressed member, but that both psychiatric groups differed from controls. However, among offspring of a depressed parent, marital discord appeared to mediate behavior problems in school as perceived by teachers and peers. Thus, parental pathology may be seen as contributing to marital dysfunction and a less than optimal emotional climate in the home which, in turn, is reflected in impaired school functioning and peer relationships.

Findings from the Rochester Child and Family Study (Baldwin, Cole, & Baldwin, 1982) likewise implicate family variables other than specific diagnosis in child maladjustment. These investigators found that lack of parent-child reciprocity in interaction and parental unavailability were associated with poorer school functioning regardless of diagnosis. Furthermore, the typical functioning of the disturbed parent appeared to be more clearly associated with the child's functioning than the level of disturbance during an acute episode. Finally, if the child's relationship with either parent was characterized by reciprocity the child was more likely to perform adequately in school, suggesting that a positive relationship with one parent can ameliorate the possible negative consequences of parental disturbance, a finding which highlights the importance of examining the overall caretaking environment.

Among the more ambitious high risk studies is the Rochester Longitudinal Study (Sameroff et al., 1982) in which the impact of multiple risk factors on infant and child development was examined in a prospective study. This research was selected for more detailed discussion because of its prospective, longitudinal design and the inclusion of multiple, developmentally-appropriate measures focused on maternal behavior, child behavior, and mother-child interaction. This study also highlights some of the dilemmas facing child psychopathology researchers resilient enough to undertake longitudinal studies.

Risk factors examined in the Rochester study included maternal psychopathology assessed in terms of severity and chronicity as well as diagnosis, social status, race, and family size. Maternal diagnoses (schizophrenic, neurotic depressive, personality disorder, no-illness control) were based on specific criteria and a standardized assessment measure was employed; inter-rater reliability for diagnostic categories was established and was relatively high. Further, criteria for chronicity and severity ratings were operationalized on the basis of number of symptoms and frequency of psychiatric contacts. While these may seem like basic requirements in any study of psychopathology, varying and loose diagnostic practices have made cross-study comparisons a problem in some high risk research (see discussion by Winters et al., 1981).

An additional problem in much clinical child research, including high risk research, is the issue of sample representativeness. Truly representative samples are difficult to obtain and even more difficult to maintain in longitudinal studies. The nature of problems varies as a function of referral source, even within a diagnostic group, and as a function of inclusion and exclusion criteria (e.g., Mednick, 1978). Since a county-wide psychiatric register is kept in the Rochester area, Sameroff et al. (1982) were able to select pregnant women who were listed in the register, rather than rely on physician or self-referrals. However, even this system was not bias-free, since women had to be receiving prenatal care in particular facilities and some of the more severely dysfunctional pregnant women may have been missed. Despite this, the distribution of diagnoses in the sample was reasonably similar to the distribution of diagnoses in the community-at-large, suggesting that this sample was relatively representative of people seeking psychiatric services in the county. It is not clear from this report, however, how many women who were eligible for the study refused to participate; refusals undoubtedly occurred, possibly among the more severely impaired women eligible to take part.

Inherent in studies with patient populations and in studies of psychosocial risk factors are problems with correlated and confounded variables. These are a fact of life, making "clean" factorial studies an impossibility and requiring the use of multiple regression techniques to examine the relative contributions of various related factors. In the Sameroff et al. study: (a) not all diagnostic groups were equally well represented; (b) severity of illness and diagnosis were not totally independent; (c) race and social class were confounded, such that all minority group members were from the lower social classes; and (d) family size was confounded with race and social class, with poorer black families having more children than middle class white families. While diagnostic groups and no mental illness controls were relatively well matched on demographic factors such as age, parity, marital status, race, and educational level, these factors varied widely within each group. For example, women ranged in age from 15 to 46 and 26% were unmarried. It is reasonable to assume that teen-age mothers were more likely to be unmarried and poor. Poverty, marital status, and teen-age parenthood can all be construed as interacting risk factors, independent of a diagnosed mental disorder. These are the realities of risk research and artificial restriction of samples to homogeneous groups of intact or middle class families will lead to their own set of interpretive problems. These are decisions that researchers must make at the start of a study and they are partly a trade-off of "purity" for reality. Sameroff et al.'s sample appears fairly representative of mentally ill women delivering infants, but the multiple confounds mean that variables such as social class, marital status, and family size may obscure the effects of maternal mental illness.

A third major and unavoidable problem confronted by investigators willing to undertake longitudinal research is that of sample attrition. Sameroff et al. were faced with a 22% attrition between prenatal assessment and 4-month follow-up and an additional 9% by 30 months. That is, of the initial 337 women seen for prenatal assessments, only 234 were available at 30 months. While Sameroff et al. report that attrition was approximately equal across diagnostic groups and that drop-outs and remainers were similar in demographics, no specific data on characteristics of drop-outs are provided. It is interesting to note, however, that four schizophrenic women out of a sample of 29 gave their infants up for adoption. It is, therefore, likely that more severely impaired women dropped out of the study, further complicating data interpretation. Even among relatively less disturbed samples, it is not uncommon for more severely dysfunctional families to drop out of longitudinal studies (e.g., Campbell et al., in press), clearly biasing the sample even further.

Despite these unavoidable problems with sample composition and attrition, this study is a vast improvement over previous studies of infants at risk. A major plus is the use of a prospective design which permitted assessment of maternal attitudes and maternal psychopathology prior to the birth of the target child, rather than reliance on retrospective assessment which might have been contaminated by problems with recall and by postpartum difficulties;

further, careful assessment of obstetric, delivery, and neonatal complications was likewise possible and, therefore, it was not necessary to rely on retrospective reports or incomplete birth records. Neonatal behavior could also be evaluated, permitting some description of infant behavior prior to and uncontaminated by experience being raised by a mentally ill mother.

This study is also one of the few to integrate developmental psychology with a prospective study of children at risk for problems of development. A homogeneous age-group of children was assessed at important developmental transition points. The data are, therefore, available to examine within-subject changes as a function of a range of environmental risk factors. Age-appropriate measures were included, reflecting the "state-of-the-art" methods of assessing infant responsiveness and interactive capacity at birth, as well as cognitive and social-emotional development and mother-infant interaction at 4 months and 12 months. Further, measures were multidimensional and included standardized assessments of infant behavior and cognitive functioning, observational measures of mother-infant interaction and quality of attachment, and maternal report measures. Thus, assessment focused on infant, mother, and dyadic interactional variables measured over the first year, consistent with a transactional model of development. Unfortunately, the 30 and 48 month assessments rely almost exclusively on maternal reports and psychological tests. In addition, it is not clear whether infant examiners or behavioral coders were blind to mental illness status and diagnosis of the mother. If not, these data may be biased in unknown ways.

This study was geared to evaluating whether a specific diagnosis, schizophrenia, was reflected in impaired maternal functioning, delayed or atypical infant development, or dysfunctional patterns of dyadic interaction; whether severe and chronic mental illness in the mother was associated with impaired development of infant or mother irrespective of diagnosis; or whether multiple risk factors, including maternal mental illness, had a combined impact on infant and maternal behavior. Results indicated that low social class and severity of maternal pathology had a more deleterious influence on infant development and maternal caretaking than specific diagnosis. In a more recent report, Sameroff (1983) noted that risk factors had an additive and linear effect on the child's cognitive functioning at age 4 with factors such as social class, race, and family composition, as well as severity of maternal impairment, having a profound impact on outcome.

In summary, although this study is not without its interpretive problems, it has numerous strengths which make it a model of developmental psychopathology research. The prospective design and repeated multidimensional assessments exemplify the fruitful application of methods and concepts drawn from developmental psychology to questions which derive from developmental psychopathology and clinical child psychology.

SUMMARY

In this chapter I have described research issues in developmental psychology which have a bearing on the nature of research questions and the design of research studies in child psychopathology. In particular, I have emphasized the need for longitudinal designs which examine children using developmentally-appropriate measures and assess age changes within subjects. Further, I have argued that children should be studied within a family and social context and that clinically-significant behaviors are probably best studied in carefully defined clinical populations. In addition, a brief overview of the field was provided, with emphasis placed on issues of syndrome definition (a necessary first step for research progress) and the identification of factors which place infants and young children at developmental risk.

REFERENCES

Achenbach, T.M., & Edelbrock, C. (1978). The classification of child psychopathology: A review and analysis of empirical efforts. *Psychological Bulletin, 85,* 1275–1301.

Achenbach, T.M., & Edelbrock, C. (1981). Behavioral problems and competencies reported by parents of normal and disturbed children aged four through sixteen. *Monographs of the Society for Research in Child Development, 46* (1, Serial No. 188).

Ackerman, P.T., Dykman, R.A., & Peters, J.E. (1977). Teenage status of hyperactive and non-hyperactive learning disabled boys. *American Journal of Orthopsychiatry, 47,* 577–596.

American Psychiatric Association. (1980). *Diagnostic and statistical manual of mental disorders.* Washington, DC: Author.

Bakeman, R., & Brownlee, J.R. (1982). Social rules governing object conflicts in toddlers and preschoolers. In K. Rubin & H. Ross (Eds.), *Peer relationships and social skills in childhood.* New York: Springer-Verlag.

Baldwin, A.L., Cole, R.E., & Baldwin, C.P. (1982). Parental pathology, family interaction, and the competence of the child in school. *Monographs of the Society for Research in Child Development, 47* (5, Serial No. 197).

Barkley, R. (1977). A review of stimulant drug research with hyperactive children. *Journal of Child Psychology and Psychiatry, 18,* 137–165.

Barkley, R.A. (1980). Specific guidelines for defining hyperactivity (attention deficit disorder) in children. In B. Lahey & A. Kazdin (Eds.), *Advances in child clinical psychology* (Vol. 4). New York: Plenum.

Barkley, R.A. (1981). *Hyperactive children: A handbook for diagnosis and treatment.* New York: Guilford Press.

Barkley, R.A., & Cunningham, C.E. (1978). Do stimulant drugs improve the academic performance of hyperactive children? A review of outcome studies. *Clinical Pediatrics, 17,* 85–92.

Battle, E.S., & Lacy, B. (1972). A context for hyperactivity in children over time. *Child Development, 43,* 757–773.

Bosco, J.J., & Robin, S.S. (1980). Hyperkinesis: prevalence and treatment. In C. Whalen & B. Henker (Eds.), *Hyperactive children: The social ecology of identification and treatment.* New York: Academic Press.

Brim, O., & Kagan, J. (Eds.) (1980). *Constancy and change in human development.* Cambridge, MA: Harvard University Press.

Camp, B.W., Blom, G.E., Herbert, F., & van Doorninck, W.J. (1977). "Think Aloud": A program for developing self-control in young aggressive boys. *Journal of Abnormal Child Psychology, 5,* 157–170.

Campbell, S.B. (1983). Developmental perspectives in child psychopathology. In T. Ollendick & M. Hersen (Eds.), *Handbook of child psychopathology,* New York: Plenum.

Campbell, S.B. (in press). Developmental issues in children's anxieties and fears. In R. Gittelman (Ed.), *Anxiety disorders in children.* New York: Guilford Press.

Campbell, S.B., Breaux, A.M., Ewing, L., & Szumowski, E.K. (in press). A one-year follow-up of parent-identified "hyperactive" toddlers. *Journal of the American Academy of Child Psychiatry.*

Campbell, S.B., & Cluss, P. (1982). Peer relationships of young children with behavior problems. In K.H. Rubin & H.S. Ross (Eds.), *Peer relationships and social skills in childhood.* New York: Springer-Verlag.

Campbell, S.B., Szumowski, E.K., Ewing, L.J., Gluck, D.S., & Breaux, A.M. (1982). A multidimensional assessment of parent-identified behavior problem toddlers. *Journal of Abnormal Child Psychology, 10,* 569–591.

Carlson, G.A., & Cantwell, D.P. (1980). Unmasking masked depression in children and adolescents. *American Journal of Psychiatry, 137,* 445–449.

Chandler, M. (1973). Egocentrism and antisocial behavior: The assessment and training of social perspective-taking skills. *Developmental Psychology, 9,* 326–332.

Cohen, N.J., Sullivan, J., Minde, K., Novak, C., & Helwig, C. (1981). Evaluation of the relative effectiveness of methylphenidate and cognitive behavior modification in the treatment of kindergarten-aged hyperactive children. *Journal of Abnormal Child Psychology, 9,* 43–54.

Crowther, J.K., Bond, L.A., & Rolf, J.E. (1981). The incidence, prevalence, and severity of behavior disorders among preschool-aged children in day care. *Journal of Abnormal Child Psychology, 9,* 23–42.

Cunningham, C.E., & Barkley, R.A. (1979). The interactions of normal and hyperactive children with their mothers in free play and structured tasks. *Child Development, 50,* 217–224.

Douglas, V.I. (1980). Treatment and training approaches to hyperactivity: Establishing external or internal control. In C.K. Whalen & B. Henker (Eds.), *Hyperactive children: The social ecology of identification and treatment.* New York: Academic Press.

Douglas, V.I., & Peters, K. (1979). Toward a clearer definition of the attentional deficit of hyperactive children. In G. Hale & M. Lewis (Eds.), *Attention and the development of cognitive skills.* New York: Plenum.

Dunn, J., & Kendrick, C. (1980). The arrival of a sibling: Changes in patterns of interaction between mother and first born child. *Journal of Child Psychology and Psychiatry, 21,* 119–132.

Earls, F. (1980). Prevalence of behavior problems in 3-year-old children. *Archives of General Psychiatry, 37,* 1153–1157.

Eisenberg, L. (1966). The management of the hyperkinetic child. *Developmental Medicine and Child Neurology, 8,* 593–598.

Emery, R., Weintraub, S., & Neale, J.M. (1982). Effects of marital discord on the school behavior of children of schizophrenic, affectively disordered, and normal parents. *Journal of Abnormal Child Psychology, 10,* 215–228.

Feshbach, N., & Feshbach, S. (1972). Children's aggression. In W.W. Hartup (Ed.), *The young child: Reviews of research* (Vol. 2). Washington, DC: National Association for the Education of Young Children.

Forehand, R., & King, H.E. (1974). Preschool children's non-compliance: Effects of short-term behavior therapy. *Journal of Community Psychology, 2,* 42–44.

Garmezy, N. (1974). The study of competence in children vulnerable to psychopathology. In E.J. Anthony & C. Koupernik (Eds.), *The child in his family: Children at psychiatric risk.* New York: Wiley.

Garmezy, N. (1978). Observations on high-risk research and premorbid development in schizophrenia. In L.E. Wynne, R.L. Cromwell, & S. Matthysse (Eds.), *The nature of schizophrenia: New approaches to research and treatment.* New York: Wiley.

Garvey, C. (1977). *Play.* Cambridge, MA: Harvard University Press.

Gittelman-Klein, R., Klein, D.F., Abikoff, H., Katz, S., Gloisten, C., & Kates, W. (1976). Relative efficacy of methylphenidate and behavior modification in hyperkinetic children: An interim report. *Journal of Abnormal Child Psychology, 4,* 361–379.

Gottesman, I.I. (1978). Schizophrenia and genetics: Where are we? Are you sure? In L.C. Wynne, R.L. Cromwell, & S. Matthysse (Eds.), *The nature of schizophrenia: New approaches to research and treatment.* New York: Wiley.

Goyette, C.H., Conners, C.K., & Ulrich, R.F. (1978). Normative data on revised Conners Parent and Teacher Rating Scales. *Journal of Abnormal Child Psychology, 6,* 221–236.

Grunebaum, H., Cohler, B.J., Kauffman, C., & Gallant, D. (1978). Children of depressed and schizophrenic mothers. *Child Psychiatry and Human Development, 8,* 219–228.

Hampe, E., Noble, H., Miller, L.C., & Barrett, C.L. (1973). Phobic children one and two years post-treatment. *Journal of Abnormal Psychology, 82,* 446–453.

Hartup, W.W. (1974). Aggression in childhood: Developmental perspectives. *American Psychologist, 29,* 336–341.

Harvey, P.D., Weintraub, S., & Neale, J.M. (1982). Speech competence of children vulnerable to psychopathology. *Journal of Abnormal Child Psychology, 10,* 373–388.

Henker, B., & Whalen, C.K. (1980). The changing faces of hyperactivity: Retrospect and prospect. In C.K. Whalen & B. Henker (Eds.), *Hyperactive children: The social ecology of identification and treatment.* New York: Academic Press.

Herjanic, W.R., & Reich, W. (1982). Development of a structured psychiatric interview for children: Agreement on diagnosis comparing child and parent interviews. *Journal of Abnormal Child Psychology, 10,* 307–324.

Hetherington, E.M., Cox, M., & Cox, R. (1978). The aftermath of divorce. In J.H. Stevens & M. Matthews (Eds.), *Mother-child, father-child relations.* Washington, DC: National Association for the Education of Young Children.

Kendall, P.C., & Finch, A.J. (1978). A cognitive-behavioral treatment for impulsivity: A group comparison study. *Journal of Consulting and Clinical Psychology, 46,* 110–118.

Klein, A.R., & Young. (1979). Hyperactive boys in their classroom: Assessment of teacher and peer perceptions, interactions, and classroom behaviors. *Journal of Abnormal Child Psychology, 7,* 425–442.

Kovacs, M. (1980). Rating scales to assess depression in school-aged children. *Acta Paedopsychiatry, 46,* 305–315.

Krouse, J.P., & Kauffman, J.M. (1982). Minor physical anomalies in exceptional children: A review and critique of research. *Journal of Abnormal Child Psychology, 10,* 247–264.

La Greca, A.M., & Santogrossi, D.A. (1980). Social skills training with elementary school children: A behavioral group approach. *Journal of Consulting and Clinical Psychology, 48,* 220–228.

Lahey, B.B., Green, K.D., & Forehand, R. (1980). On the independence of ratings of hyperactivity, conduct problems, and attention deficits in children: A multiple regression analysis. *Journal of Consulting and Clinical Psychology, 48,* 566–574.

Lambert, N.M., Sandoval, J., & Sassone, D. (1978). Prevalence of hyperactivity in elementary school children as a function of social system definers. *American Journal of Orthopsychiatry, 48,* 446–463.

Lefkowitz, M.M., & Burton, N. (1978). Childhood depression: A critique of the concept. *Psychological Bulletin, 85,* 716–726.

Leon, G.R., Kendall, P.C., & Garber, J. (1980). Depression in children: Parent, teacher, and child perspectives. *Journal of Abnormal Child Psychology, 8,* 221–236.

Loney, J. (1980). Hyperkinesis comes of age: What do we know and where should we go? *American Journal of Orthopsychiatry, 50,* 28–42.

Loney, J., Kramer, J., & Milich, R. (1980). The hyperkinetic child grows up: Predictors of symptoms, delinquency, and achievement at follow-up. In K.D. Gadow & J. Loney (Eds.), *Psychosocial aspects of drug treatment for hyperactivity.* Boulder, CO: Westview Press.

Loney, L., Langhorne, J.E., & Paternite, C.E. (1978). An empirical basis for subgrouping the hyperkinetic/minimal brain dysfunction syndrome. *Journal of Abnormal Psychology, 87,* 431–441.

Loney, J., & Milich, R. (1981). Hyperactivity, inattention, and aggression in clinical practice. In M. Wolraich & D.K. Routh (Eds.), *Advances in behavioral pediatrics* (Vol. 2). Greenwich, CT: JAI Press.

Mash, E.J., & Mercer, B.J. (1979). A comparison of the behavior of deviant and nondeviant boys while playing alone and interacting with a sibling. *Journal of Child Psychology and Psychiatry, 20,* 197–208.

McCall, R.B. (1977). Challenges to a science of developmental psychology. *Child Development, 48,* 333–344.

McCall, R.B. (1981). Nature-nurture and the two realms of development: A proposed integration with respect to mental development. *Child Development, 52,* 1–12.

McCall, R.B., Eichorn, D.B., & Hogarty, P.S. (1977). Transitions in early mental development. *Monographs of the Society for Research in Child Development, 42,* (3, Serial No. 177).

Mednick, S.A. (1978). Berkson's fallacy and high-risk research. In L.C. Wynne, R.L. Cromwell, & S. Matthysse (Eds.), *The nature of schizophrenia: New approaches to research and treatment.* New York: Wiley.

Mednick, S.A., & Schulsinger, F. (1968). Some premorbid characteristics related to breakdown in children with schizophrenic mothers. In D. Rosenthal & S. Kety (Eds.), *The transmission of schizophrenia.* Elmsford, NY: Pergamon Press.

Milich, R., & Landau, S. (1982). Socialization and peer relations in hyperactive children. In K.D. Gadow & I. Bialer (Eds.), *Advances in learning and behavior disabilities* (Vol. 1). Greenwich, CT: JAI Press.

Milich, R., Landau, S., Kilby, G., & Whitten, P. (1982). Preschool peer perceptions of the behavior of hyperactive and aggressive children. *Journal of Abnormal Child Psychology, 10,* 497–510.

Milich, R., & Loney, J. (1979). The role of hyperactive and aggressive symptomatology in predicting adolescent outcome among hyperactive children. *Journal of Pediatric Psychology, 4,* 93–112.

Milich, R., Loney, J., & Landau, S. (1982). Independent dimensions of hyperactivity and aggression: A validation with playroom observation data. *Journal of Abnormal Psychology, 91,* 183–198.

Neale, J.M., & Weintraub, S. (1975). Children vulnerable to psychopathology: The Stony Brook High-Risk Project. *Journal of Abnormal Child Psychology, 3,* 95–114.

O'Leary, K.D. (1980). Pills or skills for hyperactive children? *Journal of Applied Behavior Analysis, 13,* 191–204.

Oltmanns, T.F., Weintraub, S., Stone, A.A., & Neale, J.M. (1978). Cognitive slippage in children vulnerable to psychopathology. *Journal of Abnormal Child Psychology, 6,* 237–246.

Overton, W.F., & Reese, H.W. (1972). Models of development: Methodological implications. In J.R. Nesselroade & H.W. Reese (Eds.), *Life-span developmental psychology: Methodological issues.* New York: Academic Press.

Paternite, C.E., & Loney, J. (1980). Childhood hyperkinesis: Relationships between symptomatology and home environment. In C. Whalen & B. Henker (Eds.), *Hyperactive children: The social ecology of identification and treatment.* New York: Academic Press.

Patterson, G.R. (1976). The aggressive child: Victim and architect of a coercive system. In E.J. Mash, L.A. Hamerlynck, & L.C. Handy (Eds.), *Behavior modification and families.* New York: Brunner/Mazel.

Patterson, G.R. (1980). Mothers: The unacknowledged victims. *Monographs of the Society for Research in Child Development, 45* (Serial No. 186).

Paulauskas, S.L., & Campbell, S.B. (1979). Social perspective-taking and teacher ratings of peer interaction in hyperactive boys. *Journal of Abnormal Child Psychology, 20,* 233–246.

Peed, S., Roberts, M., & Forehand, R. (1977). Evaluation of the effectiveness of a standardized parent training program in altering the interaction of mothers and their non-compliant children. *Behavior Modification, 1,* 323–350.

Pekarik, E.G., Prinz, R.J., Liebert, D.E., Weintraub, S., & Neale, J.M. (1976). The Pupil Evaluation Inventory: A sociometric technique for assessing children's social behavior. *Journal of Abnormal Child Psychology, 4,* 83–97.

Pelham, W., & Bender, M.E. (1982). Peer relationships in hyperactive children: Description and treatment. In K.D. Gadow & I. Bialer (Eds.), *Advances in learning and behavioral disabilities* (Vol. I). Greenwich, CT: JAI Press.

Petti, T.A. (1981). Depression in children – A significant disorder. *Psychosomatics, 22,* 444–447.

Piaget, J. (1952). *The language and thought of the child.* London: Routledge & Kegan Paul.

Plomin, R., & Foch, T.T. (1981). Hyperactivity and pediatrician diagnosis, parental ratings, specific cognitive abilities, and laboratory measures. *Journal of Abnormal Child Psychology, 9,* 55–64.

Prinz, R.J., Connor, P.A., & Wilson, C.C. (1981). Hyperactive and aggressive behaviors in childhood: Intertwined dimensions. *Journal of Abnormal Child Psychology, 9,* 191–202.

Prior, M.R. (1979). Cognitive abilities and disabilities in infantile autism: A review. *Journal of Abnormal Child Psychology, 7,* 357–380.

Quay, H.C. (1977). Measuring dimensions of deviant behavior: The Behavior Problem Checklist. *Journal of Abnormal Child Psychology, 5,* 277–288.

Quay, H.C. (1979). Classification. In H.C. Quay & J.S. Werry (Eds.), *Psychopathological disorders of childhood* (2nd ed.). New York: Wiley.

Quay, L., & Weld, G.L. (1980). Visual and auditory selective attention and reflection-impulsivity in normal and learning disabled boys at two age levels. *Journal of Abnormal Child Psychology, 8,* 117–126.

Richman, N., Stevenson, J., & Graham, P.J. (1982). *Preschool to school: A behavioural study.* London: Academic Press.

Rie, H.E., & Rie, E.D. (1980). *Handbook of minimal brain dysfunction: A critical review.* New York: Wiley.

Robins, L.N. (1966). *Deviant children grown up.* Baltimore: Williams & Wilkins.

Robins, L.N. (1979). Follow-up studies. H.C. Quay & J.S. Werry (Eds.), *Psychopathological disorders of childhood* (2nd ed.). New York: Wiley.

Rolf, J.E. (1976). Peer status and the directionality of symptomatic behavior: Prime social competence predictors of outcome for vulnerable children. *American Journal of Orthopsychiatry, 46,* 74–88.

Rolf, J.E., & Hasazi, J.E. (1977). Identification of preschool children at risk and some guidelines for primary prevention. In G.W. Albee & J.M. Joffe (Eds.), *Primary prevention of psychopathology: Vol. I. The issues.* Hanover, NH: University Press of New England.

Rosenbaum, A., O'Leary, K.D., & Jacob, R.G. (1975). Behavioral intervention with hyperactive children: Group consequences as a supplement to individual contingencies. *Behavior Therapy, 6,* 315–323.

Rosenthal, R.H., & Allen, T.W. (1978). An examination of attention, arousal, and learning dysfunctions of hyperkinetic children. *Psychological Bulletin, 85,* 689–715.

Ross, D.M., & Ross, S.A. (1982). *Hyperactivity: Theory, research, and action* (2nd ed.). New York: Wiley.

Rubin, Z. (1980). *Children's friendships*. Cambridge, MA: Harvard University Press.

Rutter, M. (1981). Stress, coping, and development: Some issues and some questions. *Journal of Child Psychology and Psychiatry, 22,* 323–356.

Rutter, M., Tizard, J., & Whitmore, K. (1970). *Education, health and behaviour*. London: Longman.

Sameroff, A.J. (1983, April). *Sources of continuity in parent-child relations.* Paper presented at the Society for Research in Child Development, Detroit.

Sameroff, A.J., & Chandler, M.J. (1975). Reproductive risk and the continuum of caretaking casualty. In F.D. Horowitz (Ed.), *Review of child development research* (Vol. 4). Chicago: University of Chicago Press.

Sameroff, A.J., Seifer, R., & Zax, M. (1982). Early development of children at risk for emotional disorder. *Monographs of the Society for Research in Child Development, 47* (7, Serial No. 199).

Sameroff, A.J., & Zax, M. (1973). Perinatal characteristics of the offspring of schizophrenic women. *Journal of Nervous and Mental Disease, 157,* 191–199.

Sameroff, A.J., & Zax, M. (1978). In search of schizophrenia. Young offspring of schizophrenic women. In L.C. Wynne, R.L. Cromwell, & S. Matthysse (Eds.), *The nature of schizophrenia: New approaches to research and treatment.* New York: Wiley.

Sandberg, S., Rutter, M., & Taylor, E. (1978). Hyperkinetic disorder in psychiatric clinic attenders. *Developmental Medicine and Child Neurology, 20,* 279–299.

Sandberg, S.T., Wieselberg, M., & Shaffer, D. (1980). Hyperkinetic and conduct problem children in a primary school population: Some epidemiological considerations. *Journal of Child Psychology and Psychiatry, 21,* 293–312.

Schroeder, S.R., Milar, C., Wool, R., & Routh, D.K. (1980). Multiple measurement, transituational diagnosis, and the concept of generalized overactivity. *Journal of Pediatric Psychology, 5,* 365–376.

Shepherd, M., Oppenheim, B., & Mitchell, S. (1971). *Childhod behaviour and mental health.* New York: Grune and Stratton.

Smith, P.K., & Green, M. (1975). Aggressive behavior in English nurseries and play groups: Sex differences and response of adults. *Child Development, 46,* 211–214.

Spring, C., Greenberg, L.M., & Yellin, A.M. (1977). Agreement of mothers' and teachers' hyperactivity ratings with scores on drug-sensitive psychological tests. *Journal of Abnormal Child Psychology, 5,* 199–214.

Sroufe, L.A. (1979). The coherence of individual development: Early care, attachment, and subsequent developmental issues. *American Psychologist, 34,* 834–841.

Stewart, M.A., Cummings, C., Singer, S., & De Blois, C.S. (1981). The overlap between hyperactive and unsocialized aggressive children. *Journal of Child Psychology and Psychiatry, 22,* 35–46.

Stewart, M.A., De Blois, C.S., & Cummings, C. (1980). Psychiatric disorder in the parents of hyperactive boys and those with conduct disorder. *Journal of Child Psychology and Psychiatry, 21,* 283–292.

Thompson, R.J., & Bernal, M.E. (1982). Factors associated with parent labeling of children referred for conduct problems. *Journal of Abnormal Child Psychology, 10,* 191–202.

Trites, R.L., Dugas, E., Lynch, G., & Ferguson, H.B. (1979). Prevalence of hyperactivity. *Journal of Pediatric Psychology, 4,* 179–188.

Urbain, E.S., & Kendall, P.C. (1980). Review of social-cognitive problem-solving interventions with children. *Psychological Bulletin, 88,* 107–143.

Vaughn, B., Egeland, B., Sroufe, L.A., & Waters, E. (1979). Individual differences in infant-mother attachment at 12 and 18 months: Stability and change in families under stress. *Child Development, 50,* 971–975.

Wallerstein, J.S., & Kelly, J.B. (1980). *Surviving the break-up: How parents and children cope with divorce.* New York: Basic Books.

Weintraub, S., Neale, J.M., & Liebert, D.E. (1975). Teacher ratings of children vulnerable to psychopathology. *American Journal of Orthopsychiatry, 45,* 838–845.

Weintraub, S., Prinz, R., & Neale, J.M. (1978). Peer evaluations of the competence of children vulnerable to psychopathology. *Journal of Abnormal Child Psychology, 6,* 461–473.

Weiss, G., Hechtman, L., & Perlman, T. (1978). Hyperactives as young adults: School, employer, and self-rating scales obtained during ten-year follow-up evaluation. *American Journal of Orthopsychiatry, 48,* 438–445.

Wenar, C. (1982). Developmental psychopathology: Its nature and models. *Journal of Clinical Child Psychology, 11,* 192–201.

Werner, H., & Kaplan, B. (1964). *Symbol formation: An organismic-developmental approach to language and the development of thought.* New York: Wiley.

Werry, J.S. (Ed.). (1978). *Pediatric psychopharmacology: The use of behavior modifying drugs in children.* New York: Brunner/Mazel.

Werry, J.S., & Quay, H.C. (1971). The prevalence of behavior symptoms of younger elementary school children. *American Journal of Orthopsychiatry, 41,* 136–143.

Whalen, C.K., & Henker, B. (1980). The social ecology of psycho-stimulant treatment: A model for conceptual and empirical analysis. In C.K. Whalen & B. Henker (Eds.), *Hyperactive children: The social ecology of identification and treatment.* New York: Academic Press.

Winters, K.C., Stone, A.A., Weintraub, S., & Neale, J.M. (1981). Cognitive and attentional deficits in children vulnerable to psychopathology. *Journal of Abnormal Child Psychology, 9,* 435–454.

Part 4
GENERAL ISSUES

13

The Evaluation of Research: An Editorial Perspective

Sol L. Garfield

INTRODUCTION

Practically all the research conducted in any field usually goes through some form of evaluation. The evaluation may occur at the beginning of the research process or it may come after the actual investigation has been completed. There also may be more than one period of evaluation. It would appear, then, that evaluation is a regular part of the research enterprise and can occur at different stages as well as under different auspices.

Probably the first serious exposure to research evaluation that most clinical psychologists have is when they are preparing the research proposal for their doctoral dissertation. The focus here is on the evaluation of the design of the proposed study and whether the study is feasible and worth doing. Clearly, this is an exceedingly important aspect of research and research evaluation for it has to do with the potential value of the study as well as its feasibility. Both aspects are important. A proposed study may appear to be of potentially great significance but it may not be possible to carry it out with the time and resources available. On the other hand, a potential study may be completed with ease and dispatch, but be of little significance. If more researchers paid serious attention to such matters, a significant amount of effort and eventual frustration might be avoided. However, with the pressure on individuals to secure doctoral degrees and to publish reports of research, such desirable changes are not very likely to occur.

Generally, however, when we talk of evaluating research, we usually have reference to a completed research project or to a scholarly and critical review of the research literature on a specific topic. In both such instances an editorial evaluation may be involved. In most instances, when an investigator has completed a research project, he/she will usually want to publish a report of the project so that the findings become available to other investigators in the area and make their contribution to the accumulated body of knowledge. Although there may be other reasons for wanting to see one's work published and to see one's name in print, the basic and accepted reason for scientific and scholarly publication is the contribution of new knowledge. Whether or not everyone really believes this, it does serve as the guiding principle for editors of high quality scientific journals.

Since the usual and ultimate outlet for a research investigation is some form of publication, it is important for the researcher to be well informed concerning what constitutes good research as well as the requirements for preparing a potentially publishable manuscript. Each particular scientific or professional field has its own specialized criteria for evaluating research, but there are many commonalities among them. These include the importance of the research carried out, the adequacy of the research design, and the manner in which the research was conducted and evaluated. All of these are of some significance, and the research investigator needs to pay attention to all of them. A deficiency or limitation in any one aspect can seriously affect how the research project will be appraised. For example, a potentially important project on the possible genetic factors in schizophrenic disorders can be dismissed completely if there are serious defects in the research design or in the manner in which the research was conducted. In a similar fashion, a very carefully designed and well conducted study of a seemingly trivial and unimportant topic also will not receive much serious or positive attention. A very well designed study comparing the number of fingers possessed by patients diagnosed as having unipolar depression as contrasted with the number manifested by cases of bipolar depression would probably not be viewed very favorably, even if the samples contained 100,000 cases and the latest statistical techniques were used.

A final point to be made in this introductory section is that research findings also have to be communicated clearly and effectively. The research process usually begins with the planning of a research project to answer some question or test some hypothesis in which the investigator is interested and culminates in an oral or written report of the findings secured. This latter phase of the research process generally has not received sufficient attention. If the research findings are not communicated clearly, the potential significance of the research may be misinterpreted or not fully appreciated. Furthermore, if the results of the research investigation are written up and presented in a particularly poor manner, they may never be accepted for publication in a scholarly journal. The net result is that the expected contribution from the research project is severely limited. It is important, therefore, that the investigator pay sufficient attention to this final aspect of the research process; more will be said about it later in this chapter.

EVALUATING RESEARCH

As indicated, once a research project has been completed, the usual next step is to attempt to communicate the findings to other workers in the field. One may submit a report or abstract of the study to a program committee where the intent is to present a report of the research at a professional meeting. In this instance, members of the program committee will conduct some sort of evaluation of the study and decide whether or not it should be accepted for presentation at the meeting. If judged favorably, it will be accepted for presentation at the meeting; if judged unfavorably, it will be rejected and not placed on the program.

For many individuals, this may be the first real evaluation of their research endeavor by their professional peers. It is also a clear reminder to those involved that scientific (and clinical) research is essentially an open system where one's work is judged by his/her peers. Unfortunately, the individual who has submitted his work to the program committee receives little feedback from the committee beyond the decision made. In other words, the person is simply told that the paper has been accepted for the program or has been rejected. The reasons for the latter are usually not given although it is not uncommon for the committee to try to lessen the impact of rejection by stating that so many excellent papers were submitted that they could not all be placed on the program—or offering some other kindly euphemism. Actually, it would be far better for the individual to be given a frank and honest appraisal of his/her work since the kindly, but not quite honest, appraisal does not help such individuals to evaluate their work accurately.

There is little question that all of us need to be able to appraise the value of our work realistically. As clinical psychologists, we realize that this is not easy to do and that we develop various defensive maneuvers to help us cushion the effects of negative evaluations of us or our work. Some egos are relatively fragile and cannot well endure the "slings and arrows of outrageous fortune." However, if one is involved in research, then one exposes oneself to evaluation and possible criticism. Thus, it is both important and psychologically hygienic for the researchers to be able to step back and evaluate their work as objectively and realistically as possible. If they do, they will be in a much better position to learn from their past errors and deficiences and consequently to improve the quality of their future work and the chances of its being viewed more positively.

Submitting a paper for presentation at a professional meeting, however, is just one of the important instances when one's research work will be evaluated by others. Another, and potentially more important, evaluation awaits the individual who decides to submit a report of his research project to a professional journal for possible publication. Even if a person has been successful in having one's paper accepted for presentation at a professional meeting, when he/she wants to submit the paper for possible publication in a professional journal this calls for an evaluation of the work by a different panel of individuals who have been selected as experts in the particular area of research. Consequently, another and usually more stringent evaluation of one's work is performed by the editor and reviewers of the particular journal. Although I shall say more about this later, two aspects of the journal review and decision-making process can be mentioned here. One is that the acceptance rate of manuscripts submitted to the leading journals is much lower than the acceptance rate of papers submitted for presentation at professional meetings. Thus, even if one has presented a paper at a national meeting, there is no assurance that this paper or a manuscript based on it will be accepted for publication. In essence, a different jury or group of judges will assess its merits.

A second feature of the evaluation of a manuscript submitted for journal publication which generally is quite different from that provided by a program committee is the type of evaluation received. In addition to the editorial decision made concerning the possible acceptance or rejection of the manuscript, the author is usually provided with some detailed appraisals of the manuscript which have in great part formed the basis for the editor's decision. In other words, in the case of a manuscript which has been judged not acceptable for publication, the specific deficiencies in the manuscript are described. These comments may pertain to the significance of the research conducted, problems in the research design, to the analysis of the results, or to the clarity and organization of the manuscript.

In such cases, therefore, the researcher usually receives rather detailed appraisals of his/her research report from two or more knowledgeable individuals. Although a number of persons may be angered and irritated by critical reviews which find deficiencies in their research or research reports, others do see these evaluations as an important means of improving their work. One can be defensive about negative appraisals, or one can view them for what they are—an evaluation made by individuals with some expertise. In the latter instance, the entire process can be viewed as an opportunity for learning and improvement. As indicated earlier, being able to evaluate one's own work in a reasonably objective manner is an important aspect of improving the level of one's research work, even though it may not be an easy task to perform. Now, however, let us proceed to a discussion of the process of preparing a research report.

WRITING A RESEARCH REPORT

In the preceding account, we have discussed some of the instances where one's research is evaluated and stressed the importance of being able to appraise our own work critically as well as being able to profit from the evaluations of others. In the present section, I believe it is worthwhile to present briefly some basic considerations in the preparation of a research report or manuscript, even though this topic will be described in more detail in the next chapter.

Although there is a fairly standardized format for reporting the results of a research investigation, it is primarily a general guide. In most instances the following headings are used to indicate the major sections of the report: Introduction or Statement of the problem, Method, Results, and Discussion. The would-be author, however, needs to go beyond these general headings and their sub-units. From an editor's standpoint, I would emphasize three aspects of any report as being of great importance. These would be: clarity, conciseness, and adequacy of information. I will comment briefly on each of them.

No matter how significant the results an invesigator secures, their potential importance may not be appreciated if they are not reported in a clear and comprehensible manner. Closely related is the matter of the adequacy of the information being reported. All information that is necessary to understand and evaluate the research study should be reported. Thus, in a study of the outcome of treatment, the investigator should report the pre-and posttreatment mean scores of the groups evaluated as well as the statistical tests of significance. I have been surprised at the number of individuals who simply mention the results of their statistical analyses or include tables for the analyses of variance, and in essence present no data from their study. Presenting necessary data and presenting it clearly are of basic importance. In addition, the report should be as concise and crisp as possible in terms of the information presented and the required clarity. In this writer's experience, most would-be authors are a bit too verbose, and manuscripts can be condensed noticeably without in any way reducing the quality of the report. In fact, in most instances, the quality of communication is improved.

For a number of individuals, the research conducted for their doctoral dissertation is the first research that they attempt to report by means of journal publication . Unfortunately, they have real difficulty in trying to prepare their dissertation for publication. The dissertation is usually a comprehensive document with a lengthy review of the literature and numerous tables and appendices. Compressing and condensing a 200 page dissertation into a 15 or 20 page article can be a very difficult and painful experience. But, however difficult and painful this task may be, it can, and realistically, *must* be performed.

I have emphasized the writing of the research report here because most evaluations of research are based on some written report of the research investigation. A poorly written report makes an adequate evaluation of research very difficult and, in some instances, impossible. Consequently, while designing and conducting an excellent study are clearly important as the bases for a good research report, they are not sufficient by themselves. Preparing a lucid, accurate, and informative report is also of some consequence if the relevant professional or scientific audience is to be informed of the findings and if these findings are to make their contribution to the research literature of the particular field. Unfortunately, although graduate students usually are required to take several courses in statistical methodology and research design, they apparently are given only limited instruction in preparing written research reports.

EDITORIAL GUIDELINES FOR EVALUATING RESEARCH REPORTS

Since I have been asked to contribute this chapter from the perspective of a journal editor, it would appear to be appropriate to list and discuss some of the guidelines used by my predecessors and me in editing the *Journal of Consulting and Clinical Psychology*. The following general instructions and partial list of guidelines are ones that I have adapted and revised when I began my tenure as editor.

Editorial Guidelines for Reviewers
Journal of Consulting and Clinical Psychology

In recent years, according to the observation of the previous editor of this journal, the quality of many submitted manuscripts has diminished. Whatever the cause, be it pressure to publish or a decrease in the scientific education offered graduate students in clinical psychology, it is a problem that we have to face. Consequently, reviewers must do a thorough job in evaluating the manuscripts referred to them. Not only should they recommend rejection of poor manuscripts, but hopefully, in their comments to the authors, they should point out clearly the limitations in the manuscript which contributed to their decision. This, of course, should be done in an objective and non-vitriolic manner. The purpose is to give authors adequate feedback and, again hopefully, to educate them a bit about research publication.

The following points are among the important ones to keep in mind when appraising a manuscript:

1. Is the paper appropriate for the *Journal of Consulting and Clinical Psychology* in terms of the description in the masthead?
2. Is the introduction concise and to the point? Are the hypotheses clear and reasonable?
3. Are subjects and controls appropriate for the problem and are the methods of their selection clearly stated? Are the latter appropriate? Are the *N*s sufficient?
4. Are the measures used appropriate ones and are data provided concerning their reliability and validity?
5. Are the procedures adequately described so that replications are possible?
6. Are appropriate statistics used and the assumptions for their use met?
7. Do the findings have some practical significance as well as statistical significance? Does the author pay attention to this matter by providing more information than the level of significance (e.g., the amount of variance accounted for by the findings)?
8. Is the paper reported in a concise fashion with a minimum of verbiage? Are figures and tables necessary and clearly presented? (Tables of largely non-

significant findings can be omitted and the significant few can be presented in the body of the paper.)

9. In the discussion section has the author concentrated on his/her findings and are the generalizations and conclusions tenable? Have possible limitations in the study been mentioned by the author and has he/she related these to possible discrepancies between the reported findings and those of other studies?

The above, of course, do not exhaust the list of criteria to keep in mind, but they represent important items which need consideration in most manuscripts.

Since the readers of this chapter are potential contributors of manuscripts to professional journals, it is worth elaborating a bit more on some of the items mentioned above. The first item, for example, may appear to be self-evident. However, if one is to judge from the large number of manuscripts submitted to the *Journal of Consulting and Clinical Psychology* that are clearly inappropriate for the journal, then it seems apparent that many individuals do not examine the descriptive material on the inside cover of the journal very carefully. During the past 5 years the number of inappropriate submissions each year has fluctuated from about 18 to 20% of all manuscripts submitted! This is an unexpectedly large percentage and in actual numbers has varied around a total of 200 manuscripts per year.

Consequently, before authors submit their manuscript, they should examine carefully the descriptive material presented in the journal which describes the kinds of articles published in that journal, as well as the bibliographic style required. One should also select the *most recent* issue of the journal for this purpose since both editors and editorial policies change over time. It may be somewhat surprising to the reader to know that after 5 years as editor of the *Journal of Consulting and Clinical Psychology,* I still receive a few manuscripts addressed to the previous editor of the journal. In any event, extra delays and frustrations in getting a manuscript published can be avoided by inspecting a group of potentially appropriate journals, by discussing the matter with colleagues or teachers who have published articles recently, and then selecting the journal that appears most appropriate.

As can also be noted in the list presented, several items emphasize conciseness and clarity: two of the general points mentioned earlier. Thus, no additional emphasis is required here. Several of the other points are probably familiar ones also and need little amplification here. However, some comments can be made with regard to a few of the remaining items since the problems they refer to do appear with some frequency in manuscripts submitted for publication. The matter of selecting appropriate subjects for the problem being investigated, mentioned in item 3, is one such instance. Although this also may appear somewhat surprising to some, it actually is a problem that is noted quite regularly. A number of different kinds of examples could be presented for illustrative purposes, but just two will be sufficient for our purpose here.

The selection of the proper subjects for a specific research project is an exceedingly critical matter. If one is interested in conducting a study of clinical depression, for example, it is necessary to select subjects who would be considered clinically depressed by most accepted diagnostic criteria. The diagnosis should be made by competent clinicians using a variety of diagnostic procedures which have some demonstrated reliability and validity. Only in this fashion can other investigators have confidence in the statement that depressed subjects were actually studied. Furthermore, any attempts at replication will be guided by the explicit selection criteria used. Among the common inadequacies encountered in this regard are the use of diagnoses made some time in the past; reliance on one unspecified diagnostic interviewer with no estimate of reliability; relying exclusively on a broad diagnostic label such as schizophrenia without attention to other significant variables such as age, sex, paranoid features, and premorbid status; and relying solely on one test or personality questionnaire. I have received (and not accepted for publication) at least a few manuscripts studying certain correlates or aspects of "depression," for example, in which the "depressed" subjects were students taking introductory psychology who were selected on the basis of a score on a personality questionnaire. The use of such depressed groups and such diagnostic categorizations of "depression" are simply not acceptable for research on major depressive disorders.

Securing a suitable control group is even more of a problem, depending on the topic being investigated. In some instances a "normal" or non-pathological group may be the preferred control, whereas in other instances a clinical (disordered) group is preferable. In evaluating characteristics of married couples experiencing marital difficulties, couples with satisfactory marriages may be a suitable control group. In the case of evaluating the diagnostic efficacy of a test for organic brain involvement, however, a normal control group would not be as suitable as a group of comparably disordered patients with non-organic psychopathology. In diagnostic assessment in the clinical situation, one works generally with disordered individuals, and thus the latter control group is a more meaningful one. In treatment studies, still other considerations may have to be entertained. If treatment is lengthy, it may be difficult or unethical to use a no-treatment control. An adequate attention-placebo control may be difficult to devise and may also present ethical issues. Such problems and considerations in research will of course be reflected in the conduct of the research investigation and ultimately in the report of the research. These are also factors which will be carefully evaluated by the reviewers of the research manuscript and by the editor.

Adequate description of the study is obviously quite necessary in order to evaluate it adequately and to allow for possible replication of it. In certain studies this is not a particular problem. However, in some types of studies, such as those assessing particular forms of psychotherapy, the problem is more complicated and fuller descriptions of procedures are required. Thus, if one is comparing a particular type of cognitive or behavioral therapy with a form of psychodynamic therapy, it is not sufficient to simply describe the therapy conducted as "cognitive therapy" or "cognitive restructuring" or "dynamically oriented therapy." Such descriptions are overly general and do not give an adequate description of the operations and procedures used. Admittedly, one cannot give an overly detailed and lengthy description of the therapies used for fear of making the manuscript too long. However, a brief but meaningful description can be given and a more detailed description or manual of the therapy offered to interested readers in a footnote in the manuscript. Descriptions of the therapists employed should indicate their training, experience, age, and sex as minimal information, with comparable information provided for the subjects.

As is apparent, a number of criteria are used to evaluate a research report. Although all of them are of some importance, the clinical or theoretical significance of the research reported is of great importance, and is a matter which is often neglected. If the nature of the research is of little practical or theoretical significance, then the other considerations are really of limited consequence. As mentioned earlier, a beautifully designed and carried out study which is clearly reported in exquisite style, but which is of "no redeeming social worth," has to be viewed negatively.

For such reasons, it is worth repeating some comments I previously have made concerning the clinical significance of research projects (Garfield, 1978, 1983). In much of the research literature on clinical psychology, the results are analyzed in terms of their statistical significance. Thus, one reads that the difference between the experimental group and the control group was significant at better than the .05 level. A difference at the .05 level of probability is usually the level considered for significance, and I have seen some individuals quite elated when they were able to secure such results. In most experimental studies such a finding is seen as lending support to some hypotheses or failing to support the null hypothesis. We can interpret and accept such a finding for what it is worth. Essentially, such an analysis indicates the probability that the differences secured are due to chance. A finding significant at the .05 level is considered to be a statistically significant finding because the probability is that there are only 5 chances out of 100 that the results are due to chance. The assumption is also made that comparable findings are likely to be secured if the study were to be repeated.

I have no quarrel with the necessity and importance of securing significant results in terms of probability statistics. If the results are not statistically significant, then clearly whatever differences are secured are presumed to be due to chance, and of limited value. Consequently, a first requirement is that whatever comparisons are made be statistically significant. However, this is simply a first step. The findings also need to be judged on the basis of their clinical or practical significance. A result may be statistically significant but not clinically significant. This is particularly true when large samples of subjects are used since the larger the sample the greater the opportunity for statistically significant results. With a sample size of around 1,000, a correlation of .08 can be highly significant statistically (Garfield & Kurtz, 1976).

The real issue here is in making a judgment concerning the clinical significance of a particular set of findings. The most frequently used procedure is to estimate the amount of variance explained by a particular result. If, for example, the IQ of a sample of patients is correlated .20 with the criterion of outcome used, then by squaring the correlation we secure an estimate of the variance accounted for by the IQ. In this instance, the IQ would account for only 4% of the variance in outcome.

In other instances, however, one may have to use other procedures or even to rely on clinical judgment in estimating the clinical significance of a particular finding. Although clinical judgment is subject to distortion, one should not disregard the potential positive contribution of one's higher level cognitive processes. There are many findings that are easily interpreted as being of little practical significance. Raising a person's IQ from 42 to 48, lowering an individual's score on the MMPI Depression Scale from 79 to 71, and similar findings might be statistically significant, depending on the size of the sample. However, most clinicians, I believe, would not regard such gains as really impressive.

In some cases it may be possible to compare a treated group with a normative group to see how similar the treated group is at the completion of treatment. If a group at the beginning of treatment is widely divergent from the norm but approximates the norm at posttreatment, the findings can be interpreted as being clinically significant. On the other hand, if at the end of treatment, the treated group, while showing some improvement at a statistically significant level, is still far from the norm, such limited improvement should be noted.

The point mentioned above is clearly illustrated in a recent publication by Kendall and Norton-Ford (1982), in which they summarize the results of several studies pertaining to a cognitive-behavioral treatment for teaching children self-control. In a study of relatively brief treatment the treated group showed statistically significant changes as contrasted with a control group of children. However, as a group, the former were still one standard deviation above the mean for a normal group of children. In this instance the higher score represents a greater lack of self-control. In a later study with a longer period of intervention, a similar analysis again indicated statistically significant effects for treatment. However, at this time, the comparison of the groups with the normative mean showed a somewhat larger positive change.

Although the mean of the treated groups was still above that of the normative sample, it now differed by less than a standard deviation.

The preceding discussion should provide some illustrations of procedures that can be used to make some appraisal or estimate of the clinical significance of research results. Clearly, it is important to pay attention to this aspect of one's research findings, and there has been an increased awareness of this matter on the part of editors and reviewers.

SAMPLE MANUSCRIPT REVIEWS

Now that we have noted some of the editorial criteria used in evaluating research reports submitted for publication, it may be of interest to examine some actual reviews of such manuscripts. I have selected some sample reviews and modified them in certain ways to reduce possible identification of the materials reviewed.

Manuscript Review I

Although I was quite interested in the topic of the manuscript submitted by Smith, Brown, and Black, as well as the initial description of the study, after reading the entire manuscript I was both perplexed and disappointed. I shall try to list my specific reactions as succinctly as possible.

1. Although the title of the paper suggested that early drop-out and resistance in psychotherapy would be explained as correlates of initial client disturbances, one searches in vain throughout the paper for any results on these topics. At the bottom of the first page and continuing on the next page, the authors clearly state that the goal and approach of the study was to relate data on client disturbances to "lateness, absence and drop-out from therapy." However, no such data are provided in the manuscript.

2. The authors classify less than three interviews as constituting a drop-out from therapy and three or more interviews as reflecting continuation in psychotherapy. This is an arbitrary definition even though the authors state that three sessions constitute the shortest treatment at their clinic. The potential generalizability of these results to those of other investigators is thus decidedly limited and reflects a problem in this research area whereby three interviews constitute a continuation in one study and a drop-out in another. Furthermore, no data are provided on the range or average length of treatment provided as well as related matters, nor is any infomration given concerning the kind of psychotherapy provided.

3. In a similar fashion, little adequate information is provided on the experience and training of the therapists used in this study. The authors describe

the therapists as "advanced graduate students in clinical psychology and social welfare," but "advanced graduate student" is not defined in any manner.

4. Besides the problems that have already been mentioned, it can be noted that there is an absence of data on other specific aspects of the study. We know nothing about the mean ratings provided by the subjects for the various problems and, although the authors make reference to indices of lateness, etc., no information whatsoever is provided on these topics. Furthermore, although estimates of reliability are given for the judges' ratings of total problem scores, as far as I could make out, no such estimates were given for judges' ratings of individual problem areas. However, the latter ratings were also used in the analysis reported.

5. The authors list all of the correlations which were statistically significant. However, it would be important to know also how many correlations were performed and which problems were investigated but did not produce significant findings. With a large sample size, with many computations, and with variables which may not be fully independent, it is possible to derive somewhat faulty conclusions concerning significant findings. In addition, many of the correlations which were found to be significant, appear to be very modest and account for only small amounts of variance.

6. It also seemed clear, as the authors themselves pointed out, that many of the findings were fairly obvious and not surprising. For example, the highest correlation was obtained between school problems and student status. It is indeed difficult for individuals who are not going to school to be concerned with school problems. In a similar fashion, a relationship between family problems and marital status probably could be anticipated. One would also expect that those individuals who have physical problems would exhibit the most medical expectations. I also felt that rather over-simplified interpretations were offered in interpreting some of the results secured. For example, the authors point out the relationship secured between family problems and marital status, which is a finding that could be expected. On the other hand, marital status also correlated negatively with interpersonal problems of the opposite sex. Certainly, married partners who are having family problems with their spouses would appear to be having interpersonal problems with the opposite sex, and thus one cannot take some of the results at face value.

7. On page 12, the authors state that the clients who were students did not experience severe family disturbances, and those that did, tended to be married clients. However, in Table 2, the highest correlation between family problems and the different client ratings is actually with student status.

In summary, although the title reads somewhat otherwise, the paper is a report of correlations between certain problem areas and largely demographic variables, and most of the correlations reported fall into this category. The study is not what it says it is and, for a variety of reasons which have been listed above, it is a rather disappointing paper which does not make a contribution.

Manuscript Review II

Although this manuscript has a number of interesting aspects, there are several features which are open to cricism. The most important from my viewpoint are the following:

The author treats the different therapist attributes as separate and independent variables when it is apparent that they are highly similar and thus most likely not independent. To a large extent, the findings for each are similar. All of them show a relationship to diagnosis and prognosis. A similar question can be raised about the possible correlation of the ABC Scale and the I.E. Scale. It would seem essential to compute the correlation of these two scales to see if indeed they are highly correlated.

The use of a median split with reference to these two scales also presents some real problems of both meaning and generalizability. If, as the author points out, the present sample is below the median previously reported for the ABC Scale by Simons, then does this mean that subjects in the present sample are all low in this respect? Also, just what do the designations of "high" and "low" in the present study mean? If these values are to be defined anew by each sample, it is hard to know what they signify in any general way.

The manuscript can also be criticized for failing to include and present the actual data supposedly obtained in the study. No actual data such as the means or standard deviations of the two groups of therapists that are compared are provided. Even though a difference between means may be significant at the .05 level, the actual differences secured from the variables appraised are of some importance in evaluating their practical significance.

In several places in the manuscript, the author discusses, and tends to emphasize, differences which actually were not significant statistically. It is best, I believe, to regard such findings as non-significant, and omit any extended discussion, even though we all want to make the most of our findings.

As the author mentions in his concluding sentence, the study only investigates what a sample of therapists say about themselves and not necessarily what they would actually do in the therapeutic situation. This is an important point which deserves special emphasis. How the case material was presented may also be a factor here and may have possibly influenced the results obtained. If important aspects of a potential patient (such as degree of psychopathology and motivation for treatment) are stressed, they may well exert a greater impact on the therapist than social-demographic factors, particularly when many therapists may have become sensitive to the social implications of the latter factors.

Finally, the results as presented tend at times to be difficult to grasp and potentially confusing to the reader—particularly the more complicated interaction effects. It may be possible to use some statistical analyses that will avoid the unnecessary duplication of findings of apparently correlated variables, and to pull out what potential findings of value exist. Consultation on this matter would appear to be appropriate. Fairly extensive revision of this manuscript would have to be undertaken before it might be viewed more favorably.

Manuscript Review III

I read the manuscript by Green with considerable interest. The type of program discussed and the attempts at program evaluation are clearly of some importance. At the same time, however, there are certain aspects of the report which bother me. These have to do with the general interpretation of the results secured, and the clarity and meaninfulness of the results obtained with one of the outcome measures.

Actually, two of my concerns are interrelated. These have to do with the ABC Scale as a measure of change and with the results presented in Table 1. The ABC Scale is described as a 5-point rating scale dealing with judgments of improvement. In general, because of possible halo and related effects, such rating scales frequently tend to give more positive results than do other measures of change. Furthermore, since the ABC Scale apparently contains the same type of items as the EFG Scale which was administered first, it is rather surprising that the original scale was not readministered and difference scores obtained. Global judgments of change are just not as good as the latter for appraising change. The lack of some kind of adquate control group, furthermore, greatly weakens the significance attached to the changes reported.

I also do not understand the mean scores and the differences listed for the ABC Scale in Table 2. If these are in fact mean ratings made at the end of treatment rather than difference scores, how were the "differences" computed? This is not explained and is clearly of some importance. Furthermore, if these are really mean ratings, then in spite of the obtained statistical significance, however computed, most of the values are near the midpoint of the rating scale, which supposedly signified "no change." Clearly, the amount of change appears to be small, and this rating of change probably constitutes the most important index of change. This section certainly needs clarification if the material is to be understood.

There are some other aspects of the manuscript which are also rather disturbing, particularly in relation to the decidedly positive tone conveyed throughout the manuscript. The EFG Scale, for example, actually did not differentiate between the various groups appraised, and consequently does not appear as a valid measure of the characteristics it is supposed to measure. Furthermore, there were "no significant pure type differences" on six of the seven scales developed for these purposes. Thus, with one exception, although there were supposedly pure types, the improvement reported was more generalized. The "betas" were the only ones who improved significantly more on their particular scale than the other groups. However, inspection of Table 3 indicates that the other groups had very low scores on this variable and the possibility for change, therefore, was less on this variable than for any other.

In light of the above, I believe that the author's conclusions are stated in overly positive terms, more positively than I believe is merited by the data. Incidentally, no reason is given for the reduction of the *N* from 124 to 86 for some of the analyses. Any revision of the manuscript should answer the above points in terms of additional clarity and appropriate modification. Like the author, I too believe that interventions should be tailored to meet the particular problems of specific clients, and the present report is a step in that direction. However, the findings appear quite tentative at this point.

The preceding reviews may give the reader some concrete idea of the kind of evaluations made and offered to the individuals who submit research reports for possible publication in psychological journals. The response to them varies in terms of the kinds of reviews written and the particular authors. Some authors actually respond favorably to the serious and thoughtful appraisals of their manuscript and see them as very helpful. I have actually received a few letters from authors whose manuscripts were not accepted for publication who thanked me and the reviewers for the thoughtful evaluations they received. I have also received a few rather indignant letters as well, accusing me and the reviewers of bias, poor judgment, and ignorance.

Most of us do not like to be criticized or to have our shortcomings pointed out to us. This, of course, is perfectly understandable. However, as alluded to earlier, one can learn a great deal about research and, more specifically, about one's own shortcomings in this area from paying careful attention to evaluative critiques of one's own research reports. Furthermore, the cost of such an education is very low in economic terms and most of the commentaries are offered by knowledgeable individuals in a thoughtful and informative manner.

SUMMARY

In this chapter I have tried to discuss the most important features of research reports as well as the most frequently occurring problems noted in evaluating such reports when they have been submitted for journal publication. Unlike most other materials that I have prepared for publication in books or journals, I have made little use of scholarly references and the published literature generally. Although I did not really make a serious and detailed search of possible publications on this topic, it is my impression that very little has been published dealing directly with the editorial perspective as presented here. Books on experimental psychology do offer helpful material on preparing a manuscript for publication and tend to emphasize such matters as format, clarity, and appropriate research procedures (Borkowski & Anderson, 1977; Meyers & Grossen, 1978). However, such presentations are oriented to experimental research rather than clinical research, and the particular editorial perspective emphasized in the present chapter is generally absent.

Students and future clinical psychologists do need to be familiar with the proper format and style of a research article and they are usually informed about such matters in courses in experimental psychology or research. Beyond this, it is also desirable that prospective authors prepare their manuscripts in the specific form specified by the journal to which they plan to submit their manuscripts. The American Psychological Association (1983), for example, has a *Publication Manual* which gives detailed directions for preparing manuscripts for submission to its journals. Most graduate students in psychology become exposed to this manual at some point during their graduate study. However, the kinds of issues discussed in this chapter go beyond the more conventional topic of manuscript format. Some of the actual guidelines for reviewers of the *Journal of Consulting and Clinical Psychology* have been presented along with some sample reviews. These materials, it is hoped, have helped to make the more general presentation of the editorial perspective on research publication more concrete and informative.

Finally, I would like to pass on some observations on journal publication which may be of some interest to those who are preparing manuscripts or who will be preparing them in the future. It is important that psychologists, as is also the case with lesser mortals, have realistic expectations. This is particularly so in the area of scholarly and research publication. If our expectations are set at realistic levels, our disappointments will tend to be less severe.

It is wise to know something about the base rates for accepting manuscripts just as it is desirable to know the base rates for various types of disorders in order to evaluate the diagnostic efficacy of particular techniques. Unfortunately, most journals do not publish their acceptance or rejection rates. However, the rejection rates of the journals of the American Psychological Association are published annually. In 1982, for example, the rejection rate for these journals ranged from 43% to 90%. The rate for the *Journal of Consulting and Clinical Psychology* was 85%. These percentages tend to inflate the rejection rate somewhat, however, since the authors of some manuscripts which are formally not accepted are invited to revise their manuscript and to resubmit the revised version. A number of these are eventually accepted and thus reduce the rejection rate somewhat. It may be prudent, therefore, not to expect to have your first manuscript accepted, particularly in the original version. However, there is one chance in five or so that your manuscript may eventually be accepted. If you know this, a letter of non-acceptance may not be so crushing. Remember, that other journals may view your manuscript more positively, and remember also to view this process as an opportunity for learning. If you do, you increase your chances of having your manuscript published and of adding your individual contribution to the field of psychology.

REFERENCES

American Psychological Association. (1983). *Publication manual of the American Psychological Association* (3rd ed.). Washington, DC: Author.

Borkowski, J.G., & Anderson, D.C. (1977). *Experimental psychology: Tactics of be-*

havioral research. Glenview, IL: Scott, Foresman.

Garfield, S.L. (1978). Research problems in clinical diagnosis. *Journal of Consulting and Clinical Psychology, 46,* 596–607.

Garfield, S.L. (1983). Methodological problems in clinical diagnosis. In H.E. Adams & P. B. Sutker (Eds.), *Comprehensive handbook of psychopathology.* New York: Plenum.

Garfield, S.L., & Kurtz, R. (1976). Clinical psychologists in the 1970's. *American Psychologist, 31,* 1–9.

Kendall, P.C., & Norton-Ford, J.D. (1982). Therapy outcome research methods. In P.C. Kendall & J.N. Butcher (Eds.), *Handbook of research methods in clinical psychology.* New York: Wiley.

Meyers, L.S., & Grossen, N.E. (1978). *Behavioral research: Theory, procedure, and design* (2nd ed.). San Francisco: W.H. Freeman.

14

Writing Grant Applications: Some General Guidelines

Phillip S. Strain
Mary Margaret Kerr

INTRODUCTION

The purpose of this chapter is to describe a number of procedural steps and writing techniques that we have found useful in preparing applications for research, program development, and professional training funds. We begin the chapter with a review of strategies for finding out more about the source of monies, then describe general writing style considerations, and finally offer suggestions for the content of major sections of grants.

KNOWING THE FUNDING AGENCY

It is not by accident that most successful grant applicants have a clear understanding of the structure and function of granting agencies. While it is possible to acquire from agencies an organizational or personnel chart, there is no substitute for direct contact. We recommend a once per year informational visit to potential funding sources, and the following guidelines for a visit:

(1) Make appointments well in advance, rather than "dropping in." The latter practice is typical, but rather discourteous.

(2) Inform persons in advance what you hope to find out from them. By doing so, you will likely come home with many written products of use, rather than empty-handed. This tactic will also allow you to have a personable conversation without the need for extensive note-taking.

(3) If you have a specific idea or proposal to discuss, put it in writing (briefly) and give the respondents several weeks to read your material prior to your visit.

(4) Particularly at the federal level, many granting agency personnel have impressive professional credentials, and they are privy to the latest and best ideas that your colleagues have to offer. It is, therefore, important to listen well, not just speak about your ideas. Ask people their opinions on content issues, what gaps they see in current knowledge, what priorities they would like emphasized.

(5) There are certain matters that personnel may or may not be able to discuss with you. For example, many agencies do not release funding priorities prior to formal publication (in *Commerce Business Daily* or the *Federal Register*) or discuss upcoming proposal deadlines. If you are unsure about a question, say so as a preface. In this way, you will make it clear that you are not asking for privileged information. Simply saying "Can you discuss this matter with me?" will save face for everyone.

(6) Almost all agencies rely on external reviewers (your fellow professionals) to conduct preliminary reviews on proposals, and generally these reviews closely predict ultimate funding decisions. Occasionally, you can get a list of panel reviewers that an agency uses. In addition to this, it is perfectly reasonable to ask how the panel might respond to a certain idea. While the composition of panels typically changes over a 2–3 year period, it is not unusual for a specific panel to develop a certain reputation for favoring or disfavoring a particular theoretical orientation, methodology, and the like. Most program people will speak frankly about such matters.

(7) In presenting ideas and listening to agency personnel, it is essential to avoid criticism of other professionals or their work. You may well be criticizing work funded by the agency.

(8) Often, the published guidelines that describe the components of a proposal are not fully elaborated. Your meeting is an excellent opportunity to inquire about information that the panel and the agency would like to see in a proposal. For example, many proposals are required to have a section describing the potential impact of the project. For some reviewers and agencies, cost savings (e.g., defering institutionalization with a novel daily treatment for schizophrenics) are the raison d'être of impact. Other audiences are more concerned with theory building or idea organization, and still others would most want to know if the project affords previously unavailable opportunities for an underserved clinical group.

(9) The face-to-face contact you have with program personnel is an excellent opportunity to convey your enthusiasm for the project. It is most often the case that agencies have many excellent proposals and scant dollars to award. The excitement, energy, and interest you show can only improve your chances of receiving support.

(10) If you are a novice in the proposal writing arena, you may want to ask program personnel for a copy of an examplary proposal. Some proposals are in the public domain and some agencies will provide them upon request.

(11) If you so choose, it is quite appropriate to volunteer your services as a reviewer. However, be advised that this is an enormously time-consuming job. It is also the best way we know to become well acquainted with agencies and the better ideas in the field.

(12) In summary, before you end your visit try to obtain the following:

(a) list of currently funded projects,
(b) list of reviewers,
(c) guidelines for proposals,
(d) guidelines or criteria for reviewers,
(e) upcoming deadlines, and
(f) current funding priorities.

GENERAL WRITING/FORMAT CONSIDERATIONS

The writing style, format, and esthetics of a proposal are of enormous importance. In these areas, it is important to keep in mind that reviewers will likely be reading hundreds, possibly thousands, of pages over a brief span of time. Any efforts you can make to ease that burden are likely to be rewarded.

Reducing the amount of jargon is one of the best ways to improve communication and enhance funding opportunities. Jargon is particularly dysfunctional in a grant proposal because: (a) it is very likely that some of the reviewers will interpret your ideas incorrectly; and (b) particular jargon is usually associated with certain theoretical orientations that may be offensive to members of the review panel. If you must use highly specialized terms, it is a good idea to offer working definitions for the reader. Proposal writers also get into trouble when they use technical terms in a colloquial fashion (e.g., "We plan to reinforce skill training with homework exercises for couples.").

After several years of graduate training, it is often difficult to discriminate jargon from non-jargon. We, therefore, advise that you have an English major read your proposal with particular concern for clarity of language use.

The "reviewability" of your proposal can be greatly enhanced by altering the type, spacing, and presentation of material to highlight important points, set-off various sections of an application, and generally to save reviewers from visual monotony.

If the granting agency permits, we suggest double spacing of an application. The judicious use of capitals, bold face, and italics will also improve the visual display and help to highlight relevant sections of the proposal. For example, we recommend highlighting, in a visual sense, sections such as: (a) list of project objectives; (b) numbers or statements that reflect the impact of the project (e.g., 75 depressed patients to be treated); (c) quotes or other references as to the feasibility, quality, or importance of the work you are proposing; and (d) any innovative ideas, procedures, treatments that are proposed.

Other ways of improving the "reviewability" of a proposal include:

(1) For lengthy proposals, bind the application or use a spiral binder.
(2) Use tabs or titled, contrasting colored sheets to mark the beginning of major sections.

(3) Use figures and tables to illustrate complex data or time-sequenced activities to be conducted.
(4) Use the active voice throughout the proposal.

SPECIFIC PROPOSAL COMPONENTS

In the sections which follow, we review guidelines for writing the major sections that are included in most grant proposals. Specific sections to be reviewed include: abstract, budget, statement of need or problem, objectives, procedures, and dissemination.

Writing an Abstract

Most often abstracts are written at the last minute, in states of exhaustion and/or panic, and they suffer accordingly. In point of fact, this is one of the most vital components of your application. Abstracts are used to *screen out* of the review process proposals that do not seem appropriate to the agency or the current priorities. They are used also as an internal means of communication between program staff responsible for the review of the application and their supervisions; and, they are used as "executive summaries" or "legislative reports" for governing, law-making, and appropriations bodies. The old adage of making a good first impression applies to abstract writing.

Effective abstracts usually contain the following elements:

(1) The purpose of the proposed program,
(2) The problem(s) to be addressed and the need for this particular effort,
(3) The major objectives of the project,
(4) The proposed plan of activity, and
(5) The expected outcomes and potential significance.

For psychology-oriented applications it is often essential to describe the target population in some detail. The abstract should also make specific reference to agency priorities that the application addresses.

In summary, the abstract should communicate the major importance and content of your ideas. The goal is to make the reviewer want to read more about this exciting project! Try to keep your abstract to one page or less.

Budget Writing

In almost all instances, the funding agency or your institution will have a certain format to follow and forms to complete as a part of this section. Additionally, you should have some good guess (sometimes an actual dollar figure) as to the total dollar request that is possible under a specific competition. Before describing specific items for inclusion we will describe some general considerations in budget development:

(1) In many competitions, certainly those involving a contract rather than a grant, the cost is often the deciding factor between technically equivalent proposals.

(2) In days *past*, a typical budget strategy was to ask for more than one needed, with the expectation that cuts by the agency would result in a satisfactory level of funding. Today, however, a "fat budget" is a high-risk to the applicant. We strongly recommend requesting no more than what is needed to do the work.

(3) Budgets should be developed in concert with your agency's financial specialists. These individuals often know how to save you money, making the application more competitive.

(4) For all budgets, large or small, we recommend including a cost-efficiency section to the application. In this section you can explain how you decided upon a staffing pattern that is less costly than other alternatives; how the quality of personnel justify the costs; if applicable, how the agency is contributing financially to the project; and, what cost savings may accrue from funding this project.

The central feature of your budget is the justification. In the example provided in Figure 14.1, we present sample items from a successful application to establish an early intervention program for autistic-like children.

Major sections in the budget justification presented above include: personnel, fringe benefits, travel, equipment, supplies, duplication, postage and telephone and rationale for overall dollar request. For each of these sections, several critical features should be noted.

In the personnel section, each participant should be described in terms of his or her percent *effort* on the project and the percent of *salary support* requested. The responsibilities for each person should also be included. For staff not yet identified (e.g., Master Teacher in Figure 14.1), it is essential to describe the qualifications needed to fill a certain role. Keep in mind that the language used to describe the activities of staff should relate directly to the goals and objectives of the project.

The fringe benefits section is rather straightforward. It describes your institution's current level of extra-salary support for personnel. Rates are subject to frequent change, so it is essential to check with fiscal personnel to confirm the correct figure.

Travel requests are often subject to budget cuts, usually because of insufficient justification. In the case of local (in-town) travel, it is advisable to pre-

Personnel:

Project Director: Phillip S. Strain, Ph.D., Associate Professor of Psychiatry and Special Education; Director, Mellon Evaluation Center for Children and Adolescents—25% effort will be devoted to the project. Salary support is requested at 10%. Dr. Strain will be responsible for the overall fiscal management of the project; coordinating the evaluation of adult and child behavior change; coordinating the dissemination and demonstration aspects of the project; and for all personnel management.

Master Teachers: Bonnie V. Jamieson, M.Ed., and Marilyn J. Hoyson, Ph.D.—100% effort each will be devoted to the project. Salary support is requested at 100% each. Ms. Jamieson and Dr. Hoyson will provide direct education services to six autistic-like children. Their duties include development of IEPs; development and implementation of instructional programs; supervision of aides, student teachers, and interns; collection of child outcome data; dissemination of products; and presentation of workshops to trainees.

Parent Trainer: Linda K. Cordisco, Ph.D.—Salary support is requested at 100%. Dr. Cordisco will be responsible for the development, implementation and monitoring of parent training programs in school, home and community settings. Her duties include development of individualized instructional programs for each family; direct training of families in school, home and the community; monitoring of training data on families; and development of service delivery options for families leaving the program.

Teaching Aides: Karen A. Gable and Kurt B. Loell—Salary support is requested at 50% each. Ms. Gable and Mr. Lowell will conduct individual and small group instructional sessions; collect child outcome data on these sessions; and provide reliability checks on outcome measures.

Project Secretary: Kathleen L. Edwards—Salary support is requested at 50%. Ms. Edwards will be responsible for completing numerous record-keeping and clerical tasks related to project operations. Her duties include fiscal record keeping; typing of project manuscripts; keeping employee time records; copying materials for project staff; and maintaining correspondence files.

Fringe Benefits:

Fringe benefits are requested at 24% of salaries and wages, which is the University of Pittsburgh's current rate, effective July 1, 1982.

Travel:

In order to disseminate the outcome data and curriculum materials generated by LEAP, we are requesting $2,000 to help defray the cost of travel to national meetings, such as: Council for Exceptional Children, HCEEP Project Director's Meeting, Association for Advancement of Behavior Therapy, and National Association for the Education of Young Children.

Equipment:

Funds are requested in the amount of $1,045 for purchase of the following items: Zenith 19(219) Video Terminal ($825) and Anderson Jacobson 242 Acoustic Coupler (AJ242) at $220. This equipment will have on-site access to the University of Pittsburgh computer facility and will allow more efficient and rapid management and analysis of project data. ***(continued)***

FIG. 14.1. Sample Budget Justification

FIG. 4-1. *(continued)*

Supplies:

Funds in the amount of $500 are requested for the purchase of necessary project-related office supplies. Based on our experience with similar projects, this amount should adequately cover the following: stationery and envelopes for correspondence to schools, parents and colleagues; memoranda sheets; pens and pencils; typewriter elements; writing pads; calendars; staples, paper clips and other such sundries.

Other Expenses:

Local Travel: Funds to local travel are requested in the amount of $3,360 to help defray travel costs incurred by the Parent Trainer who will be conducting and monitoring intervention programs in the home and various community settings. Costs are calculated as follows: 24 trips/wk. @ 20 miles/trip × 35 wks. × .20¢/mile = $3,360.

Education Curriculum Materials: $1,500 is requested for the purchase of necessary materials to be used with the project children. The materials (suitable for ages 2–5) which we anticipate purchasing include: stacking rings; graduated size blocks; coloring and similar art supplies; toy cars and trucks; miniature kitchen items; matching color, animal, number and word-recognition materials; felt board materials; "Lego" games; and academic-oriented curricula (e.g., DISTAR).

Duplicating: $1,500 is requested to help offset the cost of photocopying instructional materials, forms, reports and correspondence for the project. Specific items that require extensive duplicating include: Advisory Committee agenda; minutes and project materials for review; observational data collection protocols; family screening and assessment protocols; professional papers and presentations; and correspondence.

Postage and Telephone: $1,500 is requested to help defray mailing and telephone costs related to communications with parents/guardians, teachers, cooperating agencies, and state, regional and local officials. Mailing costs ($750) include brochure dissemination; responding to information requests; disseminating papers and reports regarding this project; correspondence with referral sources; and correspondence with Advisory Board members. Besides basic telephone costs, the amount of $750 will cover long-distance service for communication with SEP, Professional and Advisory Board members, and other colleagues around the country who are involved in similar projects.

Rationale For Overall Dollar Request: In considering the staff structure of this project, and the number of autistic-like children to be served, the following factors were of primary importance: (a) follow-up data on this population shows that interventions which cover a typical school day for 9 months a year are not effective, and (b) data presented by the National Society for Autistic Children reveal that 95% of adult autistic persons are presently institutionalized. Considering these factors, we concluded that nothing less than intensive, comprehensive, "full waking-hour" services over 11 months per year should be provided. To train parents, to train other agency personnel, and most important, to offer a functional educational curriculum, is an expensive option. However, using the most conservative economic formula (i.e., not adjusting for inflation), if only one of the target children does not require institutional services (computed on the Commonwealth median of 18,000/year), then the cost/benefit ratio of this project will be 1 : 3, or three dollars saved for every one spent. Should only one target child be mainstreamed for his or her school years, then the cost/benefit ratio will increase to 1 : 4.

sent the formula used to calculate the total request. As in the example in Figure 14.1, include the number of trips to be made and where, the distance for each trip and the established institutional rate for reimbursement. For each out-of-town trip request, the specific cost of transportation (e.g., coach air fare), the per diem and number of days, other expenses (e.g., convention registration), and purpose of the travel, should be provided. To further support out-of-town travel requests, we suggest adding a specific dissemination objective to the proposal.

Equipment purchases on grants and contrasts are carefully scrutinized, particularly at the federal level. The request must be linked directly to the goals and objectives of the project. Additionally, the specific units desired should be identified by manufacturer name, product number, and current cost.

Most projects require an account under which routine office supplies can be purchased. The example provided in Figure 14.1 shows a number of legitimate items that are purchased typically under this category. Please note that office supplies do not include such non-expendable items as desks, chairs, and typewriters. These items, however difficult to justify successfully, would be included under Equipment. Many funding agencies *expect* the applicant to provide these basic items.

A traditional "budget buster" on many projects is the cost of duplicating. If your work demands extensive duplicating (i.e., multiple mailings to recruit subject or subjects' responses to questions, photocopying of protocols, filing monthly or quarterly reports to the granting agency, and so forth), each of these major expenditures should be enumerated in the justification. Occasionally during a budget negotiation, we have been asked to explain how a particular expenditure level for duplicating was determined. Typically, we have satisfied this concern by adding a statement to the justification that the level requested is based upon prior experience with similar projects.

Expenses for postage and telephone use can vary tremendously across projects and project years. It should be kept in mind that monies for these expenditures are *not* designed to cover basic office correspondence and communication. Requests in this area should highlight those project objectives (e.g., dissemination of information obtained to national audiences) and project activities (e.g., conferring with advisory committee members) that require mailings and telephone use.

One, if not the most important, component in the budget justification is a general rationale statement to support the overall dollar request. Depending upon the focus of the application, there are a number of arguments that can be used to justify the total request, including: (a) analysis of cost savings that may result from clients' improvement and reduced need for services, (b) applicants' financial contributions to the project, (c) particular cost-effectiveness made available by use of volunteers, students, etc., and (d) fiscal monitoring procedures to prevent cost overrruns.

Statement of Need or Problem

The major goal in this section of the application is to convince reviewers and the funding agency that the problems you are addressing are vital to them and to society. Some agencies and specific competitions indeed require that the statement actually include data to document need. Such data might include: (a) estimate of the number of potential clients or subjects in the immediate area; (b) availability of other service options for said clients; (c) numbers of licensed therapists, teachers, etc., for client group; and (d) outcome data on clients that show a clear need for new alternatives and information.

As a general rule, we advocate what may be described as a global-to-specific tactic for demonstrating need. For example, many psychology-related applications address, however indirectly, issues of national import (e.g., prevention of environmentally-influenced retardation, management of criminal behavior, psychological consequences of economic depression). In these cases, it is advisable to address the dimensions of the problem at a national level first. However, few proposals will ever represent a scope that can reasonably hope to address a pervasive, national problem in its entirety. Therefore, it is also necessary to specify the individual element(s) of the national problem that the project will address. The need for specificity is essential. By analyzing the elements of a said significant problem, by examining attenuate methodological issues, and by suggesting a considered solution, the Statement of Need can effectively convey your experience, competence, and capability to execute the project.

On the basis of composite guidelines for reviewers of applications, we recommend the following additional components for Statement of Need:

(1) Discussion of how the project will meet the specific need(s).
(2) Brief review of prior literature to support the proposal's solution to the problem(s).
(3) Presentation of material that shows that you and the applicant organization have a history of experience and commitment to the problem(s).
(4) Listing of funding agency priorities that the application may address.

Objectives

There is great variability in the style and content of objectives across research, demonstration, and training proposals. In spite of the heterogeneity of objectives, a few general guidelines are applicable:

(1) Objectives should together address all the relevant outcomes of the project.
(2) Objectives should follow logically from the Statement of Need.
(3) Objectives should be stated briefly.

(4) Objectives should be clearly obtainable within the timeline, personnel, and budgetary reality of the project.
(5) Objectives should be listed by order of importance or impact.
(6) Objectives should be stated in measurable terms.

In demonstration/service proposals, it usually is necessary to reference Objectives to means for their measurement. Table 14.1 is a partial listing of objectives and their measurement, complete with a timeline and designation of staff responsible for each objective. This table is from a funded proposal to the Department of Education to establish a preschool intervention program for autistic-like preschool children.

Proposals for training monies are also required to ground their objectives to measurement methods. In Table 14.2 we present a sample of Objectives from a funded application to train graduate students in single case research designs and procedures.

In examination of Tables 14.1 and 14.2, it is suggested that Objectives are not merely a shorthand mode of communicating the intent of your project; rather, they are the basis upon which you and others will evaluate the impact and effectiveness of your project.

Procedures

The Procedures section of proposals is the most heavily weighted portion when funding decisions are made. Essentially, the Procedures should, as thoroughly as possible, indicate how the project will meet its objectives. Once again, we are concerned with a proposal section that must vary greatly across demonstration/service, training, and research efforts. Still, a number of general suggestions can be made:

(1) Procedures should be included to meet *each* stated objective.
(2) Many reviewers know from first-hand experience that, "the best-laid plans" often fall through. Therefore, it is essential that the Procedures convey an understanding of the potential pitfalls in the area of work, along with plans to address the problems.
(3) For multi-year or particularly complex projects, the Procedures should contain a timeline of activities. Table 14.3 provides a sample timeline of activities from a program development proposal.
(4) Procedures should describe the rationale for selecting the particular approach to the research, program development, or training effort.
(5) Although it may not be a required component, we strongly suggest that the Procedures end with a concise statement of the potential significance of the proposed work.

In the sections below, we offer suggestions for the content of several "generic" Procedures sections.

Table 14.1. Major Objectives of Project, Activities to Meet Objectives, Persons Responsible, and Measurement Methods

Objectives	Activities to Meet Objectives	Person(s) Responsible	Measurement Methods
(1) To develop an efficient system of screening and referral such that 3–5-year-old, autistic-like children are referred in a timely fashion for educational treatment.	(1a) Write and disseminate PSAs	(1a) Principal investigator, Public Relations Office WPIC	(1a) Permanent product as specified in timeline
	(1b) Write and distribute brochures to medical professionals	(1b) Principal investigator, project secretary, project manager	(1b) Permanent product as specified in timeline
	(1c) Distribute screening forms to area pediatricians, child psychiatrists, PTAs, LEAs	(1c) Project manager, project secretary	(1c) Percent of pediatrician, child psychiatrist, PTA, and LEAs reached by distribution (goal being 90% coverage)
	(1d) Develop and field-test curriculum package for child psychiatrists in residence	(1d) Teacher coordinator, project manager, principal investigator	(1d) Percent of trainees scoring above 90% on criterion-based assessments
	(1e) Prepare and distribute child reports to referral sources	(1e) Project manager, master teacher, project secretary	(1e) Permanent product sent 2 weeks or less after referral is made
		(1a–e) Principal investigator	(1a–e) Overall measurement procedure for this objective will be an analysis of the proportion of estimated autistic-like children age 3–5 referred for services during the first year of operation

(2) To develop a series of observational and interview techniques to be used in assessing target children's home, community, and future educational settings in order to develop functional curriculum targets and intervention techniques.	(2a) Construct and field-test interview procedures across various settings	(2a) Principal investigator, project manager, master teacher, parent trainer	(2a) Established reliability across interviewers at or above 80% on three separate interviews
	(2b) Construct and field-test observational procedures across various settings	(2b) Principal investigator, project manager, master teacher, parent trainer	(2b) Established reliability across observers at or above 80% on three separate observational sessions
	(2c) Construct IEP for each child based upon information derived from interviews and observations	(2c) Project manager, master teacher, aides, parent trainer, parents	(2c) Permanent product (IEP) completed and implemented 4 weeks following acceptance into the program
	(2d) Conduct social validity checks on child progress (assess parent, teacher, peer opinions regarding behavior change)	(2d) Project manager, parent trainer	(2d) Degree of concordance between treatment levels of target behaviors and social agents' opinions regarding significance of behavior change (2a–d) Overall measurement procedure will be the assessed correlation between the target child's meeting empirically derived objectives and increased access to community placements

(continued)

Table 14.1. Major Objectives of Project, Activities to Meet Objectives, Persons Responsible, and Measurement Methods *(continued)*

Objectives	Activities to Meet Objectives	Person(s) Responsible	Measurement Methods
(3) To socially and instructionally integrate six autistic-like children in a preschool class with six normally developing children of the same age range (3–5 years).	(3a) Implement interdependent group contingency for all classroom children	(3a) Master teacher, teacher aides, parents	(3a) Percent of target behavior met for each child during interdependent group contingency sessions
	(3b) Implement Peer Imitation Training (PIT) sessions	(3b) Master teacher, teacher aides, parents, peers	(3b) Comparison between baseline and treatment levels of appropriate behavior imitation using multiple baseline across behaviors design
	(3c) Implement social behavior training during free-play	(3c) Master teacher, teacher aides, parents, peers	(3c) Comparison between baseline and treatment levels of positive social behavior using multiple baseline across behaviors/subjects designs
	(3d) Implement extra-school programming for target children	(3d) Parent trainer, parents	(3d) Comparison between baseline and treatment levels of target behaviors using multiple baseline across settings/behaviors designs
	(3e) Implement IEPs for target children related specifically to community integration	(3e) Master teacher, teacher aides, parents, peers	(3e) Comparison between baseline and treatment levels of target behaviors using multiple baseline across behaviors/subjects designs

Table 14.2. Research Training Competencies

Competency Cluster	Specific Objective	Didactic Method	Evaluation Procedure
(1) Reading Research Critically	(1a) To read and analyze all sections of a published research paper, according to a predetermined format.	Lecture	Permanent Product (pp) 10 analyses completed satisfactorily.
	(1b) To use reference materials and available colleagues to answer questions regarding research papers.	Tutorial library activity	Permanent Product (pp) 10 analyses completed satisfactorily, with self-report on use of resources.
	(1c) To conduct a comprehensive computer and library search of research within a specified area.	Library activity	Permanent Product (pp) two satisfactory computer searches incorporating at least 50 abstracts.
	(1d) To write in accepted format, a thorough review of a research paper for a journal.	Tutorial following lecture	pp: two reviews judged satisfactory by editor of a research journal.
	(1e) To provide corrective feedback to another trainee regarding his/her review of a manuscript.	Independent activity under supervision	pp: edited/marked copy of trainee's review evaluated by a journal editor.
	(1f) To develop a module of instruction that trains persons to read and review research critically, with resulting accomplishment of objectives (1a–d) by those persons.	Independent activity, with consultation	Successful completion of module by three persons with no prior training.

(continued)

Table 14.2. Research Training Competencies *(continued)*

Competency Cluster	Specific Objective	Didactic Method	Evaluation Procedure
(2) Using Measurement Systems	(2a) To use a frequency count procedure to observe/measure social behaviors, obtaining at least 85% inter-rater agreement on at least three different target behaviors.	Lecture, followed by field-based application of each procedure under supervision. (2a–2e)	pp: Submission of reliability figures on at least three protocols using each procedure. (2a–2e)
	(2b) To use a duration measure, obtaining at least 85% inter-rater agreement on at least three different target behaviors.		
	(2c) To use a non-continuous interval measure, obtaining at least 85% inter-rater agreement on at least three different target behaviors.		
	(2d) To use a continuous interval record measure, obtaining at least 85% inter-rater agreement on at least three different target behaviors.		

(2e) To calculate inter-observer agreement using the four measures specific in 2a–2d. Obtaining at least 85% inter-rater agreement on at least three different target behaviors.		
(2f) To select the best measurement system for recording at least 10 different social/classroom behaviors. Obtaining at least 85% inter-rater agreement on at least three different target behaviors.	Tutorial	(pp) Ten appropriate selections submitted as class assignment.
(2g) To design direct observational records for use in measuring the behaviors designated in (2f). Obtaining at least 85% inter-rater agreement on at least three different target behaviors.	Tutorial	Submission of protocols deemed acceptable by Supervisor.
(2h) To train at least three persons without specific prior experience to use the protocol designed in (2g), with at least 85% inter-observer agreement.	Small group instruction under faculty supervision.	Submission of completed observer records with reliability prescribed.

(continued)

Table 14.2. Research Training Competencies *(continued)*

Competency Cluster	Specific Objective	Didactic Method	Evaluation Procedure
	(2i) To provide corrective feedback to a trainee who is attempting to master objectives (2f–h), with resulting accomplishment of those objectives by the trainee. Obtaining at least 85% inter-rater agreement on at least three different target behaviors.	Tutorial under faculty supervision	Documentation of completion of objectives (2f–h) by supervisee.
(3) Research Design	(3a) To describe the purposes and features of the following research designs: I. reversal II. withdrawal-of-treatment III. multiple-baseline IV. changing criterion V. simultaneous treatment	Textbook assignments (Hersen & Barlow; Kazdin; & Sidman texts); lectures	Written exam, score of 90% or better.
	(3b) To choose correctly a research design, given a hypothetical research problem.	Simulation exercises; lecture; textbook	Written exam, score of 90% or better.
	(3c) To select a research design for a problem in the trainee's own field of research experience.	Tutorial	Submission of design section of research proposal, with acceptable evaluation by supervisor.

	(3d) To present a course lecture and/or self-teaching module to at least two trainees, on each of the above-listed research designs.	Trainee presentation, developed under faculty supervision	Score of 90% or better by each person in class, on a research design exam.
	(3e) To provide corrective feedback to another trainee attempting to master objectives (3b–c).	Trainee supervision, with consultation from faculty member	Accomplishment of objectives, (3b–c) by person being supervised.
(4) Summary and Display of Data	(4a) To describe the following methods of displaying data gathered through a research activity: I. chart of raw scores II. equal-interval graph III. semi-logarithmic graph IV. summary table.	Lecture, with audiovisual aids	Written exam, score of 90% or better.
	(4b) To visually summarize data, using hypothetical examples, in each of the methods.	Simulation exercise	Written exam, score of 90% or better.
	(4c) To display data gathered in trainee's own research field experience.	Tutorial	Submission of display deemed acceptable by faculty member.
	(4d) To conduct and describe appropriate nonparametric analyses in order to describe data gathered by trainee.	Lecture; possible coursework outside institute; simulations	Submission of results section (written) deemed acceptable by faculty member.

(continued)

Table 14.2. Research Training Competencies *(continued)*

Competency Cluster	Specific Objective	Didactic Method	Evaluation Procedure
	(4e) To assist another trainee attempting to master objectives (4b–d).	Supervision with faculty assistance	Mastery of objectives (4b–d) by Supervisee
(5) Implementing research in least restrictive environments.	(5a) To obtain approval of the appropriate Human Use Committees, by submitting an acceptable program of research and of informed consent.	Independent study of HUC guidelines; simulation exercises	Documentation of HUC approvals necessary to conduct research.
	(5b) To obtain cooperation of participating school(s) or other agencies, as reflected by letter of support for research and participation of staff and/or subjects.	Independent activity with faculty supervision	Support letter; subjects recruited.
	(5c) To assist another trainee in accomplishing objectives, (5a–5b).	Supervision, with accomplishment of (5a), (5b) by supervisee. Faculty consultation	
(6) Writing research papers.	(6a) To use APA style in writing research reports, as well as to proofread one's own writing for APA style errors.	Textbook (APA style manual; Chicago manual of style; Strunk & White); simulation activities in proofreading.	By written exam, score of less than five style errors per manuscript.

	(6b) To write a research description based on hypothetical examples.	Simulation exercises	Grade of "pass" by journal editor/faculty member.
	(6c) To write a description of trainee's own research project.	Independent writing, under faculty supervision.	Acceptance of paper in peer-review journal.
	(6d) To provide corrective feedback to trainee attempting objective (6c).	Supervision activity with faculty consultation.	Acceptance of manuscript (as in [6c]) of supervisee.
(7) Presenting research	(7a) To write an acceptable research presentation for a national conference.	Independent activity with supervision.	Acceptance of paper/presentation through a peer-review process.
	(7b) To develop suitable audio-visual aids for conference presentation.	Independent activity with supervision.	Acceptance of paper/presentation through a peer-review process. Supporting statement from a media or a-v specialist.
	(7c) To modify proposal and to present research applications to a state, local, or national teachers' and/or parents' group.	Independent activity, with assistance from teachers on the staff of the University or its school programs.	Acceptance of paper/presentation through a peer-review process. Support documented by teacher/or parent.

Table 14.3. Timeline for Major Activities of the Project[1]

Major Activities by Objectives	Months During July 1, 1981–June 30, 1982											
	1981						1982					
	J	A	S	O	N	D	J	F	M	A	M	J
Objective One:												
(1a) Write and disseminate PSAs	X					X						X
(1b) Write and distribute brochures	X	X										
(1c) Distribute screening forms	X	X										
(1d) Develop and field-test curriculum package for child psychiatrists	X	X	X	X								
(1e) Prepare and distribute child reports to referral sources			X	X	X	X	X	X	X	X	X	X
Objective Two:												
(2a) Construct and field-test interview procedures	X	X										
(2b) Construct and field-test observational procedures	X	X	X									
(2c) Construct IEP for each child		X	X	X	X	X	X	X	X	X	X	X
(2d) Conduct social validity checks					X	X	X	X	X	X	X	X
Objective Three:												
(3a) Implement interdependent contingency					X	X	X	X	X	X	X	X
(3b) Implement PIT sessions			X	X	X	X	X	X	X	X	X	X
(3c) Implement social behavior training			X	X	X	X	X	X	X	X	X	X
(3d) Implement extra-school programming			X	X	X	X	X	X	X	X	X	X
(3e) Implement community integration portion of IEP				X	X	X	X	X	X	X	X	X
Objective Four:												
(4a Develop and implement orientation modules	X	X	X	X	X	X	X					
(4b) Develop and implement exit modules	X	X								X	X	X
(4c) Conduct in-school parent training			X	X	X	X	X	X	X	X	X	X
(4d) Conduct home/community parent training				X	X	X	X	X	X	X	X	X

[1]In the timeline offered above, starting and completion dates for each major activity are designated by the "X" marked under the appropriate month abbreviation.

Table 14.3. Timeline for Major Activities of the Project *(continued)*

Major Activities by Objectives	Months During July 1, 1981–June 30, 1982											
	1981						1982					
	J	A	S	O	N	D	J	F	M	A	M	J
Objective Five:												
(5a) Provide center-based training for "receiving" teachers										X	X	X
(5b) Provide on-site training for "receiving" teachers											X	X
(5c) Provide follow-up consultation to "receiving" teachers												X
Objective Six:												
(6a) Implement child psychiatric evaluations		X	X	X	X	X	X	X	X	X	X	X
(6b) Implement neuropsychiatric assessments		X	X	X	X	X	X	X	X	X	X	X
(6c) Implement pediatric assessment of referral system		X	X	X	X	X	X	X	X	X	X	X
Objective Seven:												
(7a) Assess observer agreement			X	X	X	X	X	X	X	X	X	X
(7b) Assess social validity of outcome data					X	X	X	X	X	X	X	X
(7c) Implement multiple baseline designs			X	X	X	X	X	X	X	X	X	X
(7d) Implement 6-month follow-ups	To be done after 1981–1982 funding period											
Objective Eight:												
(8a) Pre-test families upon program entry		X	X	X	X	X	X					
(8b) Re-test families prior to exit											X	X
(8c) Perform statistical comparisons												X
(8d) Conduct 6-, 12-, 18-month follow-ups	To be done after 1981–1982 funding period.											
Other Activities:												
(9a) Hire staff	X	X										
(9b) Convene Advisory Council	X					X						X
(9c) Recruit non-handicapped children	X	X										
(9d) Purchase all materials	X	X										
(9e) Conduct visitors programs			X	X	X	X	X	X	X	X	X	X

Population Served/Subjects. As one might imagine, there is always a great amount of scrutiny given to the description of subjects in the proposed review process. At a minimum, this section should include: (a) rationale for selecting particular kinds of subjects, (b) statement of the availability of necessary subjects, (c) inclusionary and exclusionary criteria for participation, (d) recruitment procedures, (e) how sub-groups for study purposes will be formed, and (f) statement regarding your intent to comply with institutional policy regarding the protection of human (or animal) subjects.

Several authors (e.g., Hall, 1977) have cautioned proposal writers of the growing skepticism with which review panels judge the availability of subjects for psychological research and treatment program efforts. It is, therefore, advisable to document via letters from referral agents, other professionals, "expert witnesses," even potential subjects, the claims made about subject availability.

Finally, we recommend that the myriad issues that arise from subject attrition be addressed. This should include a discussion of how the author plans to prevent attrition.

Data Collection Instruments and Procedures. Almost all psychology-oriented proposals will contain procedures for assessing changes in the behavior, attitude, or knowledge of participants. In describing assessment methods, we recommend inclusion of the following information:

(1) A brief rationale for selecting each instrument *and* procedure for data collection.
(2) Where new, unfamiliar, or as yet unevaluated instruments are used, provide a detailed explanation of the advantages of these protocols over more accepted alternatives.
(3) Individuals who will collect the data and any special training or capabilities they possess.
(4) Schedules by which the data will be collected; and, if appropriate, a discussion of methodological problems that are created (e.g., practice effects) or solved (e.g., validity of behavior sample), by multiple and repeated measures.

Data Analysis. This section of an application is often high-risk. Especially for research applications, one can count on having a methodologist (or two) provide a critical review. The matter becomes high-risk in the sense that there are often many alternative forms of data analysis available to answer a specific question, and opinions about the "rightness" of one approach may be deeply held. As a result, we suggest presenting alternative methods (where applicable) along with some consideration of relative strengths and weaknesses. By adopting this approach you can help convince reviewers of the breadth of expertise available and clearly show that you have given thoughtful consideration to the limitations of your data set.

Within the behavioral sciences it is very typical to analyze data that may be described as second-order. That is, sub-scales may be pooled, categories of behaviors collapsed, and data sampling periods grouped to answer specific questions. In these instances we advise including a brief section on data reduction procedures in order to convince reviewers that the eventual unit of analysis is compatible with and meets the assumptions of the planned analytic methods.

Dissemination

Federal agencies are increasingly under fire from their appropriations sources to document the impact of their dollars. As a result, there is a renewed interest in and sympathy toward applications that offer a careful plan for disseminating the results of the project. In many cases, being productive in the traditional scholarly mode (e.g., publications in peer-reviewed journals) is a necessary, but not a sufficient, plan for dissemination.

Several application packets now call for a separate "Dissemination" section. Whether or not this is part of the application packet or not, we suggest including the following information in a dissemination plan:

(1) The target audience(s) for dissemination materials and a rationale for the selection.
(2) Specific goals for dissemination which may include: awareness of the project, information exchange with persons conducting similar work, stimulate similar projects and use of products developed, and support or alter policy decisions.
(3) Specific dissemination products and processes to be used. These may include: newsletters, public service announcements, news releases, media presentations, manuscripts submitted to professional journals, executive and/or legislative summaries, conference presentations, chapter and book manuscripts, and site visits for interested parties.

SUMMARY

Writing grant applications is very much like sitting through Ingmar Bergman's film *Scenes From a Marriage* with an ex-spouse. To be sure, both endeavors demand fortitude and persistence, both create a good dose of visceral responding, both linger in one's mind far beyond a useful point of contemplation, and both are once-in-a-life-time events for many. *Surviving* your first, second, third, and thirteenth application should be a high priority.

We think there are a number of important keys to survival. First, it must be recognized that the vast majority of proposals competing at a given time will not be funded. There are several competitions of which we are aware where the odds of funding are less than 5 in 100. Those odds mean that many outstanding ideas will not receive support the first time around. However, persistence is often rewarded in the grant-getting business. Persistence may take several forms, including: (a) revising according to review comments and resubmitting to the same competition, (b) resubmitting the same or altered application to a different agency or competition, and (c) resubmitting the same application to the identical competition.

Second, the importance of planning ahead cannot be emphasized too strongly. Hastily prepared proposals are seldom worth the postage to send them to the granting agency; such incomplete or poorly conceived work may leave reviewers with an impression of your competence that is less than ideal. There are, of course, some competitions (usually contracts) that demand a rapid response. In the vast majority of these cases, only experienced grants-persons and well-established institutions have a realistic chance to produce a competitive proposal.

A third and final key to grant writing survival is to create a rigorous, internal review process for your applications. While most institutions have internal review committees, the feedback received from these groups often comes too late to make substantive changes, and may not provide the most informed opinions available. We have profited greatly from informal review networks, with hand-picked colleagues providing consultation and feedback on specific issues.

REFERENCE

Hall, M. (1977). *Developing skills in proposal writing.* Portland, OR: Continuing Education Publications.

Author Index

Subject Index

About the Editors and Contributors

ABOUT THE EDITORS

Alan S. Bellack, (Ph.D., Pennsylvania State University, 1970) is Professor of Psychiatry at the Medical College of Pennsylvania and was formerly Professor of Psychology and Psychiatry and Director of Clinical Psychology Training at the University of Pittsburgh. He is President-elect of the Association for Advancement of Behavior Therapy, and a Fellow of Division 12 of APA. He is co-author and co-editor of 12 books including: *The Clinical Psychology Handbook, International Handbook of Behavior Modification and Therapy, Research and Practice in Social Skills Training,* and *Introduction to Clinical Psychology.* He has published numerous journal articles and has received several NIMH research grants on social skills, behavioral assessment, and schizophrenia. With Hersen, he is editor and founder of the journals *Behavior Modification* and *Clinical Psychology Review.* He has served on the editorial boards of numerous journals and has been a consultant to a number of publishing companies and mental health facilities as well as NIMH.

Michel Hersen (Ph.D., State University of New York at Buffalo, 1966) is Professor of Psychiatry and Psychology at the University of Pittsburgh. He is the Past President of the Association for Advancement of Behavior Therapy. He has co-authored and co-edited 33 books including: *Single-Case Experimental Designs: Strategies for Studying Behavior Change (1st & 2nd editions), Behavior Therapy in the Psychiatric Setting, Behavior Modification: An Introductory Textbook, Introduction to Clinical Psychology, International Handbook of Behavior Modification and Therapy, Outpatient Behavior Therapy: A Clinical Guide, Issues in Psychotherapy Research, Handbook of Child Psychopathology, The Clinical Psychology Handbook,* and *Adult Psychopathology and Diagnosis.* With Alan S. Bellack, he is editor and founder of *Behavior Modification* and *Clinical Psychology Review.* He is Associate Editor of *Addictive Behaviors* and Editor of *Progress in Behavior Modification.* Dr. Hersen is the recipient of several grants from the National Institute of Mental Health, the National Institute of Handicapped Research, and the March of Dimes Birth Defects Foundation.

ABOUT THE CONTRIBUTORS

Frank Andrasik, Ph.D., is presently an Associate Professor and Associate Director of the Center for Stress and Anxiety Disorders of the Department of Psychology at the State University of New York at Albany. His major research interests fall within the area of Behavioral Medicine, with a special focus on assessment and treatment of stress-related disorders. He serves as Associate Editor for the journal *Behavior Therapy* and is a recipient of a Research Career Development Award from the National Institute of Neurological Communicative Disorders and Stroke.

John G. Arena, Ph.D., is Director, Biofeedback and Psychophysiological Disorders Clinic, Veterans Administration Medical Center, Augusta, Georgia and Assistant Professor of Psychiatry and Health Behavior, Medical College of Georgia, Augusta, Georgia. His major areas of interest and expertise are (1) applications of psychophysiological interventions such as biofeedback and relaxation therapy to chronic pain, the anxiety-based disorders, hypertension, Raynaud's Disease and other psychophysiological disorders; (2) psychophysiological assessment; (3) psychological and behavioral assessment of chronic pain; (4) medical psychology consultation.

J. Gayle Beck, Ph.D., has recently completed her doctoral degree from the State University of New York at Albany and is an assistant professor of Psychology at the University of Houston. Her major areas of interest include psychophysiological study of sexual dysfunction and the anxiety-related disorders, specifically panic disorder. Her publications have appeared in *Journal of Abnormal Psychology, Psychophysiology, Behaviour Research and Therapy,* and *Clinical Psychology Review.*

Juris I. Berzins, Ph.D., is a Professor of Psychology at the University of Kentucky. His major areas of interest include: Psychotherapy research, sex roles, and personality. He is a Fellow of Division 12 (Clinical) of the American Psychological Association, former Director of Graduate Studies in the Department of Psychology at the University of Kentucky, 1974–83 and a former Member of the Kentucky State Board of Examiners of Psychologists.

Evelyn Bromet, Ph.D., is an Associate Professor of Psychiatry and Epidemiology at the University of Pittsburgh. She directs the Psychiatric Epidemiology Training Program funded by the National Institute of Mental Health and is co-director of a program in Psychiatric Statistics conducted jointly with Carnegie-Mellon University. Dr. Bromet has conducted research on the mental health effects of the stresses associated with the accident at Three Mile Island on adults and children and on psychosocial and neuropsychological outcomes associated with stress and neurotoxic exposure in the workplace.

Susan B. Campbell, Ph.D. is currently an Associate Professor of Psychology at the University of Pittsburgh. Her major interest area is developmental psychopathology; her research has focused on the early identification and follow-up of hyperactive children with an emphasis on their social development. Dr. Campbell's current research, a longitudinal study of hard-to-manage preschoolers, is funded by an NIMH grant.

Lori Dodson, Ph.D., is in the School Psychology Program of the Department of Educational Psychology, University of Arizona. Her major areas of expertise are school psychology and applied research.

Michael D. Franzen, Ph.D., was a post-doctoral fellow in clinical neuropsychology at the University of Nebraska Medical Center at the time this chapter was written. He is currently assistant professor of Behavioral Medicine and Psychiatry at West Virginia Medical Center and assistant professor of Psychology at West Virginia University. His research interests are in psychometric evaluation of neuropsychological tests and in scale construction in neuropsychological assessment.

Sol L. Garfield, Ph.D., is Professor of Psychology at Washington University in St. Louis. His major areas of interest are clinical psychology and psychotherapy research. He has received numerous honors, including: Distinguished Contribution to Clinical Psychology award, Division of Clinical Psychology, APA, 1976; and the APA Distinguished Professional Contribution to Knowledge Award, 1979.

Charles J. Golden, Ph.D., is professor of Medical Psychology at Nebraska Psychiatric Institute, the University of Nebraska Medical Center. His major research interests are in the area of scale construction of neuropsychological tests. He was the recipient in 1981 and again in 1982 of awards from the National Academy of Neuropsychologists in recognition of his contributions to the field.

Martin Harrow, Ph.D., is Director of Psychology at Michael Reese Hospital and Medical Center in Chicago, and Professor in the Department of Psychiatry and the Department of Behavioral Sciences at The University of Chicago. A former chess master, he has engaged in extensive research on long-term adjustment and thought disorder in schizophrenia and affective disorders, and has published over 100 articles in these and related areas. He currently holds large research grants from the National Institute of Mental Health and the MacArthur Foundation, and is Director of the Chicago Followup Study.

William Ickes, Ph.D., is Associate Professor of Psychology at the University of Texas at Arlington. His research interests in the area of personality-social psychology focus specifically on how people's personality traits and other dispositions influence the compatibility or incompatibility of their dyadic relationships. He is the editor of a forthcoming book entitled *Compatible and Incompatible Relationships* and is co-editor (with J. Harvey and R. Kidd) of the three-volume series *New Directions in Attribution Research.*

Francis J. Keefe, Ph.D., is Associate Professor of Medical Psychology in the Department of Psychiatry of Duke University. He has been an Associate Editor of *Behavior Therapy*, and has published widely in the area of behavioral medicine.

Mary Margaret Kerr, Ph.D., is Assistant Professor of Psychiatry and Special Education, University of Pittsburgh, School of Medicine, Western Pennsylvania Institute and Clinic, 201 DeSoto Street, Pittsburgh, PA. Her major areas include: interest in behavioral disorders, teacher training, consultation and adolescence. She was named in *Who's Who in Biobehavioral Sciences*, and held graduate assistantships at The American University and at Duke University.

Thomas R. Kratochwill, Ph.D., is Professor and Director, School Psychology Program, University of Wisconsin-Madison. His major areas of interest include behavior therapy with children and applied research methodology. He has numerous publications and received the Lightner Witmer Award from APA Division 16 in 1977.

Michael F. Pogue-Geile, Ph.D. is a Senior Psychologist at Michael Reese Hospital and Medical Center and a Research Associate, Assistant Professor in the Department of Psychiatry at The University of Chicago. His major research interests are in schizophrenia and behavior genetics, with an emphasis on methodological issues. He has published on these topics and was awarded the Theodosius Dobzhansky Award from the Behavior Genetics Association for his dissertation research. He received his Ph.D. from Indiana University in 1981.

Lee Sechrest, Ph.D., has recently moved to the University of Arizona, where he is Professor and Head of the Department of Psychology. Prior to that he was Director of the Center for Research on the Utilization of Scientific Knowledge, The Institute for Social Research, The University of Michigan. Even earlier, he taught at Florida State University, Northwestern University, and Pennsylvania State University. Ever since receiving his Ph.D. at Ohio State, he has been concerned to try to apply the findings of basic psychology to the practice of therapy.

Stacy Mott, Ph.D., is in the School Psychology Program of the Department of Educational Psychology, University of Arizona. Her major areas of expertise are: School psychology and applied research.

Robert Sawicki, Ph.D., was a post-doctoral fellow in clinical neuropsychology at the University of Nebraska Medical Center at the time this chapter was written. He currently is on the staff at Indianapolis Community Hospital. His research interests are in neuropsychological assessment and rehabilitation.

Philip S. Strain, Ph.D., is Associate Professor of Psychiatry and Special Education, University of Pittsburgh, School of Medicine, Western Pennsylvania Institute and Clinic, 201 DeSoto Street, Pittsburgh, PA. His major areas of interest include: Single subject research design, behavior disorders in preschool children mainstreaming and social skills training. In 1980 he was awarded the Outstanding Research Presentation at the Association for Advancement Behavior Therapy.

Harvey A. Skinner, Ph.D., is a Senior Scientist and Head of Assessment Research at the Addiction Research Foundation, Toronto; Associate Professor in the Department of Preventive Medicine and Biostatistics, University of Toronto; Associate Professor in the Department of Measurement, Evaluation and Computer Applications, Ontario Institute for Studies in Education. His major research interests include: assessment of alcohol/drug problems, applications of microcomputers in health care, lifestyle screening, multivariate techniques, classification of mental disorders, personality measurement, family assessment.

Pergamon General Psychology Series

Vol. 42. FAIRWEATHER *et al.*--*Creating Change in Mental Health Organizations*
Vol. 43. KATZ & ZLUTNICK—*Behavior Therapy and Health Care: Principles and Applications*
Vol. 44. EVANS & CLAIBORN—*Mental Health Issues and the Urban Poor*
Vol. 45. HILLNER—*Psychology of Learning: A Conceptual Approach*
Vol. 46. BARBER, SPANOS & CHAVES—*Hypnosis, Imagination and Human Potentialities*
Vol. 47. POPE—*The Mental Health Interview*
Vol. 48. PELTON—*The Psychology of Nonviolence*
Vol. 49. COLBY—*Artificial Paranoia—A Computer Simulation of Paranoid Processes*
Vol. 50. GELFAND & HARTMANN—*Child Behavior Analysis and Therapy, Second Edition*
Vol. 51. WOLPE—*Theme and Variations: A Behavior Therapy Casebook*
Vol. 52. KANFER & GOLDSTEIN—*Helping People Change: A Textbook of Methods, Second Edition*
Vol. 53. DANZIGER—*Interpersonal Communication*
Vol. 54. KATZ—*Towards the Elimination of Racism*
Vol. 55. GOLDSTEIN & STEIN—*Prescriptive Psychotherapies*
Vol. 56. BARLOW & HERSEN—*Single-Case Experimental Designs: Strategies for Studying Behavior Changes, Second Edition*
Vol. 57. MONAHAN—*Community Mental Health and the Criminal Justice System*
Vol. 58. WAHLER, HOUSE & STAMBAUGH—*Ecological Assessment of Child Behavior: A Clinical Package for Home, School, and Institutional Settings*
Vol. 59. MAGARO—*The Construction of Madness—Emerging Conceptions and Interventions into the Psychotic Process*
Vol. 60. MILLER—*Behavioral Treatment of Alcoholism*
Vol. 61. FOREYT—*Behavioral Treatments of Obesity*
Vol. 62. WANDERSMAN, POPPEN & RICKS—*Humanism and Behaviorism: Dialogue and Growth*
Vol. 63. NIETZEL, WINETT, MACDONALD & DAVIDSON—*Behavioral Approaches to Community Psychology*
Vol. 64. FISHER & GOCHROS—*Handbook of Behavior Therapy with Sexual Problems. Vol. I: General Procedures. Vol. II: Approaches to Specific Problems*
Vol. 65. HERSEN & BELLACK—*Behavioral Assessment: A Practical Handbook, Second Edition*
Vol. 66. LEFKOWITZ, ERON, WALDER & HUESMANN—*Growing Up To Be Violent: A Longitudinal Study of the Development of Aggression*
Vol. 67. BARBER—*Pitfalls in Human Research: Ten Pivotal Points*
Vol. 68. SILVERMAN—*The Human Subject in the Psychological Laboratory*
Vol. 69. FAIRWEATHER & TORNATZKY—*Experimental Methods for Social Policy Research*
Vol. 70. GURMAN & RAZIN—*Effective Psychotherapy: A Handbook of Research*
Vol. 71. MOSES & BYHAM—*Applying the Assessment Center Method*
Vol. 72. GOLDSTEIN—*Prescriptions For Child Mental Health and Education*
Vol. 73. KEAT—*Multimodal Therapy with Children*
Vol. 74. SHERMAN—*Personality: Inquiry & Aplication*
Vol. 75. GATCHEL & PRICE—*Clinical Applications of Biofeedback: Appraisal and Status*

Vol. 76. CATALANO—*Health, Behavior and the Community: An Ecological Perspective*
Vol. 77. NIETZEL—*Crime and Its Modification: A Social Learning Perspective*
Vol. 78. GOLDSTEIN, HOYER & MONTI—*Police and the Elderly*
Vol. 79. MIRON & GOLDSTEIN—*Hostage*
Vol. 80. GOLDSTEIN *et al.*—*Police Crisis Intervention*
Vol. 81. UPPER & CAUTELA—*Covert Conditioning*
Vol. 82. MORELL—*Program Evaluation in Social Research*
Vol. 83. TEGER—*Too Much Invested to Quit*
Vol. 84. MONJAN & GASSNER—*Critical Issues in Competency-Based Education*
Vol. 85. KRASNER—*Environmental Design and Human Behavior: A Psychology of the Individual in Society*
Vol. 86. TAMIR—*Communication and the Aging Process*
Vol. 87. WEBSTER, KONSTANTAREAS, OXMAN & MACK—*Autism: New Directions in Research and Education*
Vol. 88. TRIESCHMANN—*Spinal Cord Injuries: Psychological, Social and Vocational Adjustment*
Vol. 89. CARTLEDGE & MILBURN—*Teaching Social Skills to Children: Innovative Approaches*
Vol. 90. SARBIN & MANCUSO—*Schizophrenia: Medical Diagnosis or Moral Verdict?*
Vol. 91. RATHJEN & FOREYT—*Social Competence: Interventions for Children and Adults*
Vol. 92. VAN DE RIET, KORB & GORRELL—*Gestalt Therapy: An Introduction*
Vol. 93. MARSELLA & PEDERSEN—*Cross-Cultural Counseling and Psychotherapy*
Vol. 94. BRISLIN—*Cross-Cultural Encounters: Face-to-Face Interaction*
Vol. 95. SCHWARTZ & JOHNSON—*Psychopathology of Childhood: A Clinical-Experimental Approach*
Vol. 96. HEILBRUN—*Human Sex-Role Behavior*
Vol. 97. DAVIDSON, KOCH, LEWIS, WRESINSKI—*Evaluation Strategies in Criminal Justice*
Vol. 98. GOLDSTEIN, CARR, DAVIDSON, WEHR—*In Response to Aggression: Methods of Control and Prosocial Alternatives*
Vol. 99. GOLDSTEIN—*Psychological Skill Training: The Structured Learning Technique*
Vol. 100. WALKER—*Clinical Practice of Psychology: A Guide for Mental Health Professionals*
Vol. 101. ANCHIN & KIESLER— *Handbook of Interpersonal Psychotherapy*
Vol. 102. GELLER, WINETT, EVERETT—*Preserving the Environment: New Strategies for Behavior Change*
Vol. 103. JENKINS—*The Psychology of the Afro-American: A Humanistic Approach*
Vol. 104. APTER—*Troubled Children/Troubled Systems*
Vol. 105. BRENNER—*The Effective Psychotherapist: Conclusions from Practice and Research*
Vol. 106. KAROLY & KANFER—*Self-Management and Behavior Change: From Theory to Practice*
Vol. 107. O'BRIEN, DICKINSON, ROSOW—*Industrial Behavior Modification: A Management Handbook*

Vol. 108. AMABILE & STUBBS—*Psychological Research in the Classroom: Issues for Educators and Researchers*
Vol. 109. WARREN—*Auditory Perception: A New Synthesis*
Vol. 110. DiMATTEO & DiNICOLA—*Achieving Patient Compliance: the Psychology of the Medical Practitioner's Role*
Vol. 111. CONOLEY & CONOLEY—*School Consultation: A Guide to Practice and Training*
Vol. 112. PAPAJOHN—*Intensive Behavior Therapy: The Behavioral Treatment of Complex Emotional Disorders*
Vol. 113. KAROLY, STEFFEN, O'GRADY—*Child Health Psychology: Concepts and Issues*
Vol. 114. MORRIS & KRATOCHWILL—*Treating Children's Fears and Phobias: A Behavioral Approach*
Vol. 115. GOLDSTEIN & SEGALL—*Aggression in Global Perspective*
Vol. 116. LANDIS & BRISLIN—*Handbook of Intercultural Training*
Vol. 117. FARBER—*Stress and Burnout in the Human Service Professions*
Vol. 118. BEUTLER—*Eclectic Psychotherapy: A Systematic Approach*
Vol. 119. HARRIS—*Families of the Developmentally Disabled: A Guide to Behavioral Interventions*
Vol. 120. HERSEN, KAZDIN, BELLACK—*The Clinical Psychology Handbook*
Vol. 121. MATSON& MULICK—*Handbook of Mental Retardation*
Vol. 122. FELNER, JASON, MORITSUGU, FARBER—*Preventive Psychology: Theory, Research and Practice*
Vol. 123. CENTER FOR RESEARCH ON AGGRESSION—*Prevention and Control of Aggression*
Vol. 124. MORRIS & KRATOCHWILL—*The Practice of Child Therapy*
Vol. 125. VARNI—*Clinical Behavioral Pediatrics: An Interdisciplinary Biobehavioral Approach*
Vol. 126. RAMIREZ—*Psychology of the Americas: Mestizo Perspectives on Personality and Mental Health*
Vol. 127. LEWINSON & TERI—*Clinical Geropsychology: New Directions in Assessment and Treatment*
Vol. 128. BARLOW, HAYES, NELSON—*The Scientist Practitioner: Research and Accounability in Clinical and Educational Settings*
Vol. 129. OLLENDICK & HERSEN—*Child Behavioral Assessment: Principles and Procedures*
Vol. 130. BELLACK & HERSEN—*Research Methods in Clinical Psychology*
Vol. 131. GOLDSTEIN & HERSEN—*Handbook of Psychological Assessment*